Manual of

CLINICAL TRAUMA CARE

The First Hour

Manual of
CLINICAL TRAUMA CARE
The First Hour

SUSAN BUDASSI SHEEHY, RN, MSN, MS, CEN, FAAN
Director of Nursing, Emergency Department
Brigham & Women's Hospital
Boston, Massachusetts

JOSEPH S. BLANSFIELD, RN, MS, CS, CEN
Trauma Coordinator, Boston Medical Center
Boston, Massachusetts

DIANNE M. DANIS, RN, MS, CEN
Trauma Nurse Coordinator
Beth Israel Deaconess Medical Center
Boston, Massachusetts

ALICE A. GERVASINI, PhD, RN
Trauma Coordinator, Massachusetts General Hospital
Boston, Massachusetts

THIRD EDITION

with 189 illustrations

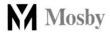
Mosby

St. Louis Baltimore Boston Carlsbad Chicago Minneapolis New York Philadelphia Portland
London Milan Sydney Tokyo Toronto

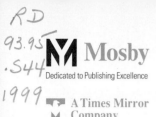

Mosby
Dedicated to Publishing Excellence

A Times Mirror
Company

Publisher: Nancy L. Coon
Managing Editor: Lisa Potts
Developmental Editor: Aimee E. Loewe
Project Manager: Patricia Tannian
Senior Production Editor: Melissa Mraz Lastarria
Book Design Manager: Gail Morey Hudson
Manufacturing Manager: Karen Lewis
Cover Design: Teresa Breckwoldt

THIRD EDITION

Composition by Clarinda Company
Printing/binding by R.R. Donnelley & Sons Company

Mosby–Year Book, Inc.
11830 Westline Industrial Drive
St. Louis, Missouri 63146

Library of Congress Cataloging in Publication Data

Manual of clinical trauma care: the first hour/Susan Budassi Sheehy . . . [et al.].—3rd ed.
   p.   cm.
   Rev. ed. of: Manual of clinical trauma: the first hour/Susan
Budassi Sheehy, Cindy LeDuc Jimmerson. 2nd ed. c1994.
   Includes bibliographical references and index.
   ISBN 0-323-00305-2
   1. Wounds and injuries—Nursing—Handbooks, manuals, etc.
2. Emergency nursing—Handbooks, manuals, etc.   I. Sheehy, Susan
Budassi.   II. Sheehy, Susan Budassi—Manual of clinical trauma care.
   [DNLM: 1. Wounds and Injuries—nursing handbooks.   2. Emergency
Nursing handbooks.   WY 49M293 1999]
   RD93.95.S44   1999
   617.1'026—dc21
   DNLM/DLC
   for Library of Congress   98-26666
                                                              CIP

98   99   00   01   02   /   9   8   7   6   5   4   3   2   1

Contributors

CAROLE C. ATKINSON, RN, MS, C
Trauma Nurse Coordinator
Children's Hospital
Boston, MA

MARY-LIZ BILODEAU, RN, MS, CS, CCRN
Critical Care Clinical Nurse Specialist;
Nurse Practitioner, Burn Service
Massachusetts General Hospital
Boston, MA

ANNE PHELAN BOWEN, RN, MS
Outreach Nurse
Trauma Program
Children's Hospital
Boston, MA

WILLIAM T. BRIGGS, RN, BS, CEN, CCRN
Nurse Manager
Emergency Service
Lawrence General Hospital
Lawrence, MA

PATRICIA J. BRUESKE, RN, MN, CFNP, CEN
Administrative Nurse Specialist
City of Houston, Emergency Medical Services
Emergency Nurse Practitioner
Hermann Hospital Medical Center
Houston, TX

KATHLEEN J. BURNS, RN, MS, CS
Acute Care Nurse Practitioner
Trauma Nurse Coordinator
Massachusetts General Hospital
Boston, MA

LORELEI B. CAMP, RN, MS, CCRN
Trauma Coordinator
Fletcher Allen Health Care
Burlington, VT

MAUREEN CULLEN, RN, MS, CCRN, CEN
Flight Nurse
Boston Medflight
Boston, MA;
Trauma/EMS Coordinator
Anna Jaques Hospital
Newburyport, MA

MARY M. CUSHMAN, BSN, RN, CEN
Trauma Coordinator
Baystate Medical Center
Springfield, MA

DEBORAH A. D'AVOLIO, RN, CS, MS
Director
Abuse and Trauma Intervention Program
Department of Ambulatory Care and Prevention
Boston, MA

BARBARA A. FOLEY, RN, BS
Associate Executive Director
ENCARE
Alexandria, VA

NICKI GILBOY, RN, MS, CEN
Nurse Educator
Emergency Department
Brigham & Women's Hospital
Boston, MA

JUDITH STONER HALPERN, RN, MS, CEN
Editor
International Journal of Trauma Nursing
Kalamazoo, MI

PATRICIA A. HUGHES, RN, MS, CS
Trauma Nurse Coordinator
University of Massachusetts Medical Center
Worcester, MA

MARY G. KENNEDY, RN, MS, CCRN, EMT-P
Trauma/Burn Program Manager
Brigham & Women's Hospital
Boston, MA

MARK C.N. LIBBY, RN, BSN, CCRN, CFRN, EMT-P
Trauma Coordinator
Department of Traumatology & Emergency Medicine
Hartford Hospital
Hartford, CT

LUANN LOUGHLIN, RN, MS, FNP-C, CEN
Director
Health Services
Massachusetts Mutual Life Insurances
Springfield, MA

CATHERINE MITCHELL McGRATH, RN, MSN
Clinical Nurse
Emergency Department
South Shore Hospital
South Weymouth, MA

ANDREA NOVAK, RN, MS, CEN
Director
Interdisciplinary Education
Fayetteville Area Health Education Center
Fayetteville, NC

JANET L. ORF, RN, MS, CCRN, CEN
Flight Nurse
Boston Medflight
Boston, MA

MICHAEL J. PINEAU, RN, MS, CEN
Trauma Coordinator
Bridgeport Hospital
Bridgeport, CT

GAIL E. POLLI, RNCS, MS
Director
Psychiatric Emergency Services
South Shore Hospital
South Weymouth, MA

GREG SCHNEIDER, RN, BSN, EMT-P, CCRN
Flight Nurse
Boston Medflight
Emergency Nurse
Beth Israel Deaconess Medical Center
Boston, MA

STEVE TALBERT, RN, MSN
Flight Nurse
University of Kentucky
Air Medical Service
Lexington, KY

LINDA TATKO COOPER, RN, MS, CEN
Clinical Nurse Specialist
Emergency Services
Baystate Medical Center
Springfield, MA

E. MARIE WILSON, RN, MPA
Chief
Systems Department
Connecticut Office Emergency Medical Services
Hartford, CT

To my son
JOHN
who has been a constant source of
encouragement, joy, and love.

SBS

To my wife
PAT
and daughters
BRITTANY and MARIEL
for your patience and understanding while
Dad was doing *his* homework.

JSB

This book is dedicated to my
COLLEAGUES and MENTORS
in emergency, flight, and trauma nursing,
and to my ENA and trauma coordinator network—
expert and caring nurses all.

DMD

To my son
CHRISTOPHER and EXTENDED FAMILY
who have always been there for me,
especially if I can't keep all the balls in the air at the same time.

AAG

Preface

It seems like yesterday that the original *Manual of Clinical Trauma Care: The First Hour* manuscript was being sent off to the publisher, and now the third edition is going into print. We are excited about this edition for many reasons. First, we have had the opportunity to work together—three trauma nurse coordinators and a director of nursing from four of the best and busiest academic medical centers and level I trauma centers in the world. With our backgrounds and experiences came contacts with some of the best trauma nurses in the world. We have asked those nurses to help us with this edition to revise chapters and write new ones so that we can bring you the most current and thorough information possible.

We hope that you will find this manual useful in your daily practice and helpful to you in understanding processes and procedures. The format of this manual has remained the same, because the feedback we have received from previous editions tells us that you have found it useful.

As always, we welcome your comments and critique.

Acknowledgments

This edition of the *Manual of Clinical Trauma Care: The First Hour* has had many contributors in many ways. We would first like to thank all of the authors and chapter revisors who have been most gracious with their time and talents. A very heartfelt thanks goes out to Leta Stoddard, who, once again, has proven to be the driving force behind this manual. Her diligence with deadlines, and her patience with those of us who are not good with deadlines, has been much appreciated. She has made sure that every "t" is crossed and every "i" is dotted. We could not have pulled this edition together without her.

A note of gratitude is essential for our families who have understood our need for quiet times and concentrated work times to complete this project.

And, last but not least, to each other for that "extra boost" when energy was low, for making a commitment to this project, and for making it happen.

The Editors of the third edition of *Manual of Clinical Trauma Care: The First Hour* would like to acknowledge the following authors who contributed to the second edition of this book:

Lisa McCabe, RN, MS, ANP

Lisa Schneck Hegel, RN, MS, ANP, CEN

Marie Bakitis Whedon, RN, MS, OCN

We would also like to acknowledge a coeditor of the first edition, Janet Marvin and coeditor of the first and second editions, Cindy LeDuc Jimmerson.

Contents

PART IV
SPECIAL POPULATIONS

PART V
CLINICAL SKILLS AND PROCEDURES

PART I

Trauma Care Systems

CHAPTER 1

The Model Trauma System

E. Marie Wilson

INTRODUCTION

Trauma is a disease characterized by injury to the body caused by intentional or unintentional acute exposure to mechanical, thermal, electrical, or chemical energy. Trauma classifications also include injuries caused by the absence of essentials such as heat or oxygen.[1] Burn injuries are identified as trauma although frostbite is not. All trauma is injury-based, but all injuries are not considered trauma.

Trauma is a public health problem of endemic proportions. It is the leading cause of death for those under 44 years of age. In 1995 the National Safety Council reported their data for unintentional injuries, not including homicide or suicide rates. There were 93,300 deaths or 35.5 per 100,000 population during 1995. In that same year there were 19,300,000 disabling injuries reported. The 1995 cost of injuries totaled $434.8 billion, of which $75.1 billion was for medical care and $222.4 billion was accounted for in lost wages and productivity.[2]

In the 30 minutes it takes to read this chapter, 6 people will be killed and 810 will suffer disabling injury at a societal cost of $24,900,000.

HISTORICAL PERSPECTIVE

The modern science of trauma care owes much of its history to innovations made in time of war or other conflicts. From the Knights Hospitaler of the Crusades, to the ambulances of Dr. Laverriey in the Napoleonic Wars, to the helicopters of the Korean and Vietnam Wars, trauma care has progressed most when necessity forced the search for answers.

In the United States, it was not until the 1966 publication of *Accidental Death and Disability: The Neglected Disease of Modern Society* that trauma was generally recognized as a disease entity worthy of specialized study and the development of trauma-specific treatment, rehabilitation, and prevention studies.[3] In 1973 Dr. R A Cowley described the "golden hour," within which

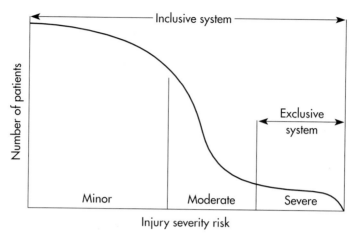

Fig. 1-1   Trauma care system. (From Bureau of Health Services Resources, Division of Trauma and Emergency Medical Services: *Model trauma care system plan,* Rockville, MD, 1992, US Department of Health and Human Services.)

time lies the best chance for optimal outcomes for trauma victims.[4] Drs. West and Trunkey reported the results of a comparison study of outcomes in the trauma patient population from two counties in California. One county had organized a systems approach to the management of trauma patients while the other had not. They concluded that the degree of organization of a trauma system directly influenced the incidence of "preventable" trauma deaths.[5]

More recently, in 1985 the Committee on Trauma Research of the National Academy of Science published *Injury in America* describing the dimensions of the problem and calling on Congress for additional resources to combat this increasing public health threat. The Centers for Disease Control in Atlanta established a division of trauma and funding was allocated to establish Injury Control Programs at selected facilities across the country.

TRAUMA SYSTEM DEVELOPMENT

In some areas of the country trauma care has been organized in a systematic way that ensures that all trauma patients are treated optimally in accordance with established standards. Unfortunately, systems are not consistent across regions or states. Some have only focused on Level I or Level II trauma centers and their catchment areas. This type of organization is reflective of an exclusive system that encompasses only critical trauma patients and those facilities that care for them. Facilities that are bypassed or not included in the system and those patients with less severe injuries are not captured in the review process for quality issues or for demographics with respect to the magnitude of trauma in a community (Fig. 1-1).

In 1990 the Trauma Care Systems Planning and Development Act was passed. This identified the need and mandated the development of a model

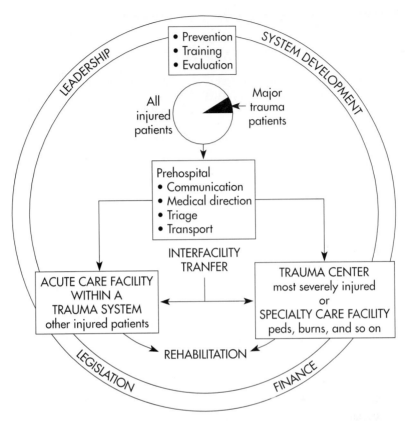

Fig. 1-2   Inclusive trauma system: Model Plan. (From Bureau of Health Services Resources, Division of Trauma and Emergency Medical Services: *Model trauma care system plan,* Rockville, MD, 1992, US Department of Health and Human Services.)

plan to assist communities/regions in the organization of trauma systems.[6] The model plan represents an inclusive trauma care system integrating multiple facilities and personnel in the management of all injured patients in a defined region or state (Fig. 1-2). Inclusive trauma systems are usually statewide in scope and administered by a government agency or private organization with legislatively delegated authority. All facilities are considered important partners in caring for trauma patients. Inclusion in the planning and implementation of systematized trauma care usually elevates the level of care in all facilities and holds them accountable for meeting system standards.

The attributes of an inclusive system are those factors that optimize patient care:

1. Designation of facilities equipped and committed to providing specialized care for critical trauma patients.

BOX 1-1

TRAUMA FACILITY VERIFICATIONS

Level I   Regional resource trauma center. Provides total care for all
trauma including cardiac, hand, microvascular, pediatric, and
infectious disease. In-house general surgeon. Education and
research essential.

Level II   Definitive trauma care center. Can manage the majority of critical trauma patients. Cardiopulmonary bypass not essential.

Level III   Community trauma facility. Transfer agreements and standardized treatment protocols required. Can assess, resuscitate, do
emergency operations, and transfer. General surgeon
promptly available.

Level IV   Remote trauma facility. Provide advanced life support before
transfer. Commitment to excellent trauma care within the
limits of its resources.

---

2. Triage of patients to appropriate facilities according to predetermined
criteria that consider physiologic, anatomic, mechanism of injury, and
co-morbid factors.
3. Expeditious transfer of critical patients who meet trauma triage criteria from community hospitals to trauma centers.
4. Internal quality improvement process for optimizing clinical care.
5. Collection of a minimum data set at a central point to monitor performance throughout the system.

Designation of facilities as trauma centers requires legislative authority.
Often the designation process includes a hospital verification of compliance
with established criteria as published by the American College of Surgeons
(Box 1-1). Although the ACS may verify a facility at a certain level, it is the
legislated authority that designates facilities within a trauma system.

Triage to the appropriate facility is the key to getting "the right patient to
the right facility in the right time." Destination hospital triage is a function of
medical control to ambulance providers, either by standing orders or direct
voice communication (Box 1-2). Triage protocols consider the physiologic and
anatomic findings first. The mechanism of injury is considered unreliable by
itself, but should raise an index of suspicion about the potential for hidden
problems. Co-morbid factors such as age (Box 1-3) and medical history
should also be considered but are not primary elements in triage decisions.

Trauma patients who meet triage criteria should be transferred to the appropriate designated facility. This transfer must be accomplished expedi-
tiously. For interfacility transfers, the initial workup should only include
those tests that are essential in determining criticality. Once the decision to
transfer is made, it is not necessary to assess the full extent of all injuries. The
care givers should stabilize the patient, identify, and arrange for an expedi-

---

BOX 1-2

GUIDELINES FOR FIELD TRIAGE OF ADULT TRAUMA PATIENTS

Adult patients who exhibit one or more of the following physical or physiologic findings shall be transported directly to an Adult Trauma Center by ALS personnel, or by BLS personnel under the direction of their medical control.

Physiologic and Physical Criteria include the following:

- GCS less than 14
- Systolic blood pressure of 90 mmHg or less
- Respiratory rate less than 10/minute or greater than 28/minute
- Penetrating injuries of the head, neck, or torso
- Suspected fracture(s) of two proximal long bones
- Flail chest
- Suspected fracture(s) of the pelvis, except those resulting from a simple fall from standing height
- Multiple system trauma that involves two at more regions of the body
- Suspected injury(ies) to the spinal cord or limb paralysis
- Amputation(s), except those that involve digits of the hand or foot
- Second- and third-degree burns that are greater than 20% Body Surface Area or burns that involve the airway, face, hands, or genitalia (transport to a Burn center)

Patients in traumatic cardiopulmonary arrest, who display no sign of life at the scene, shall be transported to the closest emergency department.

---

tious transfer. Copies of all tests and the prehospital record should be sent with the patient. A verbal report from both the referring physician and nurse should be communicated to the receiving team.

ADMINISTRATIVE COMPONENTS TO SUPPORT THE PATIENT CARE CONTINUUM

To coordinate various aspects of the inclusive system, administrative components need to provide the following:

- Education
- Data collection
- Quality improvement (QI)
- Research
- Public education and prevention
- Legislation

BOX 1-3

GUIDELINES FOR FIELD TRIAGE OF PEDIATRIC TRAUMA PATIENTS

Pediatric patients (12 years of age or less) who exhibit one or more of the following historical, physiologic, or physical findings shall be transported directly to a Pediatric Trauma Center.

Physiologic and Physical Criteria
- Systolic blood pressure less than normal range for age
- Compromised respiratory status, as evidenced by one or more of the following: respiratory rate less than normal range for age, capillary refill time greater than two seconds, decreased mental status, cyanosis
- Failure to respond to verbal or painful stimulation
- Penetrating injuries of the head, neck, or torso
- Suspected fracture(s) of two proximal long bones

- Flail chest
- Suspected fracture(s) of the pelvis
- Multiple system trauma that involves two or more regions of the body or major blunt trauma to the chest or abdomen
- Suspected injury(ies) to the spinal cord or limb paralysis
- Amputation(s), except those of the hand or foot
- Second- and third-degree burns that are greater than 10% Body Surface Area or burns that involve the airway, face, hands, or genitalia (transport to a Burn Center)

  Children in traumatic cardiopulmonary arrest, who display no sign of life at the scene, shall be transported to the closest emergency department.

Education

All of the disciplines that provide trauma care need specialized education beyond what is required in their basic educational program. Professional organizations and educational facilities offer specialized courses for trauma care practitioners. Seminars are offered throughout the country by a variety of specialty groups. Even in courses for generalists, trauma warrants particular mention so that all members of the team can function to support the patient's needs.

Data collection

Many facilities maintain internal trauma registries to track patient outcomes. These data banks should contain information about the patient from time of incident to the time of reentry to the community. Ideally, a computer link between various data sources such as police departments, ambulance companies, inpatient acute care facilities, rehabilitation units, skilled care facilities, and others, allows for a comprehensive look at the patient across the continuum from an outcome and quality improvement perspective.

Quality improvement

Every organization participating in trauma care needs a method for assuring quality care. Maintaining a computerized trauma registry is the basis for an internal QI Program. The QI program encompasses a peer-review/Morbidity and Mortality component along with reviews of institution specific audit filters identified to improve the quality of care. Quality assurance presumes an ever-narrowing spiral as the components of care are improved and the standard is reset.

Research

The knowledge base of trauma care is constantly growing. It is the responsibility of all practitioners involved in trauma care or system development to pose the questions that will lead to improved patient care.

Public education and prevention

The most cost effective treatment for trauma is the prevention of the incident. When caring for trauma patients, practitioners along the continuum of care have the opportunity to teach the patient, family, and friends, about trauma prevention and high-risk behavior. In the community those who treat trauma patients enjoy enhanced status as "tellers of truth" when they talk to audiences about the causes of the injuries encountered on a daily basis. Many organizations conduct educational programs for civic and school groups, adjusting the message to the needs of the target audience.

Legislation

The need for strong legislative support in the establishment and maintenance of Trauma Systems within Emergency Medical Services is paramount. The designated authority and funding source for a state-wide trauma system needs to be built into a legislative process to ensure the viability of the model plan.

SUMMARY

Trauma is a unique disease entity that is dependent on close cooperation and collaboration between a diverse group of practitioners for optimal outcomes. A trauma system is only as good as the EMS system that supports it. If the EMS system is supported by the community at large, and provides an organized approach to trauma care, optimal outcomes are attainable.

REFERENCES

1. Committee on Trauma, American College of Surgeons: *Resources for optimal care of the injured patient*, Chicago, 1993, American College of Surgeons.
2. National Safety Council: *Accident facts, 1996 Edition*, Itasca, IL, 1996, National Safety Council.
3. National Academy of Sciences, National Research Council: *Accidental death & disability: the neglected disease of modern society*, Washington, DC, 1966, US Government Printing Office.
4. Cowley RA: The resuscitation and stabilization of major multiple trauma patients in a trauma center environment, *Clin Med* 83:14, 1976.
5. West JG, Trunkey DD, Lim RC: Systems of trauma care: a study of two counties, *Arch Surg* 114:455-459, 1979.
6. Bureau of Health Services Resources, Division of Trauma & Emergency Medical Services: *Model trauma care system plan*, Rockville, MD, 1992, US Department of Health & Human Services.

CHAPTER 2

Hospital Systems of Care

Patricia A. Hughes and **Dianne M. Danis**

As outlined in Chapter 1, trauma care is optimally provided within an inclusive regional system that encompasses prehospital, acute care, and rehabilitative components. This chapter discusses acute care facilities and the personnel, equipment, and resources necessary for trauma centers of any level, focusing primarily on the requirements related to emergency departments.

The concept of "commitment" to excellence in trauma care cannot be overemphasized. Within hospitals that aspire to be trauma centers the commitment must be both personal and institutional. Institutional commitment means that the hospital administration supports adequate personnel and resources on a 24-hour basis, along with priority access to these resources for major trauma patients. Institutional commitment also applies to providing continuing education for clinicians and to fulfilling a leadership and service role in the community in both trauma care and injury prevention activities. Personal commitment demands that physician, nursing, and support personnel agree to provide dedicated and immediate availability 24 hours a day, as well as to participate in educational, quality improvement, injury prevention, and research activities.

TRAUMA CENTER CATEGORIZATION

The trauma care system has evolved to include different levels of trauma centers, based on need, geography, population density, and each facility's capabilities and resources. It is estimated that only 10% to 15% of all injured patients require the resources of the highest level trauma center, with the remainder of care being provided at other acute care facilities within the system.

The American College of Surgeons (ACS) has developed criteria and standards for Levels I through IV trauma centers. Many state, regional, or local systems apply the ACS criteria, modify the ACS criteria, or develop their own designation criteria. In the absence of a statewide system, some hospitals are simply self-designated or remain undesignated but still receive trauma patients.

Designation *versus* verification

In formal trauma systems each trauma care facility is officially *designated* by a regulatory body (frequently a state or regional emergency medical services [EMS] agency) according to commitment, capabilities, and resources. Trauma center *designation*, a governmental process, differs from ACS *verification*. Verification, conducted by ACS surveyors, is an on-site review of the trauma center's commitment, resources, personnel, education, research, and clinical care through special emphasis on quality improvement activities and outcome measures. The individual trauma center's role within the regional or statewide system and community is examined as well.

A verification site visit may be part of a state or regional designation process, but may also be voluntary on the part of a trauma center desiring to demonstrate excellence in trauma care.

Trauma center levels

The following definitions of trauma facility categories are those developed by ACS, outlined in their publication *Resources for Optimal Care of the Injured Patient: 1993*.[1]

Level I

The Level I trauma facility may also be termed a *regional resource trauma center*. It is typically a tertiary care hospital that can provide immediate, 24-hour, comprehensive care of the trauma patient through all phases of care (resuscitation through rehabilitation). This includes state-of-the-art diagnostic equipment and all surgical and nonsurgical subspecialty services. The Level I center must also have adequate depth in personnel and resources to be able to manage several patients simultaneously. The Level I trauma center should serve a leadership role at the local, regional, and state levels in quality improvement, education, training, systems development and evaluation, injury prevention, and research. The ACS document outlines essential and desirable criteria for equipment, personnel, quality improvement, research, education, and injury prevention.

Level II

The Level II trauma facility is also an acute care hospital that provides immediate, 24-hour, definitive care for all injuries and severities. Some Level II centers may not be able to provide definitive care for more complex injuries (e.g., replantation, cardiac surgery) or be able to provide the tertiary-level of surgical critical care. In that case, an agreement for rapid transfer to a Level I center must be in place. Level II centers frequently provide the bulk of trauma care in a community, and still have responsibilities for education, injury prevention, quality improvement, and research.

Level III

The Level III trauma facility is typically a hospital in a community that does not have a Level I or II center immediately accessible. Although this facility will manage minor trauma independently, in more severely-injured patients it will provide emergent assessment, resuscitation, stabilization, and rapid transfer to a Level I or II facility. Level III facilities must be able to perform emergency surgery, and therefore general surgeons must be promptly available. Protocols and agreements for the rapid transfer of patients to a Level I or II facility must be in place.

Level IV

The Level IV facility is found in rural or remote areas where no other level of care is available. The Level IV facility may not even be a hospital and may have limited or no physician coverage. The primary function would be emergent resuscitation and transfer. Standard treatment protocols and transfer agreements developed in collaboration with a Level I or II center are essential.

SPECIALTY TRAUMA CENTERS

Pediatric trauma care

Severely injured children require appropriate acute and rehabilitative care to improve survival and minimize long-term disability. ACS verifies pediatric trauma centers as either Regional Pediatric Trauma Centers (Level I centers only) or Adult Trauma Center with Pediatric Commitment (Levels I or II).[1]

Trauma centers that make the commitment to care for injured children must possess additional specialized resources. Personnel requirements include a multidisciplinary team approach and ideally a pediatric surgeon (or a general surgeon with expertise and experience in the management of children), as well as other surgical subspecialties and medical and nursing personnel with expertise in the care of injured children.

Burn centers

Of the more than 500,000 persons who experience burn injuries every year, 70,000 require hospitalization. Of that group, 20,000 require the services of a center that can provide specialized acute and rehabilitative burn management. Therefore, as in the larger trauma population, an inclusive system of care must provide for the entire spectrum of burn injury.

Institutions that make the commitment to provide burn care follow criteria developed by the American Burn Association.[2] These include education, quality improvement, research, and injury prevention responsibilities. There is also a burn center verification process available through the ACS. Burn centers are typically located within Level I or II trauma centers because of the resource intensity and specialized surgical critical care required.

TRAUMA RESUSCITATION TEAM

The trauma resuscitation team is the core of an institution's trauma care program. The team should operate according to the fundamental philosophy of a trauma resuscitation as a coordinated, standardized, multidisciplinary team process.

Although the composition of the trauma team may vary in different institutions and at varying trauma center levels, certain personnel are necessary to provide appropriate evaluation and resuscitation. These include:

- Trauma Surgeon/Team Leader (Attending surgeon or PGY4 or higher level surgical resident)
- Additional physician assistance (Surgery, Emergency Medicine, Anesthesia, Radiology)
- Primary registered nurse
- Additional nursing assistance (associate, "circulating," and/or recording nurse)
- Radiology technician
- Respiratory therapist (as necessary)

The number of team members and the exact composition of the team should be determined by the needs of each facility. ACS[1] and the Emergency Nurses Association[3,4] both offer resources to assist in developing the team. However, every team should have **one** clearly identified physician team leader who orchestrates a rapid, organized, and efficient resuscitation. Team members must be clear about their roles and responsibilities and perform them rapidly and simultaneously, with minimal direction and discussion.

Trauma team activation

Criteria for activating the trauma team, and communication systems for notifying members of the trauma team to respond to the emergency department, varies among different institutions and trauma center levels depending on capabilities and resources. Many trauma centers and regional trauma systems follow or modify ACS criteria[1] as guidelines for determining when the trauma team needs to be activated (see Chapter 5).

Some trauma centers have further refined their trauma team system to incorporate a "tiered" response with the goals of more appropriately utilizing resources, allocating staff, and reducing costs. In a nontiered response system the full trauma team is activated for every trauma patient. In a tiered response, selected team members respond based on prehospital report of injuries and severity, the full team responds for patients with major trauma, and a smaller team for less severely injured patients. Alternatively, the initial evaluation of trauma patients may be conducted by Emergency Medicine physicians with response by the Trauma Team for patients who meet predefined criteria. Criteria for activating the trauma team should be collaboratively and clearly defined by a multidisciplinary trauma center administrative committee, and must adhere to state and regional regulations, as well as ACS verification standards.

The system for activation of the trauma team usually includes a multiple page beeper (voice or digital) system that announces either the arrival or the "ETA" of a trauma patient. Early notification is important, so that the team can be prepared and assembled before the patient's arrival. However, the trauma team system must also be able to function efficiently in the absence of any advance warning.

Resuscitation roles and responsibilities

The first step in the evaluation and resuscitation of a trauma patient is for the team to receive a rapid and concise report from the prehospital provider. This should occur while simultaneously moving the patient onto the hospital trauma stretcher, gaining exposure to the patient, and initiating the primary survey.

Trauma resuscitation evaluation and intervention traditionally follow the recommendations of the Advanced Trauma Life Support Course[5] (ATLS). The Trauma Nursing Core Course[6] (TNCC) teaches a similar approach. Both advocate a step-wise, standardized, and organized multidisciplinary team approach, prioritizing care by utilizing "primary" (airway, breathing, circulation, and disability assessment, coupled with immediate intervention for life-threatening conditions) and "secondary" (head-to-toe identification of all other non–life-threatening injuries) surveys. This approach to evaluation and resuscitation enhances efficiency and minimizes delayed or missed diagnoses. Chapter 15 covers the specifics of the trauma evaluation and resuscitation.

Every trauma center should develop roles and responsibilities for each trauma team member, covering all the activities and tasks that need to be carried out during a resuscitation.

TRAUMA ROOM

The trauma resuscitation area should be designed to meet the needs of the major trauma patient by providing immediate access to all of the equipment necessary to perform a rapid and efficient resuscitation. The trauma resuscitation room or bay must be equipped and standing at the ready (or be **immediately** available) at all times to receive trauma victims (ideally two to three at once), with or without advance notice. A discrete, dedicated, and fully equipped resuscitation area for pediatric patients is also necessary, either contained within the larger trauma space, or located in another part of the emergency department.

The space for trauma resuscitations must be able to accommodate the entire trauma team, as well as necessary equipment such as ventilators, x-ray machines, and ultrasound machines. Adequate lighting, the ability to rapidly warm the resuscitation area, telephone lines (including "hot lines" to blood bank, operating room, trauma surgeons, etc.), computer terminals, an intercom system, and communication boards mounted in visible places (for communicating and documenting patient information, on-call schedules, standard drug doses and formulas, and other useful information) are important considerations.

The following equipment and procedure trays and sets should be clearly marked and strategically placed adjacent to the location where the procedure is likely to be performed:

- airway management
- phlebotomy
- intravenous line placement
- tube thoracostomy
- urinary catheter kit
- gastric tube equipment
- diagnostic peritoneal lavage
- pericardiocentesis
- open thoracotomy
- cervical spine skeletal traction
- pelvic fixators
- laceration stapling/suturing kits

Nurses and physicians awaiting a patient's arrival should always further prepare the area, being sure that equipment and supplies are ready for the specific type of patient expected. The resuscitation bay should be cleaned and restocked rapidly after every resuscitation and each shift.

Access to the resuscitation area should be strictly limited to those team members who will play an active role in the resuscitation. Many centers employ some type of physical barrier to clearly define essential versus nonessential resuscitation personnel, for example, a yellow line on the floor. Anyone who crosses this line must have a legitimate reason for doing so, and must don universal precautions garb (i.e., fluid-impervious gowns, gloves, mask, protective eyewear). The importance of "crowd" and noise control cannot be overemphasized. Only the team leader should speak, directing the flow of the resuscitation, giving orders, and requesting information from team members. The primary nurse keeps the team leader apprised of the status of the patient and collaborates to implement the plan of care. Emergency department (ED) nurses are in a good position to create the appropriate "culture" for resuscitations, one that encourages collaborative team work, is sensitive to and respects patients and families, and preserves confidentiality.

TRAUMA CARE DOCUMENTATION

The thorough, accurate, and legible documentation of all phases of the trauma patient's care is, of course, important for many reasons. In addition to allowing quality assessment/improvement (QA/I) activities, a good record also supplies data needed for the trauma registry, supports maximal financial reimbursement, and provides adequate legal justification for care that was (or was not) provided. Another important aspect of trauma documentation, but beyond the scope of this chapter, is the preservation of forensic evidence.

It is recommended that a separate flow sheet be designed specifically for documenting trauma care to capture all necessary data for QA/I and legal purposes. Reviewing examples from other institutions can be helpful.[3] The flow sheet should be "user friendly" to expedite and facilitate the capture of information. Even though it is recommended that there be a dedicated nurse recorder present during resuscitations, volume or staff limitations may not allow this at all times. A form that contains features such as check off lists, boxes, easily calculated scores (e.g., Glasgow Coma Score [GCS]), anatomic diagrams to identify injury sites, and yes/no options makes documentation easier.

The emergent nature of trauma care certainly presents obstacles to documenting care at the time that it occurs, but nurses should not feel absolved from the responsibility of completing a sound record. It is acceptable to complete or amend records as long as the appropriate notations are made to indicate when and by whom the additions were made.

Trauma documentation should include, at minimum, the following:

- Time of arrival, procedures, significant events, and disposition to other diagnostic and/or definitive care areas; and, importantly, the notification and arrival times of the trauma team, trauma attending surgeon, and other subspecialists such as neurosurgery or anesthesia.
- Key prehospital information: mechanism of injury, field interventions, patient responses.
- Patient health history: past medical history, medications, allergies.
- Initial and frequent vital signs and GCS scores.
- Results of the primary and secondary surveys with pertinent positive and negative findings.
- All treatments, procedures, significant events, and patient responses.
- All medications and fluids given before arrival and in the emergency department.
- All lab and x-ray results.
- All team members present, family, and others.
- Patient belongings, forensic evidence collected.

Some trauma centers create separate physician and nursing forms, dividing up the data documentation burden. Any system that works well is acceptable. It is also recommended that trauma flow sheets be produced on multiple-copy paper to provide extra copies in the event of lost forms or for use by the trauma registry.

Regular QA/I monitoring should be performed collaboratively by the trauma nurse coordinator and ED nursing staff to ensure compliance and to identify areas that require further education and/or counseling.

TRAUMA QUALITY IMPROVEMENT

An effective QA/I program for trauma care and trauma care systems is essential (and is mandated by the ACS verification standards). The most common reason cited for the failure of an ACS verification review is the lack of an adequate QA/I program. The trauma QA/I program is multifaceted. It incorporates peer review and credentialing, continuous and periodic monitoring of process and outcome indicators, mortality review, and other QA/I activities. While using ACS and other resources as a foundation,[1,5] the program should be carefully designed to address the unique aspects of the individual facility.

The goal of any QA/I program is to improve patient outcome. In the same way that there must be institutional and personal commitment to being a trauma center, there must be mutual respect for, and commitment to, the quality improvement program by all who participate in the trauma care system. Nurses in all areas of the trauma center play a key role in defining a patient-focused QA/I program, identifying deviations from standards, and monitoring compliance with protocol or policy changes. Emergency department nurses have a critical role in effecting changes in practice to improve patient outcome. The trauma nurse coordinator will work closely with the ED nursing staff in this endeavor.

Quality assessment/improvement indicators

The ACS provides a list of standard audit filters.[1] Some of the indicators that apply specifically to the resuscitation phase of care include:
- All trauma deaths (including a determination of preventability, potential preventability, or nonpreventability of the death).
- Patients with a GCS score less than 14 who do not receive a head computed tomography (CT) scan.
- Patients with a GCS score less than or equal to 8 who leave the emergency department without a definitive airway.
- Patients with abdominal injuries and hypotension (<90 mmHg) who do not undergo laparotomy within 1 hour of arrival.
- Patients with an epidural or subdural hematoma who undergo craniotomy more than 4 hours after arrival.
- Patients with an open tibial fracture, excluding a low-velocity gunshot wound, and an interval of longer than 8 hours between arrival and the initiation of débridement.
- Documentation of trauma surgeon and subspecialist notification and response times.

Videotaping trauma resuscitations

The videotaping of trauma resuscitations for quality improvement review and provider education has been used in many trauma centers for the past several years.[7,8]

Videotaping can be a valuable adjunct to the trauma QA/I program. The ability to watch actual resuscitations is a powerful teaching tool. Also, trauma videotapes allow the lessons learned during a trauma resuscitation to be disseminated among many clinicians.

The prospect of being videotaped can be intimidating and may lead to resistance among staff. How the program is presented is very important in eliciting cooperation and willing participation. A nonthreatening, collaborative approach is essential.

Videotape reviews can improve resuscitations in the following areas:

- Prehospital report and patient entry
- Primary and secondary survey: performance and completeness
- Treatment priorities and decision making
- Procedures and techniques
- Universal precautions compliance
- System breakdowns: improving efficiency, eliminating delays
- Team leadership: organizational and communication skills
- Teamwork: improving communication and collaboration
- Clinical scenarios: correlating book learning with real life

The use of videotaping carries with it some significant concerns about peer review protection and patient confidentiality. The trauma center must approach this issue with careful planning after researching hospital and state laws and regulations concerning confidentiality and peer review protection. A protocol for who will activate the camera, who will have access to tapes, and where and how long tapes will be stored must be clearly defined. The forums for review should also be clearly defined and covered under peer review laws and access to these sessions should be appropriately limited as well.

QUALIFICATIONS OF NURSES CARING FOR TRAUMA PATIENTS

Nurses play a critical role in the assessment, management, ongoing monitoring, and planning of care for trauma patients. Expert care of trauma patients requires a combination of training and education, and skill and experience.

The *Resource Document for Nursing Care of the Trauma Patient*[4] makes recommendations concerning the trauma-related expectations of emergency nursing services. Emergency nursing services should provide a trauma-related component of orientation and an annual trauma skills validation. In collaboration with the trauma program, they should participate in the trauma QA/I program and develop ED-specific trauma-related policies and procedures.

The emergency department should identify one or more trauma resource nurses. The trauma resource nurse may be a clinical nurse, clinical nurse specialist, nurse educator, or nurse manager. The trauma resource nurse possesses a special interest and expertise in trauma, serves as a consultant and role model, and works to develop the trauma skills of the rest of the staff.[4]

It is recommended that 50% of the ED nursing staff be currently verified in TNCC, the Emergency Nursing Pediatric Course (ENPC) or Pediatric Advanced Life Support (PALS), and Advanced Cardiac Life Support. At least one nurse in every trauma resuscitation should be a TNCC provider.[4]

Nurses who work in trauma center emergency departments will be expected to obtain trauma-related continuing education on an annual basis. Some of this education should be provided within the trauma center. In addition, there are many nationally accepted educational programs available to trauma nurses. These include TNCC, Course in Advanced Trauma Nursing, ATLS, ENPC, PALS, and Advanced Burn Life Support. Other educational opportunities include regional, state, and national conferences.

BEYOND THE EMERGENCY DEPARTMENT

The evaluation and management of trauma patients are far from over when the patient leaves the emergency department. The continuum of care frequently extends from the emergency department to the operating room, intensive care unit (ICU), surgical floor, and on to the rehabilitation phase, and may unfold over the next several weeks, months, or years. The care of trauma patients may require the services of every department in the hospital at one time or another, frequently on a top priority basis.

Trauma center expectations extend beyond the emergency department as well. The most important components are the trauma service, trauma chief, and trauma nurse coordinator. A trauma center must have an organized trauma service, a trauma registry, a qualified surgeon chief and surgical staff, and a trauma coordinator. The areas that care for trauma patients, particularly the operating room and ICU, are held to high expectations, similar to the emergency department, regarding personnel and resources. Additional standards apply to radiology and laboratory services and other services and departments throughout the hospital.

REFERENCES

1. American College of Surgeons Committee on Trauma: *Resources for optimal care of the injured patient: 1993*, Chicago, 1993, American College of Surgeons.
2. Guidelines for the operation of burn centers, *J Burn Care Rehabil* January/February:20A-29A, 1995.
3. *Trauma coordinators resource manual*, Park Ridge, IL, 1994, Emergency Nurses Association.
4. *Resource document for nursing care of the trauma patient*, ed 2, Park Ridge, IL, 1997, Emergency Nurses Association.
5. American College of Surgeons Committee on Trauma: *Advanced trauma life support*, Chicago, 1993, American College of Surgeons.
6. *Trauma nursing core course*, ed 4, Park Ridge, IL, 1995, Emergency Nurses Association.
7. Blank-Reid CA, Kaplan LJ: Video recording trauma resuscitations: a guide to system set-up, personnel concerns, and legal issues, *J Trauma Nurs* 3:9-12, 1996.
8. Hoyt DB, Shackford SR, Fridland PH, and others: Video recording trauma resuscitations: an effective teaching technique, *J Trauma* 28:535-540, 1988.

CHAPTER 3

Mass Casualty and Disaster Preparedness

Carole C. Atkinson

In no other situation do the concepts of interagency cooperation, communication, preplanning, and trauma team cohesion become more important than in the event of a mass casualty incident (MCI). On the local level, the principles of trauma team development, prehospital communication, and integrating community resources are truly put to the test. On a grander scale, regional, state, and federal agencies must be incorporated into the response system.

DEFINING MASS CASUALTY AND DISASTERS

A disaster situation can be defined as one in which the capacity of the daily operating system of care is exceeded. Mass casualty events or external disasters, such as the derailment of railroad cars, a terrorist attack, or an earthquake, usually result in a sudden influx of injured or ill patients into the emergency department (ED). The size of the facility and its proximity to resources such as transportation, additional personnel, and technical assistance on short notice, are factors that determine if the situation is a disaster for the institution. An internal disaster, such as medical gas failure, is a situation occurring within a hospital that disrupts normal operations of patient care. An internal incident, such as a fire, or a natural catastrophe, such as a hurricane, could also impact normal operations of a hospital and result in multiple victims. Safety and security of the patients and staff should be a priority.

INSTITUTIONAL PLANNING FOR DISASTER

A hospital wide disaster committee should be created to develop criteria for the activation of resources in the event of an internal or external disaster. Representation from all departments in the institution, not only the emergency department, is essential to efficiently organize disaster response. Institutional,

21

BOX 3-1

KEY ELEMENTS OF THE HOSPITAL DISASTER PLAN

1. Table of contents: for quick referencing
2. Definitions: to establish a frame of reference
3. Purpose and scope: to establish administrative authority
4. Plan activation: procedures for putting the plan into action
5. Notification and communication procedure: to ensure a smooth flow of information
6. Chain of command: to identify decision makers and authority figures
7. Command center: point of coordination and communication
8. Patient management plan: procedures for patient care functions
9. Patient staging area plan: readiness to receive victims, respond, and recover
   Traffic flow: systematic entry into system to prevent confusion
   Triage: classification of needs
   Decontamination: if toxic agent suspected
   Treatment areas: designated to maximize space utilization
      critical, dead, minor, fractures, pregnant, unsalvageable,
      surgical, medical, psychiatric, discharges, uninjured
10. Specialized areas: to maintain control
    family, media, employee volunteers, morgue
11. Individual departmental plans: to guide personnel
12. Internal disaster plans: individual procedures to respond to all categories of incidents
13. Evacuation plans: orderly routes to follow to secure patients and personnel
14. Interagency agreements: for specific resources, such as water suppliers or ambulances
15. Transfer criteria and agreements: for specialized treatment, such as burns or pediatrics

---

community, and regional uniqueness makes the utilization of generic disaster plans impossible (Box 3-1). Potential risk and variability of institutions require individual plan development for response to all potential causes of disasters (Box 3-2). The responsibilities of the hospital disaster committee include the following:

- Define what would be a disaster for the hospital.
- Review standards and guidelines developed by the Joint Commission on Accreditation of Healthcare Organizations (JCAHO) and local regulators addressing emergency preparedness.
- Create, review, and update the hospital plan as the institution changes, regulations are amended, or a flaw in the plan is identified.
- Assist each department with clarifying the roles of responders and predetermining leadership within the department.

BOX 3-2

POTENTIAL CAUSES OF DISASTERS

External Events

Natural

Earthquake

Tornado

Hurricane

Flood

Storm

Fire

Manmade

Terrorism; such as the Oklahoma
City or World Trade
Center bombing incidents

Transportation related: such as
airplane crash or railroad car
derailment

Nuclear/Biological/Chemical
(NBC) materials incident: such
as Chernobyl

Mass gathering: hysteria or
unrest

Internal Events

Electrical power failure: medical
equipment shutdowns, as well
as electronic information
systems

Water loss: heat, steam, and
vacuum

Fire/explosion: potential situation
for evacuation, as well as
victims

Loss of medical gases: oxygen
and air primarily for life
support

Flood

Chemical or radiation release

Bomb threat/explosion

Violence/hostagetaking

Elevator emergencies

Inability of staff to reach hospital

- Create a uniform format for each departmental plan; include external resources for personnel, equipment, and supplies.
- Create a concise notification system to contact on-duty and off-duty personnel.
- Integrate the local, regional, and state plans into the design of the hospital plan.
- Participate in the development of the local, regional, and state disaster plans.
- Orient, educate, and reeducate all personnel to disaster activation protocols.
- Conduct and evaluate drills testing the system; amend and improve the plan
- Critique activations of the disaster plan within the institution and community

COMMUNITY PLANNING FOR DISASTER

Resources beyond local responders may be necessary for some mass casualty incidents. Team leadership, predetermined during community planning, directs and delegates which agencies or positions have responsibility during an incident for such things as triage, extrication, decontamination, and initial treatment at the disaster site. Determining the need for supplemental resources to assist with disaster site activities is a key element of the community plan, but these resources must be identified ahead of time and assimilated into the plan. The ED will continue resuscitation and provide definitive care efficiently, only if they have understood and incorporated the initial community response into their disaster plan. At any time during the disaster, or in the hours, days, or weeks following the disaster, victims may present to the ED without the benefit of emergency medical services (EMS) involvement, or seek care at other locations in the community. Therefore the goal should be to provide a coordinated, comprehensive response to their needs. Essential points for a community plan include the following:

• Collaboration with all agencies that may be called on to respond in a disaster, including police, fire, EMS, hospitals and urgent care centers, Red Cross, utility companies, and the state/federal emergency management agency.
• A clear understanding by all agencies of what communication system will be used and who will conduct the central communications.
• A clear understanding by all agencies of the incident command system (ICS) and the leadership hierarchy.
• Participation by all agencies in regular sessions to create a plan, simulate the plan, and revise the plan for the community or region.
• A system for ongoing communication and reporting of activities in the aftermath of the disaster so that necessary services may be enhanced.

CONDUCTING A DISASTER DRILL

Annual evaluation of institutional response to disasters or emergencies is a requirement of JCAHO. The management plan for the facility describes actions to be taken for external and internal disasters, and outlines implementation of the educational component for personnel, as well as performance standards and evaluation criteria. The plan must be interpreted by the institution to fulfill Standard EC.1.6: A management plan addresses emergency preparedness. Disaster drills are executed by facilities to meet these requirements. The quality and effectiveness of the drill as an educational and evaluation tool is determined by the attitudes of the organizers and the participants. If the activity is taken seriously by all the stakeholders, helpful information about emergency procedures can be shared, inconsistencies and inadequacies in the plan can be identified, and suggestions for improvement and revisions can be made. Below are a few tips that may make the drill process successful.

• Put the plan on paper first; be certain that all participating agencies have clearly defined roles and procedures to follow.
• Include all agencies in planning the disaster drill, from outcomes and goals for the exercise, to choosing the scenario, site, date, and time of the drill.

- Conduct intradepartmental instruction for response so that each staff member has a clear understanding of his or her role in the drill; be certain to identify terminology that differentiates the drill from an actual event.
- Conduct an announced drill before an unannounced drill; although it may sound contradictory, actual events are infrequent, so having the opportunity to walk through the process is essential.
- In each department preassign an objective "observer," not involved with operational duties at the time of the drill, to provide feedback on their function.
- On completion, provide a mechanism, either on paper or an open forum, for each department to evaluate their part of the drill.
- Provide an opportunity for a representative from each department to participate in a hospital wide evaluation of the drill as close to the conclusion of the drill as possible and distribute a summary report internally of the evaluation results, identifying changes to incorporate into the disaster response procedure.
- Include all agencies in a discussion and critique of the drill, again as close to the end of the drill as feasible while impressions are fresh.
- Provide the community planning group with a summary report, including goals and outcomes met; make recommendations for amendments of the community drill process.
- Now, schedule an unannounced community-wide disaster drill. Invite the press to cover the exercise and use the opportunity to educate the community while working collaboratively with the media.

There is much to be learned from the actual and simulated disaster experiences that have been published in nursing, emergency medicine, and hospital administration journals. A review of this literature would be of great assistance in establishing or revising a plan. The most important concept to consider is that every plan must be written to meet the specific needs of the institution and the community. Collaborating with community members experienced in disaster response may prove to be the greatest asset in planning for the unexpected.

SUGGESTED READINGS

Joint Commission on Accreditation of Healthcare Organizations: *Hospital accreditation standards,* Oak Ridge Terrace, IL, 1997, The Commission.

Sigma Theta Tau International: *Reflections: journey of courage,* First quarter, Indianapolis, 1996, Center Nursing Press.

Morresca A, Burkel S, Lilibridge S: Disaster medicine, *Emerg Med Clin North Am* 14(2): 1996.

Sheehy SB: *Emergency nursing: principles and practice,* ed 4, St Louis, 1997, Mosby.

PART II

Clinical Principles

CHAPTER 4

Mechanism of Injury

Judith Stoner Halpern

Optimal care of a trauma patient combines a careful history with the assessment. It is crucial to identify the *mechanism* (i.e., the event that caused the injuries) and obtain details that help to estimate the severity of the incident. Certain mechanisms of injury are associated with specific patterns and may be used to predict severity of injury. The history can be used by the trauma team to anticipate the patient's needs and to plan care before his or her arrival. Providers can anticipate interventions, diagnostics, and additional personnel who may be needed. In essence, knowing the mechanism gives the trauma team the ability to act instead of react. In addition to helping with immediate planning, data collected and trended over time about certain mechanisms of injury can be used to identify high-risk populations and help direct trauma prevention programs.

HISTORY

Prehospital providers who encounter the patient at the scene of injury function as the eyes and ears for the rest of the trauma team (Fig. 4-1). They can collect pertinent, reliable details about the injuring event.

Motor vehicle crash

Important details to collect for a motor vehicle crash include:
- Speed of vehicles involved
- Size of vehicles involved
- Type of impact (e.g., frontal, lateral, sideswipe, rear, or rollover)
- Position of victim(s) in or on the vehicle(s) before *and* after the crash (e.g., driver, passenger(s), pedestrian(s)) (Fig. 4-2)
- Use of safety devices (e.g., lap belt, shoulder belt, child car seat) and if properly employed
- If air bags were deployed and approximate position of the victim(s) in relation to bag when inflated (e.g., seat distance, if safety belts were in use)

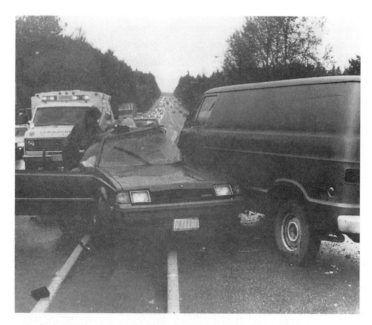

Fig. 4-1 History is important. Be sure to include the angle of impact. (Courtesy Tacoma Fire Department.)

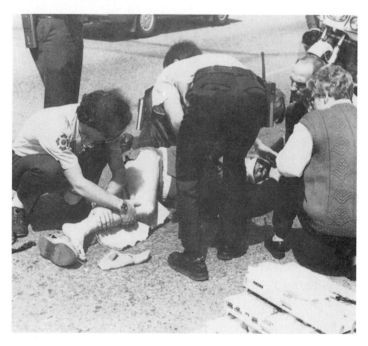

Fig. 4-2 Consider the position of the patient. (Courtesy Tacoma Fire Department.)

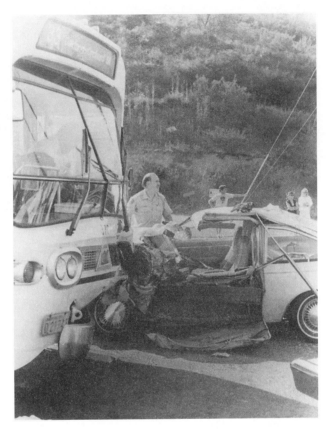

Fig. 4-3   Notice bent or broken objects. (Courtesy Tacoma Fire Department.)

- Vehicle deformity suggestive of force involved in impact (e.g., broken seat, approximate distance exterior was pushed into interior of vehicle) (Fig. 4-3)
- Structures where occupant may have made contact (e.g., broken windshield, broken rearview mirror, bent steering wheel, broken gearshift)
- Smoke or fumes at scene that may have affected injury environment
- Condition of other occupant(s) (e.g., death of another occupant is clear evidence that force was powerful enough to cause major injuries) (Fig. 4-4)

Penetrating injuries

Important details to collect for penetrating injuries include:
- Identification of number and type of wound(s), paying close attention to areas such as axilla, groin, thick or matted hair that may hide wounds; carefully preserve clothing and other potential evidence that may be used for estimating injury and/or medical-legal cases

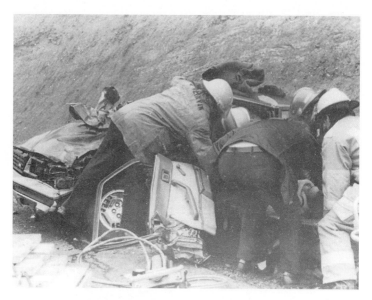

Fig. 4-4 Trauma occurs when a person experiences an acute exposure to energy. (Courtesy Tacoma Fire Department.)

- Size of wounding instrument (e.g., caliber, velocity of bullet, distance from assailant, length of knife, impaled object) and approximate direction of entrance to determine tract

Falls and jumps

Important details to collect for falls and jumps include:
- Distance of fall or jump
- Surface that victim hit (to estimate how much force was absorbed by surface)
- Area of body that made initial impact (e.g., feet first, along entire axis of body, other prominent point)
- Victim's activity before fall or jump

Fires

Important details to collect for fires include:
- Thermal or chemical injury to body structures (e.g., approximate body surface area and depth of burn, smoke or heat inhalation)
- Field therapy for surface injury
- Environment (e.g., closed space, open area with ventilation)
- Explosive forces involved (e.g., if protected from or exposed directly to blast wave, additional injury by flying debris, collapsing structures, onto what surface victim thrown)
- Potential for secondary injuries from chemicals, toxic gases, burning products, victim's attempt to escape (e.g., jump from building)

Injuries related to machines

Important details to collect for injuries related to machines include:
- Length of time since injury, extrication
- Function of machine (e.g., grinding, chopping, rotary, high-energy source)
- Potential contaminants (e.g., bacterial, animal manure, pesticides, herbicides, lubricants, fuel)

Other helpful information

It is helpful to remember that the term *injury* also includes physiologic damage caused by extremes of temperature or absence of life-sustaining substances, such as oxygen; therefore, it is also important to relate the conditions of the scene. Extreme cold or heat, wet conditions, and smoke can create additional injuries that may not be as visible.

Medical conditions and the consumption of alcohol or other drugs can significantly alter a patient's response to injury. It is especially helpful if field personnel survey the scene for evidence of the victim using medications, beverages, or illicit substances.

FORCE OF INJURY

Tissues are injured when exposed to excessive amounts of mechanical, electrical, thermal or chemical energy, and/or deprived of heat and oxygen. The injury can be a structural or physiologic disruption. Because most cases of trauma involve mechanical energy, a brief overview of several key points is provided.

Kinetic energy

The wounding potential of an event is greatly affected by the amount of kinetic energy (energy in motion) that is transferred to the victim. Kinetic energy is determined by the mass of the object in motion and its velocity or amount of acceleration. The following formula demonstrates the relationship:

$$KE = \frac{1}{2} \text{ mass} \times \text{velocity}^2$$

By this formula one can note that kinetic energy can be increased in two ways; doubling the mass results in doubling the kinetic energy; however, doubling the velocity results in quadrupling the kinetic energy.

Laws of motion

Newton's first law of motion holds that when an object is set in motion, it will remain in motion until acted on by an outside force. A person riding in a vehicle, thrown, falling, or suddenly struck by an object will remain or be set into motion and remain at that rate of acceleration until another force inhibits that motion (i.e., causes deceleration): the vehicle crashes, or the person lands on a surface. Deceleration forces cause deformation of tissue referred to as *strains*, which are classified as *tensile* (stretching), *shear* (opposing forces across an object), or *compressive* (crushing). When the deforming force exceeds the tissue's ability to regain its original shape (*elasticity*) or its ability to resist a change in shape during motion (*viscosity*), the tissue will be injured, resulting in lacerations, contusions, fractures, ruptures, and other types of injuries.[1]

The pattern of injuries noted with deceleration can be attributed to multiple factors, which include point of impact and rate of deceleration. During a motor vehicle crash (MVC), the vehicle travels at a set speed until stopped. An occupant continues to travel at that speed until an outside force or object (safety belt, air bag, or striking the vehicle interior) causes him or her to stop. Because certain organs or anatomic structures within the body are able to shift position (i.e., are not anatomically "fixed"), they continue in motion until they strike a hard interior structure or strain flexible points of attachment (e.g., the first impact is car to tree, the second impact is occupant to instrument panel, the third impact is heart to sternum). This is described as a *crash within a crash within a crash* and is used to describe the pattern of injuries seen in sudden deceleration. External injuries are directly related to the force or objects that strike the body in a sudden deceleration. Internal injuries are related to deceleration, which causes deforming forces to underlying structures and organs that are not "fixed" and therefore able to shift to be set into motion, which suddenly strike a hard interior surface and/or rupture from points of attachment (e.g., brain, heart, liver, spleen, intestine).

TYPES OF INJURY MECHANISMS

In describing the types of injury mechanisms, a distinction is made between penetrating forces and blunt forces.

Penetrating forces involve direct contact with an instrument that cuts the skin, require less energy to injure, and result in fewer body structures harmed. Penetrating injuries are the result of a stabbing, a bullet wound, a high-pressure injections, and an impaled foreign object.

Blunt forces involve compression, deformation, or sudden change in atmospheric pressure. They result in more injuries and more types of injuries, including contusions, lacerations, fractures, or ruptures of solid tissue masses. Injuries sustained with a blunt force tend to be more difficult to manage because more structures can be affected, the lack of external signs with occult injuries may delay diagnosis, and the patient may experience more complications as a result of the injury(ies).

PATTERNS OF INJURY ASSOCIATED WITH VARIOUS INJURY MECHANISMS

Motor vehicle crash

Patients who are injured as a result of an MVC can have patterns of injury that vary according to their position in the vehicle and the use of safety restraints.

Position in vehicle

The driver is at risk for striking the steering column, instrument panel, gear-shift handle, rearview mirror, windshield, the A pillar (between windshield and door), and the door. The reported patterns of injury correspond with the body parts most likely to hit these structures:
• Facial lacerations, facial bone fractures
• Scalp lacerations, skull fractures, intracranial injuries
• Spinal injuries
• Chest wall lacerations, contusions; rib, clavicle, and sternal fractures; pulmonary contusions, lacerations with corresponding pneumohemo-thorax
• Thoracic aorta laceration at area of attachment (i.e., superior to left subclavian artery)
• Abdominal wall lacerations, contusions; rupture or avulsion of liver, spleen, kidney, pancreas, bowel, bladder
• Fractured humerus, radius, ulna, wrist, hand
• Fractured pelvis; posterior hip dislocation; fractured femur, tibia, fibula, ankle, foot; ligamentous injury to knee.
• Several common patterns of skeletal injury in an MVC involve the knee striking the instrument panel (causing a patellar fracture and ligamentous disruption in the knee joint), the force transmitted along the axis of the femur (producing a posterior hip dislocation and femoral shaft fracture), or the feet becoming entangled in the floor pedals and causing fractures or strain on joints

Front-seat passengers are not exposed to the same number and type of internal vehicle structures and have a different pattern of injuries. Although they have a higher incidence of head, abdominal, and upper torso fractures, they have fewer thoracic injuries and lower torso fractures.[1]

Rear-seat passengers' incidence of severe injury can be as high as front-seat occupants if they are not restrained.

Use of safety restraints

Shoulder and lap restraints reduce the incidence and severity of injury by reducing the force with which a person strikes a surface, preventing the victim from striking multiple surfaces or preventing ejection from the vehicle (Fig. 4-5). Consequently, restrained occupants have fewer or less severe head, facial, and thoracic injuries, or upper and lower torso fractures. In a crash with significant forces or cases in which the restraints are used improperly, the restraint can produce injuries to the
  • chest (fractured ribs, lung or cardiac contusion)
  • abdomen (tear or rupture of liver, spleen, kidney, pancreas, bowel, iliac artery, or aorta)
  • cervical spine (fracture, dislocation of spine, blunt injury to cervical blood vessels) or lumbar spine (disrupted ligaments, vertebral fractures)

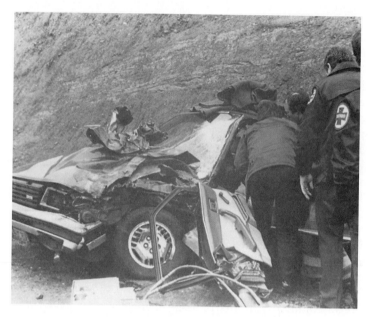

Fig. 4-5 Driver, unrestrained, sustained major trauma. (Courtesy Tacoma Fire Department.)

Air bags installed in vehicles are a supplemental restraint in frontal crashes. Some automotive manufacturers have also introduced side air bags for lateral impacts. Air bags have been associated with a reduction in the severity of brain injury and incidence of facial fractures and lacerations and lower extremity fractures.[2]

As with other types of safety restraints, air bags can also pose a risk for injury for certain high-risk individuals. Occupants who are out of position (leaning forward, riding with seat close to air bag, or unrestrained) or infants and children in car seats can be struck by the air bag or module cover. The air bag can produce *direct contact injuries* (contusions, abrasions, lacerations, fractures), trauma to internal organs (eye, heart, intraabdominal organs), and severe head and neck injuries in children.[3]

Pedestrians struck by motor vehicle

A moving vehicle strikes a pedestrian with its bumper and hood, causing the individual to lose balance or become airborne and finally land on a surface, which provides a third area of impact. The areas of impact can vary depending on the victim's height and the size of the vehicle. Typical injuries occur in a triad pattern (Fig. 4-6):

- hood strikes an adult on lower abdomen, hip, or upper femur region; a child in the head, chest, or abdominal region

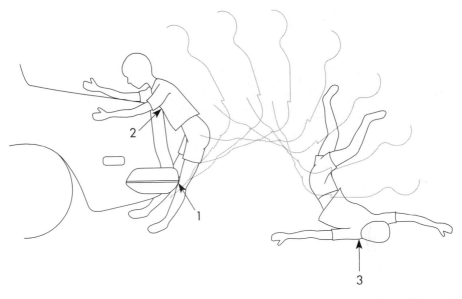

Fig. 4-6   Pedestrian struck by vehicle will typically have several points of impact. A child will be struck by the (1) bumper in the lower leg; (2) hood in the upper torso; and (3) force of impact, which will cause victim to strike the ground. This pattern of injuries is referred to as Waddell's triad. (Redrawn from Halpern JS: *J Emerg Nurs* 8:172, 1982.)

- bumper strikes adult on lower leg; child in femur or tibia/fibula region
- victim lands on hood or ground (producing head, chest and/or abdominal injuries)

If a patient presents with injuries that correspond to one or two of the above regions, the provider should be alert to the possibility of additional injuries that fit this pattern.

Cyclists

The patterns of injuries can vary between riders of motorcycles and bicycles. Motorcycles tend to be heavier and tip sideways, entrapping extremities and producing lateral injuries. Bicycles are lighter than motorcycles. The front tire catches or becomes destabilized, causing forward-leaning cyclists to be propelled forward, striking their face, head, or outstretched arms.

Falls or jumps

While an MVC represents a form of horizontal deceleration, a jump or fall creates a vertical deceleration if the person lands on the feet, buttocks, or top

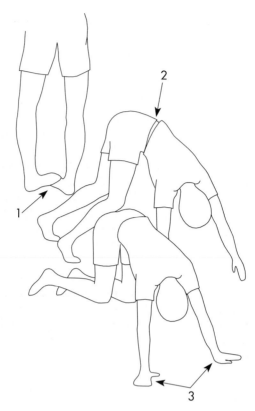

Fig. 4-7 Pattern of injuries associated with a jump or fall. (1) Victim lands on feet, causing lower-extremity injuries; (2) force causes victim to hyperflex the lumbar spine; (3) victim lands on outstretched arms, causing injury to the distal upper extremities. (Redrawn from Halpern JS: *J Emerg Nurs* 8:174, 1982.)

of skull. The mobile internal structures move up and down, stressing different points of attachment than if the motion was anterior or posterior. The patterns and severity of the victim's injuries will depend on

- distance traveled
- impact surface (i.e., energy absorbing or rigid)
- body area(s) making initial contact on impact

If the victim lands on his or her feet, buttocks, or top of head, the impacting force is transmitted along the axis of the skeleton causing

- compression fractures of the os calcis (heel); long bones of lower torso, pelvis, and lumbar spine—if person propelled forward, may stretch out arms to inhibit fall and cause bilateral wrist (Colles') fractures (Figure 4-7)
- pelvic vascular injuries

- descending aortic disruption at area of attachment (i.e., above dia-phragm)
- separation of heart from aortic valve

Penetrating wounds

Objects that penetrate the skin can produce a wide variety of injury patterns depending on the degree of penetration, the ability to release kinetic energy, and the untoward effects that the missile produces. Objects with low kinetic energy (i.e., low velocity), such as knives, produce *stab wounds* that are limited to the length of the penetrating object, direction or trajectory of the stabbing motion, and the structures that are in line with the sinus tract produced. An impaled object should be left in place whenever possible to aid in the diagnosis of the injury and to help tamponade any small, bleeding surfaces. Objects that appear to be close to a bone should be evaluated to determine if the wound constitutes a compound fracture and requires surgical débridement and infection prophylaxis.

Objects that enter the body as missiles can be classified as *gunshot wounds* or *impaled foreign objects.* Bullets produce a wide range of injuries, and wound ballistics (i.e., the study of how a missile interacts with target tissue) are dependent on characteristics of the missile, weapon, and body part(s) struck.[4] When assessing the severity of a gunshot wound, the following information should be obtained:

- caliber (size or diameter of missile)
- type of missile (potential to deform or fragment)
- type of gun
- trajectory of missile in body (structures involved)
- range (distance between victim and weapon)

Missiles produce tissue injury by two methods: *direct* (laceration, heat) or *indirect* mechanisms (cavitation, shock wave). It is difficult to predict exact internal injuries associated with a gunshot wound because kinetic energy and the tissue response vary. A low-velocity missile, which cuts or lacerates tissue, can be fatal if it strikes a highly vascular structure, such as the aorta, or inconsequential if it strikes a less vital structure. This type of missile produces little cavitation and does not exceed the tissue's elasticity.

Temporary cavitation is more of an issue with a high-velocity missile. A high-powered missile can be discharged at close range and pass through an extremity, creating just a laceration because of the high elasticity of the muscle. However, if the kinetic energy is transmitted to less-elastic tissue, that same extremity may need to be amputated because the bones are shattered and neurovascular structures destroyed beyond repair. Cavitation is most destructive in nonelastic tissue, such as bone, liver, spleen, and brain.[1]

Other types of impaled objects are dangerous because the initial appearance of the wound may not be significant. *High-pressure injection wounds* come from the inadvertent introduction of a liquid into tissue, such as in the hand. Initially, the wound appears to be a minor puncture site, painless and nonedematous. Within hours, the injected foreign substance (water, cleanser, paint, or lubricating solution) begins an inflammatory response that leads to infection and compartment syndrome. Patients with injection wounds need to be evaluated immediately for surgical exploration and débridement.

PATTERNS OF INJURY ASSOCIATED WITH KNOWN INJURIES

Patterns of injuries can also be predicted according to the anatomic area involved. When certain body areas are subjected to a sudden deceleration or compressive force, the rigid bony skeleton and mobile tissue mass can produce underlying contusions or rupture.

Scalp

Tissue is quite vascular and does not readily vasoconstrict; therefore direct pressure is required to control blood loss. Large, bulky dressings cannot generate the point-specific pressure required.

Skull

A linear fracture over the temporal region could be associated with injury to underlying middle meningeal artery and subsequent epidural hematoma. A depressed skull fracture requires significant force, therefore underlying intracranial soft tissue and dural layers may also be contused, lacerated, or contaminated.

Brain

The brain is mobile within the rigid skull, and if set into motion (acceleration or deceleration forces), can strike multiple surfaces within the skull and cause multisite contusions (i.e., coup-contrecoup mechanism). The mobile brain strains at the points of attachment, which are the veins beneath the dura (creating a subdural hematoma), brain stem, and cranial nerves.

Eye

The eye is a liquid-filled globe generally protected by the bony rim created by the facial bones. Eye trauma is the result of an object smaller than the circumference of the rim (e.g., golf club, fist, steering wheel) coming in direct contact with the eye and causing an increase in intraorbital pressure. Any pressure applied to a fluid in a container is transmitted undiminished in all directions throughout the fluid (Pascal's principle), resulting in stretching of ocular structures (e.g., retina, iris, choroid, ciliary body) and blowout fractures of the weaker medial orbital floor. Clinically, backward displacement of the eye into the orbit and possibly hypesthesia (loss of feeling) below the eye may result.

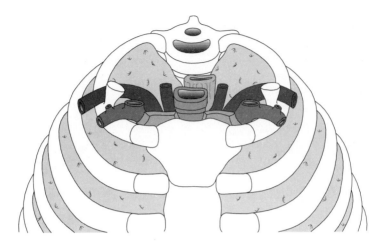

Fig. 4-8   Anatomy of root of neck showing structures that may be injured with penetrating forces to the upper torso/neck region. (Redrawn from Naclerio E: *Chest injuries, physiologic principles and emergency management,* Orlando, FL, 1971, Grune & Stratton.)

Facial bones

The bones in the face fracture from direct impact and involve multiple sites. Fracture may be suspected clinically when facial structures are edematous and asymmetric and eye movement is limited. The patient's airway can easily be compromised by hemorrhage or edema. Direct trauma to the face may precipitate intracranial and/or cervical spine injuries.

Neck

Penetrating injury of the soft tissues near the thoracic outlet (base of neck) should be carefully assessed for possible involvement of underlying structures, including apices of the lung, major vascular structures, esophagus, trachea, or cervical spine (Fig. 4-8); penetrating injury of the esophagus can produce sepsis from bacterial contamination of surrounding tissue. Cervical spine injury should be suspected with blunt forces to the neck.

Chest

Deceleration forces cause heart, aorta, and bronchus distal to the carina (point of bifurcation into left and right bronchi) to tear from points of attachment. Compressive forces can cause fractures of relatively strong skeletal structures, and underlying organ damage should be suspected when fractures are found (e.g., ribs [pulmonary contusion, injury to proximal artery, lacerated liver or spleen, ruptured diaphragm], scapula [pulmonary contusion, brachial plexus disruption], sternum [cardiac contusion, lacerated liver]). Ecchymosis or abrasion in areas consistent with the safety belt should alert clinical personnel to

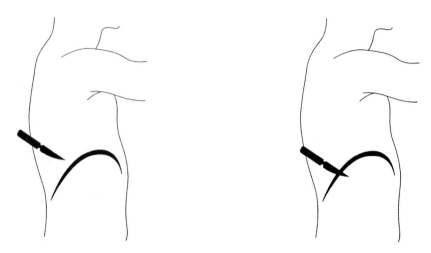

Fig. 4-9 Trajectory of stab wound to midchest region. Note possible involvement of intrathoracic and intraabdominal structures. (Redrawn from Naclerio E: *Chest injuries, physiologic principles and emergency management,* Orlando, FL, 1971, Grune & Stratton.)

the potential for pulmonary and/or cardiac contusion, or rib fracture with or without flail segment.

Abdomen

Compressive forces cause solid organs to rupture and hemorrhage if pressure is great enough; hollow organs, such as the bowel and bladder, can rupture and spill their contents at the time of injury; fractures of lower ribs may lacerate abdominal structures; ecchymosis or abrasion in areas consistent with the safety belt should alert clinical personnel to the potential for small bowel, pancreatic, and lumbar spine injury (Chance fracture).

Deceleration forces can tear the bowel at points of attachment, including the retroperitoneal duodenum and intraperitoneal small bowel. Penetrating objects may produce wounds that involve the chest wall, pleura, diaphragm, and/or multiple sites in the bowel (because of the proximity of bowel loops) (Fig. 4-9); they may produce eventual sepsis if the bowel is penetrated.

Pelvis

The pelvis is made up of multiple durable and injury-resistant bones, which protect the lower abdomen and major blood vessels. The bones and soft tissues are highly vascular and can produce a significant blood loss if disrupted. The pelvic bones form a ring, which usually disrupts in more than one area. A fractured pelvis should be considered as a sign that the victim has sustained a major force, is likely to have significant intraabdominal and bladder injuries, and has a high potential for major blood loss. Males may experience urethral disruption if a pelvic fracture causes strain on rigid soft tissues that anchor the urethra on the inferior surface of the prostate gland.

Extremities

Compressive strain on the skeleton causes forces to be transmitted along the axis of the bone to weaker, less elastic structures (joints). Fractures may appear alone or in association with ligamentous injuries in distal joints. Because many nerves and blood vessels are close to bones, the possibility of neurovascular compromise should be considered. Wounds on an extremity with a known or suspected fracture should be considered as a possible open fracture (if examined closely, clinical personnel may note golden globules, evidence of bone marrow in a wound, in serous drainage).

REFERENCES

1. Feliciano DV: Patterns of injury. In Feliciano DV, Moore EE, Mattox KL, editors: *Trauma*, ed 3, Stamford, CT, 1996, Appleton & Lange.
2. Loo GT, Siegel JH, Dischinger PC, and others: Airbag protection versus compartment intrusion effect determines the pattern of injuries in multiple trauma motor vehicle crashes, *J Trauma* 41:935-951, 1996.
3. Weintraub B: Air bag-mediated injury in the emergency department population, *Int J Trauma Nurs* 3:46-49, 1997.
4. Dufresne GW: Wound ballistics: recognizing wound potential. Part 1: characteristics of missiles and weapons, *Int J Trauma Nurs* 1:4-10, 1995.

CHAPTER 5

Prehospital Care

Mark C. N. Libby

The earliest aspect of trauma care is the prehospital phase, the period of time from the injury occurrence through recognition of the emergency situation, response, resuscitation, triage, and transportation to definitive care. Prehospital trauma care is the foundation on which subsequent elements of the trauma care system are built. A successful prehospital system integrates the public safety, public health, and healthcare systems to provide appropriate assessment, treatment, and transport of the trauma patient to an appropriate facility.

Modern civilian trauma systems have implemented many of the principles first learned by the military services during wartime. The military experience demonstrated that trauma is a time-sensitive disease. The military achieved dramatic improvements in casualty survival by providing an organized system for trauma care. Lives were saved when care was initiated in the field (at the scene) and the time from injury to definitive surgical care was decreased. As these lessons were applied to civilian practice, prehospital systems were developed that brought together education of the lay public and prehospital care providers, triage and practice guidelines, communications capabilities, and ground/air transport modes. Mature systems are now also engaged in quality improvement activities, clinical and systems research, public education, injury prevention, legislative activities, and public policy formation.

PREHOSPITAL ENVIRONMENT AND SCENE SAFETY

The prehospital environment is unpredictable at best and dangerous at worst. At all times, the personal safety of the prehospital trauma care provider must come first. Consider the risks of being called to a potentially violent event, in adverse weather and terrain, with hazardous materials and biohazards, loud noise levels, risk of fire, and anxious bystanders. In responding to a motor vehicle crash, for example, there are potential hazards from downed electric wires; spillage of hazardous chemicals, fuel, or oil; broken glass or jagged metal; blood or body fluids; the operation of hydraulic or pneumatic extrication tools; and from the risk posed by distracted motorists passing by the scene. The injury scene may also be a crime scene where critical forensic and physical evidence has to be preserved. Professionals who participate in prehospital care must be intellectually and physically capable of identifying and managing potential risks, providing direct patient care, and managing stressful situations. Collectively, possession of this set of observational, assessment, planning, and behavioral skills is referred to as "situational awareness" or "street sense."

The most important step for safety at the incident is personal preparation. The prehospital care provider must be mentally alert and have focused communication with other team members. Universal precautions must be employed, including eye protection. Personal immunization against hepatitis B and tetanus should also be current. Physical fitness and agility should be sufficient to permit the rescuer to perform tasks such as lifting and carrying equipment and patients. Protective, high-visibility clothing appropriate to the environmental risk should be employed. For example, when caring for a patient during motor vehicle crash extrication, protection consisting of a helmet with face shield, heavy gloves, boots, and firefighting coat and pants is mandatory. All medical and rescue equipment should be checked at the beginning of each shift to ensure that it is complete and functional.

INCIDENT MANAGEMENT AND WORKING AT THE SCENE

The prehospital care provider always works as part of a team. The field team is usually a multiagency effort, made up of fire/rescue, law enforcement, and emergency medical services (EMS) units. To safely and effectively coordinate the efforts of individual units as a team, most jurisdictions implement an incident management system, sometimes also known as the incident command system. Incident management is a standard method of operating at all incidents. The key element of incident management is the establishment of a command structure, regardless of whether the incident is large or small. Command is invested in the one person responsible for the outcome of the incident. The incident commander is responsible for planning (assessment of current and anticipated needs), operations (mitigation of the emergency), logistics, and administration. One of the most dangerous and counterproductive behaviors at the scene of an incident is "freelancing," when personnel do not operate as part of the team. Prehospital care providers must be willing to accept direction from the incident commander.

On arrival at the incident location, the prehospital care provider should report, by radio, to the incident commander. The scene should not be approached until it has been evaluated for life-threatening hazards and access has been granted by the incident commander. The mechanism of the event can then be assessed to estimate the transfer of force to the patient and the potential for injury. Instant or digital photography of the scene helps to document and communicate the mechanism of injury.

Once working at the scene, constant vigilance is required so that risks are identified and controlled. There should also be an early determination whether there are sufficient assets available on scene to manage the situation. This is especially important for air medical helicopter services and specialty rescue units such as confined space, heavy rescue, or hazardous materials teams.

TRIAGE AND TRANSPORT

Of the prehospital trauma care provider's many responsibilities, the triage decision is one of the most important. The task of the prehospital care provider is to identify those patients who need trauma center care. Trauma triage protocols and practices should be developed and monitored at the system level. A model approach to trauma triage has been promulgated by the American College of Surgeons (Fig. 5-1).

The greatest potential for harm comes from undertriage. *Undertriage* means that the patient's injuries were underestimated or that the patient was transported to a facility that did not have adequate resources to manage the patient. This can result in a delay in care and additional morbidity and mortality. A patient is *overtriaged* when the potential for injury is overestimated or more resources are deployed than needed. The problem with overtriage is that it incurs additional expense to the system and diverts resources away from more seriously injured patients. There is currently no triage methodology that totally avoids both overtriage and undertriage. Trauma systems developers usually agree to tolerate a certain level of overtriage to protect patients and ensure that undertriage is kept to a minimum.

The provider must assess the patient's potential for serious injury, determine the best available facility to care for the patient, consider transport time, and decide the mode of transport to that destination. The closest facility is not always the best facility. When the destination is in question, it is best to make a conservative judgment and transport the patient to a predesignated trauma center. The prehospital care provider should also consider establishing communication with the medical direction facility, describing the situation, and asking for guidance.

Many prehospital care providers now have air medical services available to them. These are helicopters or fixed-wing aircraft. Air medical transport should be considered based on the mechanism of injury, severity of the patient's injuries, the need for rapid transport, need for a higher level of care during transport, and other situational considerations. Air medical transport offers the advantages of high-level care, mobility, and speed of transport. If air medical services are available, providers must know how to access the program and should have attended a formal briefing on aircraft landing zone safety and patient loading.

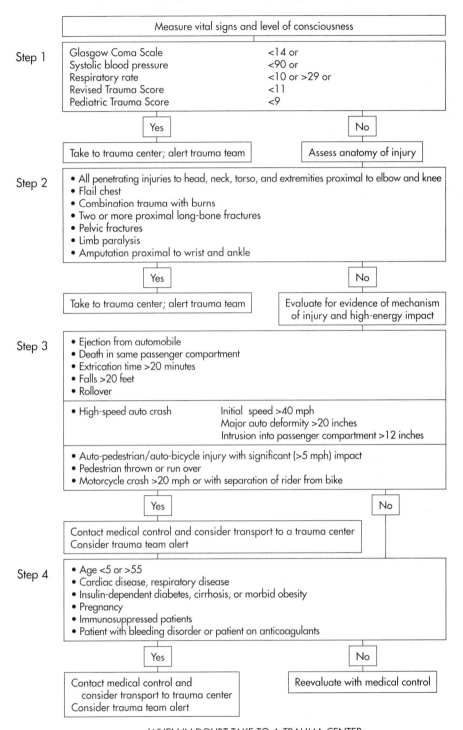

Fig. 5-1 Triage decision scheme. (From American College of Surgeons: *Resources for optimal care of the injured patient,* Chicago, 1993, American College of Surgeons.)

PREHOSPITAL TRAUMA RESUSCITATION

The goal of prehospital trauma resuscitation is to begin to identify life-threatening injuries and to initiate therapy as soon as possible, without delaying immediate transport to the trauma center. Since survival is often directly linked to the length of time from injury to trauma center care, prehospital care providers should strive to limit the time on-scene by only addressing key tasks such as airway control and immobilization of the spine. All other assessments and interventions should be performed while en route to the trauma center. Physical assessment of the trauma patient at the scene is often hampered by poor access to the patient, lack of exposure, background noise, and darkness. The clinician is therefore challenged to develop assessment skills that overcome these evaluation obstacles. Field trauma resuscitation should follow the methodical but rapid **A**irway-**B**reathing-**C**irculation format for primary survey and intervention.

The prehospital trauma care provider should first assess the patient's airway, with simultaneous control of the cervical spine. These are the two most important field interventions for decreasing trauma morbidity and mortality. If a patient cannot maintain a patent airway, the airway must be secured at once. Endotracheal intubation is the most desirable method of securing the airway. This skill, however, can be difficult in the field. At all times, there must be a backup plan to manage the airway, by either reverting to basic maneuvers or performing a surgical airway. The patency of the airway must be ensured at frequent intervals, especially when the patient is extricated or otherwise moved.

Breathing should be assessed for rate, rhythm, and adequacy of air exchange. High-concentration supplemental oxygen should be administered. Ventilation should be assisted with a bag-valve ventilator whenever air exchange is inadequate.

Circulation is assessed by checking for the presence of central pulses. Severe external hemorrhage is best managed with direct pressure to the wound. Large-bore intravenous access and infusion of fluids can be initiated while en route to the trauma center. If at any time during the resuscitation there is uncertainty about how to proceed, or if there is an interruption of the plan of care, the prehospital care provider should revert to fundamental assessments and interventions using the A-B-C format.

COMMUNICATION AND DOCUMENTATION

Many of the communications that take place in the prehospital environment occur via radio systems that serve law enforcement, fire services, and EMS. When communicating by radio, remember to:
• Speak clearly and briefly, directly into the microphone.
• Identify yourself by your service and unit number.
• Protect patient confidentiality when conveying medical information. Remember that many people, including citizens with radio scanners, are listening to these transmissions.

- Maintain professionalism; be patient when information or transmission is unclear. Never use profanity or jargon. Most systems tape all transmissions.
- Convey information in a systematic manner. Patient information should include age, gender, mechanism of injury, chief complaint, level of consciousness, brief description of suspected injuries, vital signs, interventions, and estimated time of arrival (ETA).
- Sign off to indicate the end of your transmission.

Emergency department staff receiving the radio report should expect only a general understanding of the patient's condition. Nonessential questions should be held until the patient arrives to avoid tying up the radio channel or taking the EMS provider away from the patient.

On arrival at the trauma center, the patient report is verbally given to trauma team members. The report should include any changes that occurred during transport. Because the team is simultaneously assuming care of the patient, be prepared to repeat elements of the report. Written documentation of the prehospital care episode should be prepared and placed in the patient's medical record. The prehospital care report is important for patient care, quality improvement, research, and as a legal record. It must be accurate, legible, and complete.

TEAMWORK

Hospital-based trauma team members must encourage open communication with prehospital care providers, offer guidance and educational opportunities, and listen to concerns and suggestions. Inclusion of prehospital care providers in continuing education, case reviews, quality improvement programs, and research initiatives strengthens team relationships and improves patient care. Follow-up information given to prehospital providers on the trauma patient's injuries and outcome provides feedback and closure of the episode. Because of the stressful nature of prehospital care, there should also be opportunities for a team debriefing after difficult cases.

Nurses and physicians who work in emergency departments, critical care units, or trauma units are encouraged to ride as observers with EMS teams. This offers valuable insight into the early care of trauma patients, as well as improving the relationship between prehospital and hospital personnel.

SUGGESTED READINGS

Emergency medical services agenda for the future, Washington, DC, 1996, National Highway Traffic Safety Administration.

National Flight Nurses Association: *Flight nursing: principles and practice,* ed 2, St Louis, 1996, Mosby.

Semonin-Holleran R: *Prehospital nursing: a collaborative approach,* St Louis, 1995, Mosby.

CHAPTER 6

Patient Transfer

Mary G. Kennedy

Because patient outcome may depend on rapid transport to an appropriate facility, an efficient patient transfer process is vital. The first step is to develop a comprehensive transfer plan.

This chapter discusses interfacility transfers, but *intra*facility transfers (e.g., from the emergency department [ED] to computed tomography [CT] scan, operating room [OR], or intensive care unit [ICU]) also require planning and preparation. Appropriately trained staff and the proper equipment should accompany patients whenever they are in transit.

TRANSFER PLAN

Every institution should have a transfer plan that has been coordinated between transferring and receiving agencies. Agency policies and procedures should be consistent with local or regional policies, when they exist.

The transfer plan should include the following:
- Names and contact phone numbers of receiving facilities
- Criteria defining types of patients to be transferred
- Criteria defining appropriate receiving facilities for each type of patient (trauma, burns, pediatric, etc.)
- Guidelines for the selection of the appropriate transfer mode and accompanying personnel
- Names and contact phone numbers of ambulance and helicopter services
- Communications procedures with transport services and receiving facilities
- Requirements for stabilization before transfer
- Requirements and expectations of the receiving facility
- Provisions for families and friends of the patient
- Forms for documentation before and during the transfer and documentation guidelines
- Guidelines for care en route

- Lists of equipment and supplies (or prepackaged kits) to accompany patient, if hospital personnel conduct a transfer
- Policy detailing who assumes financial responsibility for the transfer

In addition, patient care plans should be developed for patients who have sustained multiple trauma, serious single-system injuries (such as head, cervical spine, chest, or abdomen), amputations, and burn injuries. There should also be transfer care plans for infants, children, pregnant women, and elderly patients.

LEGAL CONSIDERATIONS

Important legal considerations apply to transfer situations. The Consolidated Omnibus Budget Reconciliation Act (COBRA) is a federal law enacted in 1986. COBRA was later combined with the Emergency Medical Treatment and Active Labor Act (EMTALA). The overall purpose of COBRA and EMTALA is to provide guidelines for and regulate the treatment and transfer of patients between hospitals.

The following are key points relevant to trauma patient transfers:

- Hospitals are obligated to provide *appropriate* medical screening examinations to all patients who present to their emergency department.
- The reason(s) for transfer and advantages of sending a patient to another facility must be documented clearly. Patients should only be transferred to a higher level of care, (i.e., a level III trauma center should transfer to a level I trauma center) or to a lateral level of care (i.e., the patient is followed at a specific hospital that has at least the same capabilities as the sending facility).
- Ground and air ambulances must have appropriate personnel and equipment for the transfer. The level of care provided during interfacility transfers should not fall below that level of care provided within the referring hospital. Nursing organizations such as the Emergency Nurses Association (ENA) have created specific position statements in regard to this issue. The ENA recommends that if a patient requires specialized nursing care before transfer, the same expertise should be required during transfer.[1]
- All patients must be maximally stabilized before transfer, within the capabilities of the sending facility.

Transfer documentation should include, when possible, permission to transfer the patient given by the patient or the patient's next of kin. The receiving physician's name and acceptance of the patient should also be documented.

PREPARATION FOR TRANSFER TO A TRAUMA CENTER

Decision to transfer

Each institution should develop criteria for transfer based on the availability of specific personnel, skills, equipment, or technology. It is important to be able to determine when a patient needs definitive care beyond the scope of what is available in the receiving hospital, community, or system. General guidelines concerning patients likely to require trauma center care are available from the American College of Surgeons (Box 6-1).

Modes of transport

Clinical personnel should identify the various modes of transport available to the community or facility and should be familiar with the advantages and disadvantages of each so that an informed decision can be made. Personnel should also be familiar with the means to gain access to these transportation modes and know how to access regional resource centers. It is wise to have transport policies and plans in place before the need arises. These policies and plans should be written with the mutual agreement of the referring and receiving facilities and transporting agencies.

When determining the mode of transportation that would best serve the needs of the patient, clinical personnel should consider the time required to transfer the patient; the type of equipment available; patient care and work space required; the type and capabilities of personnel involved in the transport; and other limiting factors such as weather conditions, terrain, and transport distance.

Ground ambulance

ADVANTAGES

- Usually readily available
- Can travel in most weather conditions
- Usually adequate space in which to provide patient care
- May be able to carry more than one patient or one patient plus large pieces of equipment
- Usually less noisy than aircraft
- May be staffed by advanced life support (ALS) personnel with ALS equipment
- Usually has space for additional personnel or family members

DISADVANTAGES

- Increased transport times
- Possibility of traffic collisions
- Sometimes bumpy or rough ride
- Limited access to certain terrain
- Possibility that ALS personnel and equipment are not available
- Travel on icy or muddy roads

Helicopter (rotorcraft)

ADVANTAGES

- Can travel long distances
- Relatively fast (twice as fast as ground travel for the same distances)
- May be able to land on adverse terrain that is not prepared for fixed-wing aircraft or that cannot be reached by ground vehicle

---

BOX 6-1

HIGH-RISK CRITERIA FOR CONSIDERATION OF EARLY TRANSFER

(These guidelines are not intended to be hospital-specific.)

Central Nervous System
Head injury
- Penetrating injury or open frac-
  ture (with or without cerebro-
  spinal fluid leak)
- Depressed skull fracture
- Glasgow Coma Scale (GCS)
  <14 or GCS deterioration
- Lateralizing signs
Spinal cord injury
- Spinal column injury or major
  vertebral injury

Chest
Major chest wall injury
Wide mediastinum or other signs
  suggesting great vessel injury
Cardiac injury
Patients who may require pro-
  longed ventilation

Pelvis
Unstable pelvic ring disruption
Unstable pelvic fracture with
  shock or other evidence of
  continuing hemorrhage
Open pelvic injury

Major Extremity Injuries
Fracture or dislocation with loss
  of distal pulses

Open long-bone fractures
Extremity ischemia

Multiple-System Injury
Head injury combined with face,
  chest, abdominal, or pelvic
  injury
Burns with associated injuries
Multiple long-bone fractures
Injury to more than two body
  regions

Comorbid Factors
Age >55 years
Children
Cardiac or respiratory disease
Insulin-dependent diabetics,
  morbid obesity
Pregnancy
Immunosuppression

**Secondary Deterioration (Late
Sequelae)**
Mechanical ventilation required
Sepsis
Single or multiple organ system
  failure (deterioration in central
  nervous, cardiac, pulmonary,
  hepatic, renal, or coagulation
  systems)
Major tissue necrosis

(From American College of Surgeons Committee on Trauma: *Resources for optimal care of the injured patient,* Chicago, 1993, The College.)

- May be able to fly when road conditions are poor
- Flight usually relatively smooth
- Usually staffed by ALS personnel

DISADVANTAGES

- May be limited by adverse weather conditions
- Noisy

- Very limited space in smaller models
- Weight restrictions
- Strict limits on number of crew and passengers it can carry
- May be limits on amount or size of equipment it can carry

Airplane (fixed-wing aircraft)

ADVANTAGES

- Can travel long distances at high speeds
- Usually holds more personnel and equipment than helicopter
- Usually has more patient care space than helicopter
- Cabins can usually be pressurized
- Can sometimes fly *above* the weather

DISADVANTAGES

- Not always on standby; may therefore take longer to obtain service
- Has limited landing capabilities
- Noisy
- Low humidity
- Usually most expensive mode of transportation

PHYSIOLOGIC EFFECTS OF AIR TRANSPORT AT HIGH ALTITUDES

- Possible hypoxia
- Acceleration or deceleration forces
- Gas expansion with altitude increase
- Motion sickness
- Dehydration
- Vibration or motion
- Increased noise
- Thermal changes (decreased ambient temperature at high altitudes)

Equipment considerations for transfer

- Oxygen and delivery source (including ventilator)
- Airway adjuncts
- IV fluids, equipment, and infusion pump or pumps
- Emergency medications
- Prescribed medications
- Cardiac monitor-defibrillator
- Suction
- Stabilization devices
- Pneumatic antishock garment (PASG)
- Chest tube (with Heimlich valve) attached to appropriate drainage or suction device
- Dressings
- Extra batteries

Information that should accompany the patient

Chart information transmitted to receiving facilities by facsimile machine before the patient's arrival assists the receiving team's preparation, but hard copies of this information should be included with the patient as well.

- Patient's name and age
- Patient's family's address and phone number (state whether or not members are en route and what information they have been given)
- Referring physician's name and phone number
- Receiving physician's name and phone number
- Name and phone number of contact person at referring facility
- Details of incident
- Patient assessment information
- Past medical history, medications, allergies
- Flow sheet that includes
  - Medications
  - Vital signs
  - Serial neurologic examinations
  - Any diagnostic and therapeutic interventions
  - Intake and output record
  - Laboratory results
  - Monitoring parameters
- X-rays
- Laboratory specimen results
- Pretransfer discharge note
- Time at which patient departed the referring facility
- Copies of patient's current and old medical records, if available
- Information about patient valuables (give to family when possible)

Stabilization of the patient for transport

It is essential to attempt to stabilize the patient before transport to another facility. Clinical personnel should consider not only immediate needs but also those needs that may arise *during* transport. Anticipation of potential problems is the key to a safe and smooth transfer.

It is important to strive for the minimum amount of time possible in the referral facility by deferring all nonessential tests and interventions and by developing an efficient transfer process. It is not necessary to conduct a complete patient workup before transfer. Once the need for transfer has been recognized, the patient should be stabilized and transferred as quickly as possible.

Airway

Clinical personnel should ensure that the patient has a patent airway. Endotracheal intubation is indicated if the patient has an altered level of consciousness, massive facial trauma, or difficulty handling secretions. Endotracheal intubation should also be considered when the patient has experienced smoke inhalation or has an unstable chest injury, such as a flail chest. If an airway adjunct is in place, personnel should be sure that it is secured for transport and that a spare is carried in the event of accidental removal.

Breathing

Patients should be placed on supplemental high-flow oxygen. The supply available should be sufficient to provide the patient with oxygen until arrival at the receiving facility. A full E-cylinder of oxygen lasts approximately 60 minutes at sea level if run at a 15 liter per minute flow rate.

If the patient has sustained a pneumothorax, a flutter valve or chest tube should be placed and connected to a drainage system before transfer. If suction is required, personnel should include an additional suction device on the transport equipment list. A bulb syringe can often be used as an emergency backup suction device.

Equipment should be available to provide positive pressure breathing, if the need arises.

An orogastric or nasogastric tube should be placed before transport to decompress the stomach and avoid emesis and aspiration, especially if the transport is a long distance, over rough terrain, or by air when vibration and turbulence are anticipated.

Circulation

Appropriate therapeutic interventions should be performed with the goal of maintaining an adequate pulse and blood pressure and controlling external bleeding.

Clinical personnel should initiate and/or maintain two large-bore (14 gauge if possible) intravenous lines, and warmed crystalloid solutions (usually Ringer's lactate or normal saline) should be used to maintain the systolic blood pressure above 80 mmHg. Plastic IV bags should be used to accommodate expansion and contraction of gases during high-altitude flights. If extension tubing is used, excess tubing should be coiled and taped to avoid inadvertent snagging and possible accidental removal.

At times, if local protocol dictates, a PASG may assist in stabilizing a patient for transfer. The most accepted indication is for the hemodynamically unstable patient with a serious pelvic fracture. If the PASG is not already in use, personnel should place it on or under the patient before transfer, so that it can be easily inflated if needed. Because PASG is a controversial treatment, clear direction from medical control or the referring physician is important before inflation.

If the flight is going to be long or the patient requires it for comfort or monitoring, a urinary catheter should be placed.

Personnel should anticipate heat loss during the flight and provide extra blankets for patient warmth.

Cervical spine/thoracic spine

Clinical personnel should maintain alignment of the cervical and thoracic spine by providing stabilization with immobilization devices. Placement of the patient on a backboard minimizes patient movement during the transfer, decreases the likelihood of injury, and reduces the amount of pain the patient will experience. The patient should be adequately secured so that, if emesis occurs, the patient can be turned on his or her side without compromising spinal immobilization.

Need for restraints should be evaluated before departure from the referring facility. If restraints are not used at the outset, they should be within easy reach of the attendant during transfer in case the patient's level of consciousness changes and creates a risk to treatment or his or her safety or of the transfer crew. Either physical or pharmacologic restraints may be needed.

Splints

All suspected or proven fractures or dislocations should be splinted at the joints above and below the injury sites. Personnel should check and document distal neurovascular status before and after splinting and following any movement of the patient. Traction splints may be used as appropriate.

Wound care

External bleeding can be controlled by using direct pressure. If pressure dressings have been applied, personnel should indicate it both verbally and in writing on the patient's report.

Tetanus prophylaxis or tetanus immune globulin should be administered in accordance with standard guidelines. The appropriate antibiotics should also be administered.

Burn wounds should be covered with dry, sterile dressings. Clinical personnel should avoid wet dressings because they may cause the patient to develop severe hypothermia. Pain should be controlled with IV narcotics, such as fentanyl citrate (Sublimaze).

Laboratory, x-ray, and other diagnostic studies

Some tertiary referral centers recommend that cervical spine films *not* be taken before transfer if interventions performed before and/or during transport will not change regardless of findings on the cervical spine x-rays.

RADIOGRAPHS
• Cross-table lateral cervical spine
• Chest

LABORATORY STUDIES
• Hematocrit and hemoglobin
• Urinalysis
• Arterial blood gases and oximetry

CARE DURING TRANSFER

Assessment of the patient must continue while he or she is en route. Assessment should include vital signs, oxygen saturation, end tidal carbon dioxide (if available), GCS, neurologic status, chest excursion and compliance, and any signs of tension pneumothorax.

Humidified oxygen should be given throughout the transport. If the patient is on a ventilator, settings should be monitored closely for any changes from air expansion and/or vibration. An in-line manometer should be available for frequent tidal volume checks, especially with air ambulances.

Intravenous fluids should be placed in pressure infuser devices for air transport to ensure a constant and regular rate of administration. All medications should be delivered via an infusion pump or flow regulating device. Arterial lines should be flushed and pulmonary artery catheter waveforms should be monitored to prevent inadvertent wedging of the catheter.

The transport team should be prepared to turn a patient quickly if emesis occurs, especially if there is no orogastric or nasogastric tube in place. These tubes should be vented or attached to low suction. Analgesics and sedatives should be used judiciously, based on patient needs, neurologic status, and hemodynamics. The patient and any passengers should be given safety briefings and provided with reassurance and support for the transport.

Communication

A brief, concise entry notification should be communicated to the receiving facility before arrival. This notification should include the patient's general condition, vital signs, any changes and interventions in transit, and the patient's response. An estimated time of arrival should be given and any specific requests for equipment or personnel should be stated at this time.

A written summary of events during transfer should also be given to the receiving facility. This summary should include any medications or intravenous fluids given and patient changes.

Special considerations for patients with specific injuries

- Consider positioning of the patient in the aircraft in regard to takeoff, landing, and flying angles to minimize the possibility of increased intracranial pressure.
- Consider altitude restrictions or increased cabin pressurization to decrease the likelihood of gas expansion of trapped air in body compartments and equipment (such as chest tubes, IV bags) in fixed-wing aircraft.

Eye injury

- Consider altitude restrictions or increased cabin pressurization to decrease the likelihood of intraorbital gas expansion, reduced extraocular pressure, and the possibility of vitreous or aqueous humor release through a penetrating injury.

Chest injury

- Provide for the release of trapped gases (via chest tubes) that may increase the likelihood of a tension pneumothorax. **Never clamp a chest tube during air transfer!**

Multiple trauma

- Consider the need for PASG air release during ascent (higher altitude) because of gas expansion in the suit. Consider air addition during descent because of gas contraction
- Consider bringing 2 to 4 units of blood for administration en route.

Burns

- Consider that dehydration may occur as a result of a decreased humidity factor in the aircraft; additional fluid replacement may be required.

SUMMARY

The ultimate decision to treat the critically injured trauma patient in one's own facility or to transfer the patient to a regional referral center must be made by an objective appraisal of the level of care that can be delivered within a given facility. There is an ethical and legal duty to transfer a patient to a facility where definitive care can be given whenever such a transfer is feasible and available.

REFERENCES

1. Emergency Nurses Association: *Interfacility transport of the critically ill or injured patient (position statement)*, Park Ridge, Il, 1995, Emergency Nurses Association.

SUGGESTED READINGS

American College of Surgeons Committee on Trauma: *Resources for optimal care of the injured patient: 1993*, Chicago, 1993, The College.

Emergency Nurses Association: *Care of the pediatric patient during interfacility transfer (position statement)*, Park Ridge, IL, 1995, Emergency Nurses Association.

Emergency Nurses Association: *Emergency nursing core curriculum*, ed 4, Philadelphia, 1994, Saunders.

Emergency Nurses Association: *Interfacility transport of the critically ill or injured patient (position statement)*, Park Ridge, IL, December 1995, Emergency Nurses Association.

Emergency Nurses Association: *Sheehy's emergency nursing: principles and practice*, ed 4, St Louis, 1997, Mosby.

Lee G: *Flight nursing: principles and practice*, ed 2, St Louis, 1996, Mosby.

CHAPTER 7

Shock and Fluid Replacement in Trauma

Steve Talbert

SHOCK

Shock is the inability of tissues to receive oxygen and nutrients and to rid themselves of waste products. It is inadequate tissue perfusion. Three components in the body are essential for the transport of oxygen and nutrients to the cells and waste products from the cells:

- Heart: The heart's function is to pump blood to the lungs and to other parts of the body.
- Vascular System (from the macrocosm of the great vessels to the microcosm of the arterial/capillary cellular membranes): The vascular system is the "pipes" through which blood and other fluids are transported.
- Blood: Blood is the fluid medium that contains components with oxygen, nutrient, and waste product carrying capacity.

Conditions that cause dysfunction of any of these three components may result in shock. When shock occurs, the brain, heart, lungs, kidneys, liver, and adrenal glands are affected in the following ways:

- Brain: The brain is primarily affected because it depends on glucose and oxygen to function.
- Heart: The heart muscle itself relies on the delivery of oxygen and nutrients to its cells via the coronary arteries. As blood supply to the coronary arteries decreases, the heart muscle becomes dysfunctional, and the heart ceases to function adequately as a pump, causing decrease in cardiac output.
- Lungs: Ventilation and perfusion are necessary for oxygenating hemoglobin and removing waste gases from the lungs. If shock ensues, and ventilation or perfusion does not occur, gas exchange does not take place.
- Kidneys: As blood supply through the kidneys decreases, there is a concurrent decrease in urinary output. Because the kidneys are dependent on blood flow, renal failure may also ensue.

- Liver: When severely injured, the adrenal glands are stimulated, activating the sympathetic nervous system. Epinephrine is released. When there is an excess of circulating epinephrine, glycogen stores in the liver are depleted. Also, there is a reduction in the amount of metabolic acids that are broken down in the liver, and existing metabolic acidosis becomes worse.

Monitoring parameters in shock

Pulse

As shock worsens, the pulse increases as a compensatory mechanism until catecholamines are depleted, and bradycardia is evidenced as a terminal event. Tachycardia may not be seen in an elderly patient whose catecholamine release and subsequent cardiac response are limited. Tachycardia is considered to be evidenced when the following pulse rates are present.[1]

Infants	>160 beats per minute
Preschool age children	>140 beats per minute
Preschool to puberty age children	>120 beats per minute
Adults	>100 beats per minute

Respirations

As the shock state worsens, respirations become more rapid and more shallow. This is a mechanism to improve oxygenation and compensate for the metabolic acidosis associated with shock.

Blood pressure

Blood pressure is not a reliable indicator of shock in the early stages because compensatory mechanisms may cause blood pressure to remain at a normal level for a period of time. Hypotension results from significant fluid loss or compensatory mechanism failure and is usually a late sign of shock.

Temperature

As most shock conditions worsen, temperature may remain normal or may decrease. The temperature of a patient in septic shock usually elevates.

Skin vital signs

Sympathetic nervous system activation results in peripheral vasoconstriction. The patient's skin becomes pale, cool, and clammy. Patients exhibiting these changes in skin vital signs in conjunction with tachycardia should be considered to be in shock until proven otherwise.

Jugular veins

Distended jugular veins may indicate increased intrathoracic pressure, which forces blood to "backflow" into the jugular veins and decreases filling of the right heart. Possible causes of distended jugular veins include pericardial tamponade (cardiogenic cause) and tension pneumothorax (pulmonic cause).

Flat jugular veins may indicate hypovolemia (massive hemorrhage) or vaso-dilation (anaphylactic, septic, or neurogenic shock).[2] However, pericardial tamponade or tension pneumothorax cannot be ruled out on the basis of flat jugular veins if hypovolemia is present.

Cardiac rhythm

A variety of cardiac rhythms occurs in shock states. Sinus tachycardia is the most common cardiac rhythm seen in shock. Sinus bradycardia, heart blocks, ventricular tachycardia, and fibrillation may also occur.

Level of consciousness

Patients in early shock may exhibit restlessness or anxiety. As the shock state worsens, brain tissue perfusion is compromised, resulting in a decreased level of consciousness.

Arterial blood gases

The most common arterial blood gases (ABG) finding in shock patients is metabolic acidosis (the end result of inadequate tissue perfusion and anaero-bic metabolism). Metabolic acidosis associated with shock is characterized by a low pH, normal or low $PaCO_2$, higher base deficit (more negative base ex-cess), and lower bicarbonate level. If respiratory insufficiency is present, $PaCO_2$ levels may be elevated.

Central venous pressure

Central venous pressure (CVP) (right-sided heart pressure) indirectly re-flects blood volume, vascular tone, and pump effectiveness. A normal CVP measurement is 4 to 10 cm H_2O pressure.[3] A value of less than 4 cm may be indicative of hypovolemia or vasodilation. A value of greater than 10 cm may indicate pericardial tamponade, fluid overload, pulmonary edema, tension pneumothorax, or hemothorax.[3] A central venous pressure reading may be falsely elevated secondary to use of the pneumatic antishock garment (PASG).

Arterial pressure

Arterial pressure is measured through an intraarterial line or cannula via a percutaneous puncture or a surgical cutdown site. Mean arterial pressure is normally 70 to 90 mmHg. A value of less than 70 mmHg may be indicative of vasodilation or hypovolemia.[3]

Pulmonary artery wedge pressure

Pulmonary artery wedge pressure (PAWP) is an indirect measurement of left arterial and ventricular pressure. A pulmonary artery catheter is inserted into the venous system and moved into the right atrium, through the right ven-tricle, into the pulmonary artery, and into a pulmonary capillary wedge. Pressures should be equivalent to those of the left ventricle. Normal values are 6 to 12 cm H_2O pressure.[4] Values less than 6 cm may indicate hypovolemia or vasodilation.

Urinary output

The average adult hourly urine output is 0.5 to 1 mg/kg. Less than 35 ml per hour *may* be indicative of decreased renal perfusion from hypovolemic or decreased cardiac output.

Types of shock

There are three categories of shock: hypovolemic, distributive, and cardiogenic. There are three types of distributive shock: neurogenic, septic, and anaphylactic.

Hypovolemic (hemorrhagic, low-volume) shock

Hypovolemic shock is a "fluid" problem. It is the most common type of shock caused by trauma. It can result from lacerations, disruption of internal organs and vasculature, and fractures of the long bones or the pelvis. Hypovolemic shock may also result from any condition in which fluid volume is depleted, such as a severe crush injury, massive soft tissue injury, severe burn injury, gastrointestinal bleeding, and severe dehydration. For the sake of this text, hypovolemia is discussed in terms of hemorrhage caused by trauma. The degree of shock depends on the amount of blood lost, the rate at which it was lost, the age and general physical condition of the patient, and the patient's ability to activate compensatory mechanisms.

The average amount of blood in an adult is 7% to 8% of the person's ideal body weight. A child has 80 to 90 ml of blood per kilogram of body weight.[1] The diagnosis of hypovolemic shock can be made by clinical observation, physical examination, laboratory specimen analysis, CVP measurement, arterial pressure or pulmonary capillary wedge pressure measurement, or the patient's response to fluid or blood replacement.

Neurogenic shock (spinal shock)

Neurogenic shock is a "pipe" problem caused by vasodilation. It may be the result of a severe brain stem injury at the level of the medulla, an injury to the spinal cord, or spinal anesthesia. The etiology of neurogenic shock is a loss of sympathetic tone, causing peripheral vasodilation and resulting in severe hypotension.

Neurologic shock may mask signs and symptoms of other types of shock. If neurogenic shock is present, there should be a heightened index of suspicion for undetected sources of hemorrhage. Any sources of ongoing blood loss should be identified and hemorrhage control measures initiated.

- Decreased blood pressure
- Rapid, shallow respirations or no respirations
- Bradycardia
- Paraplegia or quadriplegia
- History of recent spinal anesthesia
- History of recent major head trauma
- Priapism (sustained erection) indicating spinal cord injury
- Cool, clammy skin *above* the level of the spinal cord lesion
- Possible diaphoresis *below* the level of the lesion
- Be prepared to administer vasopressors if hypotension persists after volume resuscitation.

- Ensure ABCs
- Protect the cervical spine
- Administer IV crystalloid solutions judiciously

Septic shock

Septic shock is a "pipe" problem caused by vasodilation. It is caused by an overwhelming infection and may be the result of a suppressed immune system, a massive burn injury, or anything else that can introduce an infecting organism into a compromised victim. The most common organism is a gram-negative enteric bacillus such as *Escherichia coli, Pseudomonas,* or *Staphylococcus.* These organisms enter the vascular system and promote the release of endotoxins, which cause an interstitial fluid leak, increased vascular permeability, and vasodilation (also known as *volume shunting*), which leads to shock. It is commonly seen in extremes of age—the very young and the very old. Circulatory blood volume is usually close to normal.[1] Septic shock is not seen acutely but may be seen in delayed resuscitation situations.

- Normal blood pressure with widened pulse pressure or decreased blood pressure
- Tachycardia
- Hyperpyrexia
- Chills or tremors
- Warm, dry skin
- Nausea and vomiting
- Decreased cardiac output
- Decreased level of consciousness
- Metabolic acidosis
- Positive blood cultures

THERAPEUTIC INTERVENTIONS

- High-flow oxygen
- IV lines
- Antibiotics
- Dopamine, dobutamine, or levophed (primarily for alpha-adrenergic effects)

Cardiogenic shock

Cardiogenic shock is a "pump" problem that can occur from electrical causes (dysrhythmias), a filling defect (tamponade), or damage to the heart muscle resulting from a myocardial infarction, contusion, or rupture. Myocardial infarction is the most common cause of cardiogenic shock.[3] Myocardial infarction may result from decreased coronary artery perfusion resulting from hypovolemia.[1] When a myocardial infarction occurs, the area infarcted becomes dysfunctional. Depending on the size of the infarction, stroke volume and cardiac output may decrease with a concurrent increase in left ventricular end-diastolic pressure. As cardiac output decreases, blood pressure and tissue perfusion decrease, resulting in cardiogenic shock. It usually takes about 40% of the left ventricular myocardium to infarct before cardiogenic shock will occur.[5] Cardiogenic shock is not uncommon. It occurs in 15% to 20% of all myocardial infarction patients. Often cardiogenic shock occurs as a result of a traumatic injury, either from the injury itself or from a concurrent myocardial infarction.[5]

ASSESSMENT

- Signs of myocardial infarction
    - Chest pain
    - Nausea and vomiting
    - Syncope
- Weak or diminished peripheral pulses
- Rapid, shallow respirations
- Decreasing blood pressure
- Decreased cardiac output
- Decreased level of consciousness
- Pale, cool, clammy skin
- Decreased urinary output
- Metabolic acidosis
- PAWP >18
- Cardiac dysrhythmias
- Elevated cardiac isoenzymes
- ECG changes indicative of myocardial infarction

THERAPEUTIC INTERVENTIONS

- High-flow oxygen
- IV lines

- Inotropic agents (dopamine or dobutamine) to increase cardiac output and coronary artery perfusion
- Vasodilator agents (sodium nitroprusside or nitroglycerin) to decrease left ventricular and peripheral vascular resistance and to decrease left ventricular filling pressures, causing an increase in cardiac output
- Intraaortic balloon pump (IABP; also known as the intraaortic diastolic assist device), which inflates during diastole to increase blood flow to the coronary arteries
- Pain control (usually with narcotics)

Anaphylactic shock

Anaphylactic shock is a "pipe" problem caused by vasodilation. When a sensitized person is exposed to an antigen to which he or she is allergic, an antigen-antibody reaction occurs. This reaction releases histamine, which causes extreme vasodilation and increased capillary permeability. The resulting fluid leak into the interstitial space may cause relative hypovolemia and shock.

Common antigens to which people are allergic include:
- Hymenoptera stings (bees, wasps)
- Shellfish
- Medications
- Monosodium glutamate (often found in Chinese food)
- Environmental agents

ASSESSMENT

- Urticaria
- Edematous tongue
- Decreased blood pressure
- Tachycardia
- Bronchospasm
- Respiratory stridor
- Wheezing
- Respiratory distress
- Respiratory arrest

THERAPEUTIC INTERVENTIONS

- ABCs
- High-flow oxygen
- Epinephrine 0.1 to 0.5 ml of a *1:10,000 solution* given very slowly intravenously

    In profound anaphylactic shock, epinephrine should be given as *1:10,000 solution intravenously* (rather than a 1:1000 solution subcutaneously, to be assured that it will be absorbed rapidly).

    Propranolol (Inderal) should be available in the event of profound hypertension and tachycardia caused by the epinephrine.

- Aminophylline for bronchospasms
- Antihistamines (such as diphenhydramine [Benadryl]) to decrease circulating histamines
- Steroids to reduce inflammatory response

Classifications of shock

Shock can be classified into four categories:[1]

Class I: less than 15% blood loss

ASSESSMENT

- Slight tachycardia
- Normal blood pressure
- Normal pulse pressure
- Normal respiratory rate and depth
- Normal skin vital signs (color, temperature, moisture)
- Normal urinary output

THERAPEUTIC INTERVENTIONS

- Usually no intervention is required other than controlling obvious bleeding.

Class II: 15% to 30% blood loss

ASSESSMENT

- Tachycardia
- Slight decrease in blood pressure
- Increased respiratory rate or no change in depth
- Decreased pulse pressure or increase in diastolic pressure
- Slightly cool skin
- Normal urinary output

THERAPEUTIC INTERVENTIONS

- Oxygen
- Identify source, and control bleeding
- IV fluids
    Crystalloids: replace at 3 ml for every 1 ml of blood loss
    Blood products: replace at 1:1 ratio
- Consider the use of the pneumatic antishock garment (PASG)
- Identify the source, and control bleeding
- Consider surgical intervention

Class III: 30% to 40% blood loss

ASSESSMENT

- Tachycardia
- Anxiety, restlessness, or decreased level of consciousness
- Cool, clammy extremities
- Tachypnea

- Narrow pulse pressure
- Decreased blood pressure
- Decreased urinary output to oliguria
- Decreased CVP
- Decreased PAWP

THERAPEUTIC INTERVENTIONS

- Oxygen
- Identify source, and control bleeding
- IV lines
  Crystalloids: replace 3:1 ml
  Blood products: replace 1:1 ml
- Prepare for surgical intervention, or transfer to facility with surgical capabilities

Class IV: greater than 40% blood loss

This is a life-threatening condition.

ASSESSMENT

- Decreased level of consciousness
- Tachycardia
- Cool, clammy skin
- Severely decreased blood pressure
- Decreased urinary output to oliguria to anuria
- Decreased CVP (<5 mm); may be decreased before Class IV
- Decreased PAWP (<4 mm); may be decreased before Class IV
- Arterial blood gases: metabolic acidosis and respiratory alkalosis

THERAPEUTIC INTERVENTIONS

- Oxygen
- Identify source, and control bleeding
- IV lines; crystalloids and blood products; do not use vasopressor agents
- Requires surgical intervention
- Prepare for emergency thoracotomy (if appropriate)

The key to effective management of any classification of shock is to identify the cause and intervene appropriately. The presence of head trauma and increased intracranial pressure does not usually decrease blood pressure unless the brain stem is injured. If clinical findings do not correlate with the diagnosis, further evaluation of the patient is essential.

Clinical personnel must assess and reassess the patient frequently. The overall outcome for the patient depends on duration and severity of the shock state and rapid delivery of appropriate therapeutic interventions.

Compensatory mechanisms in shock

Sympathetic activation

Stimulation of the adrenal glands activates the sympathetic nervous system, which causes a release of catecholamine (epinephrine and norepinephrine). Catecholamines cause constriction of the peripheral vasculature and shunting of blood to vital organs (heart and brain). Other effects of catecholamine release include increasing heart rate and myocardial contractility, which improves cardiac output and increases blood pressure.

Activation of the renin-angiotensin-aldosterone mechanism

Decreased kidney perfusion activates the renin-angiotensin-aldosterone mechanism. Renin is released by the kidneys and converted in the blood to angiotensin I. Once in the lungs, angiotensin I is converted to angiotensin II. Angiotensin II has two primary actions: It acts as a vasoconstrictor, and it stimulates the release of aldosterone. Aldosterone causes increased sodium reabsorption in the renal tubules. Because water follows sodium, there is a subsequent increase in intravascular volume, resulting in increased venous return to the heart, increased cardiac output, and increased blood pressure.

Antidiuretic hormone

Antidiuretic hormone (ADH) is released by the anterior pituitary gland. It causes increased water absorption at the renal collecting duct. This release increases venous return to the heart, cardiac output, and blood pressure. *The patient's urinary output will decrease.*

Intracellular fluid shift

Fluid will shift from the intracellular and interstitial spaces to the intravascular space, thus increasing vascular volume, return of blood to the heart, cardiac output, and blood pressure. *If awake, the patient will complain of being thirsty.*

FLUID REPLACEMENT IN TRAUMA

When a severe trauma has occurred, it is essential to gain vascular access. To ensure delivery of fluid, some researchers recommend a site above the diaphragm and a site below the diaphragm, no matter what the cause of the injury.

IV sites

It is preferable to use sites that can contain a large-bore cannula and a large amount of volume at a brisk flow rate. Clinical personnel should find sites that are readily accessible and relatively easy to cannulate.
- Peripheral sites
    Arm: antecubital fossa
    Neck: external jugular vein

Foot: saphenous vein
Groin: femoral vein
Interosseous: tibial plateau (in children under 6 years of age)
- Central sites
Anterior chest: subclavian vein
Neck: internal jugular vein
- Surgical cutdown site
Foot: saphenous vein
Arm: brachial vein
Groin: femoral vein

Size of cannula

Clinical personnel must use the largest gauge and shortest length cannula possible. In the adult patient, at least a 16-gauge cannula or larger should be used and the length appropriate for the site cannulated. If a cutdown entry, a large vein site (such as the femoral vein), or a central line site is used, a number 8 French cannula or larger is preferred because it can carry a large volume of fluid.

Type of tubing

- Standard *macrodrip* tubing or high-volume trauma tubing that is capable of administering blood; *microdrip* tubing should not be used.
- Inline manual pumping devices are appropriate.
- Extension tubing is controversial because it slows the rate of delivery of fluid to the venous system.

Adjunct devices

- Pressure cuffs speed the rate of delivery.
- Some warming coils slow the rate of delivery but may be required to warm blood. High-volume fluid warmers may be used. A device is available in which the IV bag is placed in a specially designed pouch that holds a chemical hot pack and the IV tubing is covered with an insulated cover to keep fluids warm.
- If the cannula is in the saphenous vein and the PASG leg units are inflated, personnel must ensure that pressure on the IV bag is greater than that in the PASG or the IV will not run. Personnel should place a pressure cuff on the IV bag and inflate to a pressure greater than PASG pressure or until the fluid drips at an appropriate rate.

Types of fluids

In hypotensive states resulting from trauma, it is recommended that crystalloid solution be administered as indicated by the patient's hemodynamic status. Clinical personnel should consider the early administration of blood components as the need for oxygen-carrying hemoglobin becomes evident. The

American College of Surgeons Committee on Trauma (ASCOT) classifies hemorrhage and recommended fluid replacement as follows[1]:

15 to 25% blood loss	Crystalloid solution
>30% blood loss	Crystalloid solution and blood products

NOTE: Crystalloid solutions should be replaced in a 3:1 ratio with blood.

Fluids should be warmed before administration.

Crystalloids

Ringer's lactate approximates plasma electrolyte composition and plasma osmolality and is usually the recommended crystalloid solution to use.

Normal saline solution may be used initially in fluid replacement, but it may cause hyperchloremia, hypernatremia, and acidosis if large volumes are given. Its choice is usually made by physician preference. Hypertonic saline solutions may be used in selected situations.

Colloids

Colloids, such as albumin and Plasmanate, are not usually recommended, because they may increase bleeding from raw surfaces, may confuse type and crossmatch, infuse slowly, and are expensive.

Blood and blood components

Packed red cells are given to maintain hematocrit at 30% to 35%.[6] At this level, oxygen can be transported without slowing circulation time caused by increased viscosity. In massive trauma, clinical personnel should initially send blood specimens for type and crossmatch for 4 to 6 units with directions for the blood bank to always have 2 units of blood ready for use until notified that the blood is no longer needed. If 3 to 4 liters of crystalloid solution have been given and it appears that the patient continues to be hypovolemic, the administration of blood products is appropriate.

Because fresh whole blood containing red blood cells, plasma, and clotting factors is rarely readily available, blood components, such as red blood cells, are usually given.

Red blood cells (packed red cells)

Red blood cells have many of the components of whole blood, but because plasma has been extracted, the risk of transfusion reactions and transmission of infectious diseases is greatly reduced. Packed red cells also have a lesser amount of citrate, phosphate, free potassium, and debris.

Clotting factors and platelets are minimally functional or nonfunctional in packed red cells. The patient must be monitored closely for bleeding disorders as a result of massive transfusions.

O negative packed cells

If blood is required *immediately,* O negative packed red cells should be given until type-specific or type and crossmatched blood is available. O negative is known as the universal donor. If large amounts of O negative blood are given, the patient may have a reaction later when type-specific or type and cross-matched blood (to the patient's type) is given. O positive blood may be administered to males and postmenopausal females with unknown blood types without risk of significant complications.

Type-specific, uncrossmatched red cells

If blood is required, but clinical personnel can wait for laboratory processing, then type-specific, uncrossmatched blood should be given. There is a lower adverse reaction rate with this type of blood.

Typed and crossmatched blood

If blood is required and personnel can wait until typed and crossmatched blood is available, typed and crossmatched blood should be used. It is the most preferred because reactions are extremely low.

Colloidlike plasma expanders

A number of colloidlike solutions are available to expand plasma volume. Although they are not used widely in trauma resuscitation, practitioners may encounter situations in which their use is advocated. The two most common colloidlike plasma expanders are Dextran and Hydroxyethyl starch (Hetastarch). These solutions use large molecules to expand plasma volume by increasing intravascular osmolarity (oncotic pressure). Fluids are pulled from the interstitial space into the intravascular space, thereby increasing intravascular volume.

These solutions are not without risk. The most common adverse reactions include coagulopathies and anaphylactic reactions. Patients receiving colloidlike plasma expanders should be closely monitored for adverse side effects.

Massive transfusion

The definition of massive transfusion is blood replacement of 50% or more of the patient's calculated blood volume over a 3-hour period.[7] There are several problems associated with massive transfusion:
- Hypothermia can result from the cold temperature of the stored blood. Coldness increases the viscosity of blood and slows delivery rate. This can be prevented by warming the blood.
- Hyperkalemia is caused by hemolysis of red blood cells. It cannot be prevented, but close monitoring of serum electrolyes and appropriate therapeutic intervention should be undertaken if hyperkalemia occurs. It is usually a transient condition and resolves as the patient stabilizes.
- Hypocalcemia is caused by the binding capacity of citrate on calcium. It cannot be prevented, but close monitoring of serum calcium levels and

appropriate calcium replacement should occur. If citrated whole blood is administered at greater than 100 ml/minute, clinical personnel should give 10 ml of a 10% solution of calcium chloride with each 10 units of whole blood.[1]

- Acidosis is a result of the pH (7.1) of banked blood. It cannot be prevented, but close monitoring of arterial blood gases (especially pH) should be carried out, and disorders should be treated appropriately. The patient should also be monitored for dysrhythmias that are associated with acidosis.
- Alkalosis usually occurs following massive transfusion, because citrate eventually converts to bicarbonate in the liver. It cannot be prevented, but close observation of arterial blood gases (especially pH) is warranted.
- Coagulation disorders occur because of loss of clotting factors. This loss cannot be prevented, but close monitoring of prothrombin time and partial thromboplastin time is appropriate. Also, the patient should be monitored closely for bleeding. Fresh frozen plasma and platelet therapy may be required (usually 1 unit with each 10 units of whole blood).
- Debris may be present in transfused blood. Although it is not known if this debris is harmful, the use of 160 μm Micropore filters is recommended to remove microaggregates.[1] Note that the use of filters may slow the rate of delivery of the blood.

Autotransfusion

Autotransfusion may be a useful adjunct in an emergency department when there is massive blood loss into the thoracic cavity. It is not routinely used to collect blood from other body cavities in the emergency setting, because blood other than chest blood is considered contaminated. Also, if there is a known coagulation defect or if the patient has cancer, shed blood from any cavity should not be used. With autotransfusion, blood from the chest cavity is collected, filtered, anticoagulated, and reinfused into the vascular system.

Considerations of transfusion

Replenishment of red blood cells, plasma, and platelets is routine therapy for patients experiencing hemorrhagic shock. However, physiologic, cultural, and religious considerations should be noted before and during administration of these substances. Any patient receiving a transfusion is at risk for adverse physiologic reactions. Administration of type-specific or crossmatched blood reduces this risk. All patients receiving blood products should be monitored for adverse physiologic reactions.

Cultural and religious considerations generally involve refusal to have blood products transfused. Caring for patients with objections to blood transfusions as potentially life-saving treatments can be difficult. Institutional policies and protocols can facilitate the decision-making process. The wishes of competent patients or those who have expressed their wishes through legal documents (e.g., advanced directives) should be respected. If necessary, court orders may be obtained that allow medical treatment contrary to the wishes of patients or guardians in certain extreme circumstances, usually involving a patient who is a minor or a patient who is deemed not competent to make a decision for himself or herself.

REFERENCES

1. American College of Surgeons/Committee on Trauma: *Advanced trauma life support instructor manual,* Chicago, 1992, American College of Surgeons.
2. Lawrence P: *Essentials of general surgery,* Baltimore, 1988, Williams & Wilkins.
3. Sheehy SB: *Emergency nursing,* ed 3, St Louis, 1985, Mosby.
4. Sheehy SB: *Mosby's manual of emergency care,* ed 3, St Louis, 1990, Mosby.
5. Franaszek JB: Cardiogenic shock. In Rosen P and others, editors: *Emergency medicine,* ed 3, St Louis, 1992, Mosby.
6. Robinson WA: Fluid therapy in hemorrhagic shock, *CCQ* 2(4):1, 1980.
7. Davis JH: *Clinical surgery,* St Louis, 1987, Mosby.

SUGGESTED READINGS

American College of Surgeons: *Shock in advanced trauma life support,* Chicago, 1997, American College of Surgeons.

Bickell WH, Wall MJ, Pepe PE, and others: Immediate versus delayed fluid resuscitation for hypotensive patients with penetrating torso injuries, *N Engl J Med* 331:1105-1109, 1994.

Cardona VD, Hurn PD, Mason PJB, Scanlon AM, Veise-Berry SW, editors: Intral management of traumatic shock. In *Trauma nursing: from resuscitation through rehabilitation,* ed 2, Philadelphia, 1994, Saunders.

Cone A: The use of colloids in clinical practice, *Br J Hosp Med* 54-155, 1995.

Conte MA: Fluid resuscitation in the trauma patient, *CRNA* 8-31, 1997.

Emergency Nurses Association: Shock. In *Trauma nursing care course,* Park Ridge, IL, 1995, Emergency Nurses Association.

Guyton AC, Hall JE, editors: Circulatory shock and physiology of its treatment. In *Textbook of Medical Physiology,* ed 9, Philadelphia, 1996, Saunders.

Krausz MM: Controversies in shock research: Hypertonic resuscitation—pros and cons, *Shock* 3:69-72, 1995.

Shoemaker WC, Peitzman AB, Bellamy R, and others: Resuscitation from severe hemorrhage, *Crit Care Med* 24:S12-23, 1996.

Von Rueden KT, Duhnam CM: Sequelae of massive fluid resuscitation in trauma patients, *Crit Care Nurs Clin North Am* 6:463-672, 1994.

CHAPTER 8

Wounds and Wound Management

Patricia A. Hughes

Proper attention to traumatic wounds in the early phases of injury management is vital to achieving the goals of obtaining hemostasis, avoiding complications such as impaired healing and wound infection, and maximizing functional recovery. The same conscientious attention should be paid to all wounds, regardless of whether they are minor or major, because any wound infection affects the patient's overall recovery and functional outcome.

Although the ABC priorities of evaluation and resuscitative management of trauma patients are always maintained, the risk of infection should also be given careful consideration and appropriate initial treatment begun. In addition to the therapeutic interventions outlined in this chapter, this includes the strict adherence to universal precautions (gown, mask, eye protection, and gloves) for all caregivers with direct access to the patient. Routine use of this protocol provides protection for both patient and provider.

THE SKIN, INJURY, AND WOUND HEALING

The two major layers of the skin are the epidermis and the dermis. The epidermis, the outermost layer, and the underlying dermis protect the body from external pressure and injuring forces. The dermal layer also provides the skin with its strength and elasticity.

Beneath the dermis lies the subcutaneous tissue. The subcutaneous tissues play an important role in traumatic injury because of their shock absorption, insulation, nutrient storage, and body "shaping" functions. The subcutaneous tissues are vulnerable to decreases in vascular supply when blood is shunted to vital organs and can therefore be at a higher risk for impaired healing and infection. Beneath the subcutaneous tissues lie the fascia and muscle tissues.

Wounds are classified as "superficial" (involving the epidermal layer) or "full thickness" (involving the epidermal, dermal, and perhaps the subcutaneous tissue, muscle, and bone layers).

Tissue response and healing in injury

Vasoconstriction occurs immediately at the time of injury, followed by vasodilation 5 to 10 minutes later. Vasodilation results in redness with subepithelial swelling (inflammation) and hemostasis. Over the next 24 to 36 hours, the wound is cleared of cellular debris, and epithelial cells begin to migrate. Fibrin also begins to layer in the wound (fibroblast proliferation). The wound is then fortified with collagen over the next several months (epithelialization, contraction, remodeling).

Factors affecting wound healing

Many factors affect and potentially compromise wound healing:
• Age (especially the elderly)
• Impaired tissue oxygenation and perfusion
• Wound infection, contamination, or systemic sepsis
• Anemia (hemorrhagic and chronic)
• Nutritional status (malnutrition/obesity; vitamins A or C, zinc, iron, or copper deficiencies)
• Electrolyte imbalance
• Stress (physical and psychologic)
• Preexisting conditions (liver failure, vascular disease, diabetes, chronic obstructive pulmonary disease (COPD), uremia, cancer, chronic alcohol use, immunologic depression)
• Medications (especially steroids)
• Radiation, chemotherapy
• Sutures, drains, foreign bodies, packings or dressings
• Patient compliance with treatment regimen

WOUND ASSESSMENT AND MANAGEMENT

The only goal of the primary survey related to wounds is to control major hemorrhage. This can usually be accomplished by using sterile pressure dressings. The sterile dressings also protect against further contamination or injury. After the primary survey and management of life-threatening injuries is completed, clinical personnel can quickly assess all wounds and decide how they will be managed.

Assessment of traumatic wounds

Whether the patient's wounds are isolated or a result of multiple trauma, the care provider must attempt to obtain as much information as possible concerning the circumstances of the injury, because the information guides wound management decisions.

History (from prehospital report, the patient, family, or witnesses) should include[1]:
• How did the wound occur?
• What type of object caused it?

- In what environment did the wound occur (type and degree of contamination, such as feces, fresh water, road dirt, and human versus mammalian bites)?
- What interventions or treatments have already been provided?
- When did the wound occur?
- What is the patient's general physical condition? Past medical history (smoking and alcohol use, medications, allergies)?
- What is the tetanus prophylaxis status? (See Prevention of Infection starting on page 87.)
- What type of work does the patient do?
- Which is the dominant hand?

Wound assessment and documentation of information should include the following:

- Where is the wound located?
- Describe the wound using appropriate wound terminology (length, depth, and appearance).
- Is there bleeding or exudate?
- Are there any foreign bodies?
- What do the peripheral tissues look like? Can the wound edges be approximated?
- Are there any obvious underlying or associated injuries (e.g., fractures, tendon or vessel injuries)?
- Document the neurovascular status distal to the wound and the cranial nerve status in facial injuries.

Wound management considerations

Therapeutic decisions about wound management are influenced by the answers to the following questions.[2]

- Does the wound require management in the operating room?
- Are there associated injuries that will require other interventions, such as underlying fractures, visceral injuries, or brain injuries?
- Are there preexisting conditions that will impair healing?
- How should the wound be closed to best minimize infection risk and optimize healing (primary, secondary, or third-intention healing)?
- Will the patient require antibiotic therapy?
- What type of dressing care, splints, activity restrictions, and home care will the management plan require?

Wound closure options

There are several options for wound closure: closure by suture, tape, or staples (primary-intention healing); leaving the wound open to granulate and close on its own (secondary-intention healing); leaving the wound open and then closing it primarily a few days postinjury (delayed primary closure or tertiary-intention healing); or closing the wound using a skin graft or tissue flap (the timing of this procedure varies depending on the wound).

The decision whether to close a wound primarily is determined by the degree and type of contamination and the length of time from injury to treatment. If a wound is heavily contaminated (all traumatic wounds are considered contaminated), especially with the bacteria contained in feces or saliva, it may be wiser to allow the wound to heal by secondary intention. A carefully managed open wound is less likely to develop infection than a heavily contaminated, inadequately cleansed and débrided closed wound. Generally, wounds that are treated within 6 to 8 hours of injury are considered for primary closure. Wounds that have occurred more than 8 hours earlier should be considered for secondary-intention healing or delayed primary closure. Wounds of the face and scalp may be an exception to this rule because a better vascular supply to these areas reduces infection risk and because of the cosmetic considerations. Wounds that exhibit extensive soft tissue loss and cannot be closed primarily require skin grafting or flap closure.

ANESTHESIA FOR WOUND CLEANSING AND REPAIR

There are several types of anesthesia for the cleansing, débridement, and repair of traumatic injuries. This chapter focuses on the use of anesthetics commonly used in the Emergency Department (ED) setting.

Local and topical anesthetics

The most common form of anesthetic is local anesthesia delivered by subcutaneous infiltration. Commonly used agents include:
• **Lidocaine hydrochloride** (Xylocaine): the most common agent used for local anesthesia; available with or without epinephrine. Lidocaine has a rapid onset and a 30- to 120-minute duration.

NOTE: Epinephrine should not be used around the ears, nose, fingers, toes, or penis. Its use should be avoided in patients with severe peripheral vascular disease. Epinephrine has also been implicated in the increased risk of wound infection.

• **Bupivicaine** (Marcaine): rapid onset, 3 to 7 hours' duration
• **Procaine** (Novocaine): onset 2 to 5 minutes, duration 1 to 1½ hours
• **Mepivicaine** (Carbocaine): rapid onset, 2 to 2½ hours' duration
• **Tetracaine/adrenaline/cocaine (TAC):** a commonly used topical anesthetic in children; should not be used near mucosal membranes.

Regional anesthetics

Regional blocks are a useful alternative to local anesthetics for extremity wounds. Regional blocks are less painful and provide better anesthesia for the patient. They require a smaller volume of anesthetic agent. Regional blocks are administered by applying a tourniquet near the wound proximal to the body and injecting an anesthetic agent intravenously distal to the wound.

Digital nerve blocks are an injection of an anesthetic agent along a nerve course.

Conscious sedation and inhalation agents

Conscious sedation may be used in the ED for the management of painful wound cleansing or repair of lacerations. A combination of intravenous fentanyl (Sublimaze) and midazolam (Versed) is administered, with continuous hemodynamic monitoring.

A mixture of 50% nitrous oxide and 50% oxygen (Nitronox, Entonox) is an inhalational agent that the patient self-administers. It is particularly useful when a procedure will be short but may be quite painful, such as scrubbing or débridement of abrasions or burn wounds.

WOUND CLEANSING AND DÉBRIDEMENT

The importance of appropriate and thorough wound cleansing cannot be overemphasized. All traumatic wounds are contaminated. The risk of developing a wound infection is directly related to the adequacy of cleansing, irrigation, and débridement.

In general, the procedure is as follows:
1. Irrigation with 0.9% normal saline solution (the choice of solutions is debated, but normal saline is believed to be the least toxic to tissues, followed by surfactant cleansers) under pressure. Irrigation methods include:
   - A liter bag of saline IV solution with the IV tubing attached via a stop cock to a 22-gauge angiocath and a syringe, allowing the solution to be delivered under pressure[2]
   - A plastic liter bottle of normal saline irrigation solution with 8 to 12 holes cut in the sterile plastic cap, ejecting the fluid with firm pressure[2]
   - Other commercially available irrigation systems

NOTE: Irrigation with a bulb syringe does not adequately remove bacteria and microscopic debris, nor does simple gravity flow of fluid via IV tubing.

---

2. Débridement of any nonviable or necrotic tissue using a scalpel and normal saline irrigation. This may require a physician.
3. Achievement of complete wound hemostasis. The development of hematomas is a risk factor for infection. Hematomas may require a pressure dressing, closed suction drainage, or operating room management.
4. Change wet, contaminated drapes and gloves for closure.

SUTURES AND OTHER CLOSURE MATERIALS

The type of closure material selected is influenced by the location of the wound, the type of wound, the amount of tension that is applied to the wound, and the desired cosmetic result. In the acute phase of trauma management, the need to control significant external bleeding takes priority over these other factors. Skin staples are commonly used for this purpose in areas in which cosmesis is not a concern.

Suture material

Sutures are available as absorbable or nonabsorbable and monofilament or multifilament. Absorbable sutures dissolve on their own (they retain tensile strength for about 60 days), and nonabsorbable sutures need to be removed in a prescribed period of time. Absorbable, monofilament sutures are used on the deeper layers of tissue to provide closure and decrease tension on the skin surface. Nonabsorbable, monofilament sutures such as prolene, nylon, and stainless steel are the sutures of choice for primary closure of the skin because they produce less skin reaction.

General guidelines for suture removal are

Eyelids	2 to 3 days
Face	3 to 4 days
Scalp, abdomen, chest, trunk	7 to 10 days
Hands, arms, legs, feet	10 to 14 days (1 to 2 weeks longer if over active area)

Skin staples

Skin staples allow rapid skin closure. Staples are most commonly used in the trauma setting to control rapid bleeding, as well as in patients who are unstable and who will not be able to have their wounds further addressed for several hours. Staples can leave significant skin marks if not removed in 7 days or less.

Tape closure

Closure of wounds with adhesive tapes is another option that does not require anesthesia, is less time consuming, and does not leave needle marks. However, wound edge approximation may be less precise, keeping the area clean is more difficult, and patient compliance (especially in children) may be an issue.

WOUND DRESSINGS

Many wound dressings are available for use in the emergency care setting today. While the type of dressing may vary depending on the type of wound and treatment plan, the general principles and goals have remained constant. These include decreasing contamination and dehydration of the wound, providing support to the wound during granulation, and stabilizing the reapproximated wound edges.

In general, wound dressing materials can be broken down into major groups[1,2]:

• Gauze (fluffs, 4 × 4s): adherent, absorbent, occlusive

- Impregnated gauzes (e.g., Xeroform, Vaseline): nonadherent, absorbent, occlusive
- Hydrocolloid (e.g., Duoderm, Comfeel, Tegasorb, Biofilm): nonadherent, absorbent, occlusive
- Alginates (e.g., Sorbsan, Tegagal, Kaltostat): absorbent, occlusive
- Films (e.g., Op Site, Tegaderm, Bioclusive): nonabsorbent, occlusive

Traditionally, a sterile, occlusive, normal saline-moistened wet-to-dry gauze dressing has been applied to open wounds, and a dry, sterile dressing to sutured or stapled wounds. Although these methods are still widely used and effective, the hydrocolloid and alginate dressings are gaining popularity for use with both primary-closure and secondary-intention wounds. Proponents cite the advantages of more rapid healing, less frequent dressing changes, and increased ease of management.

SPECIFIC TYPES OF WOUNDS AND WOUND MANAGEMENT

Wounds are categorized by their mechanism of injury and/or depth of injury. The major types of wounds include abrasions, avulsions, amputations, contusions, crush injuries, lacerations, and punctures.

Abrasion

Loss of the epithelial layer with exposure of the dermal and epidermal layers (partial thickness skin loss) caused by friction of the skin against a hard surface or object. Abrasions are sometimes referred to as *road rash* when the mechanism involves a motorcycle or bicycle crash.

ASSESSMENT

- Assess the amount of fluid loss in large wounds.
- Assess functional capabilities.
- Assess pain control.
- Assess tetanus prophylaxis status.

THERAPEUTIC INTERVENTIONS

- May require parenteral sedation, local infiltrative, topical, or operating room anesthesia for wound cleansing.
- Cleanse wounds thoroughly by scrubbing with normal saline or surfactant-soaked sponge or brush and irrigation. Be sure to remove all debris and foreign bodies to avoid traumatic tattooing.
- Apply antibiotic ointment.
- Leave wound uncovered, or cover with nonadherent, occlusive dressing (reduces pain but increases infection risk).

PATIENT EDUCATION

- Take systemic antibiotics as directed.
- Take pain medication as directed.

- Cleanse wounds (or shower) with mild (nonperfumed) soap and water at least twice daily and as necessary to keep clean. Scarring and tattooing may be increased if crust and debris are allowed to accumulate.
- Pat dry, and apply antibiotic ointment each time.
- Call physician or return for check if increasing pus, bleeding, redness, hotness over wound, or fever occurs after the first several days.
- Return for wound check as directed.
- Keep lightly covered with clothing if out in direct sunlight; apply sunscreen whenever exposed to the sun after wounds are completely healed.

Avulsion

A full-thickness skin loss in which wound edges cannot be approximated, usually as a result of a tearing or gouging mechanism. Degloving or flap injuries are avulsions.

ASSESSMENT

- Assess amount of tissue loss, depth, functional loss, and pain status.
- Assess tetanus prophylaxis status.

THERAPEUTIC INTERVENTIONS

- Control bleeding by direct pressure.
- Administer appropriate pain medication.
- Cleanse thoroughly as described above.
- Physician will débride nonviable tissues, repair viable underlying structures, repair and/or refer for split-thickness skin graft or flap closure.
- Cover wound with appropriate sterile dressing, splints and/or ointments depending on location of wound and closure versus secondary intention.
- Tetanus prophylaxis and systemic antibiotics as appropriate.

PATIENT EDUCATION

- Take antibiotics as prescribed.
- Take pain medication as directed.
- If discharged home, wound must have daily dressing changes (type and frequency determined by wound depth, location, degree of contamination, closure versus open management), and wound check. Dressings must stay clean and dry. Determine need for home nursing visits and physical therapy if an extremity is involved.
- Return or call before scheduled follow-up for increased pain, fever, wound redness, swelling, heat or drainage (pus), development of numbness, coolness, or cyanosis if an extremity injury.

Amputation

An avulsion or crushing type of injury in which a body part is partially or completely severed or torn from the body.

ASSESSMENT

- Assess for amount of blood loss, continued bleeding, neurovascular status, and pain control.

NOTE: Time (sometimes up to 6 to 12 hours postinjury) and degree of damage to vascular and nerve structures are critical factors in replantation.

- Assess tetanus prophylaxis status.

THERAPEUTIC INTERVENTIONS

- Control bleeding with direct pressure and elevation.
- Apply moist, sterile dressing over amputation stump.
- Amputated body part should be wrapped in moist, sterile dressing; placed in plastic bag; and placed *over* ice or in an insulated cooler (do not freeze or place in water or other solutions). Assessment of amputated part for viability by a reconstructive surgeon should occur immediately.
- Administer pain medication and tetanus prophylaxis as directed.
- Partial and complete amputations require operative irrigation and débridement, repair of injury to underlying structures, and revision of stump.

PATIENT EDUCATION

- Most patients with partial or complete amputations of body parts require an inpatient stay for operative repair and/or a replantation attempt, followed by rehabilitative therapy.

Bite

Breakage of the skin caused by animal or human teeth. All bite wounds are considered contaminated.

ASSESSMENT

- Assess nature of bite: human or animal; type of animal
- Assess time of bite and location of wound (hand wounds, deep puncture wounds, and old wounds are at increased risk for infection)
- Assess tetanus prophylaxis status
- Assess rabies exposure risk for animal bites (see Prevention of Infection, page 88)

THERAPEUTIC INTERVENTIONS

- For human bites: Copious irrigation, débridement of devitalized tissue, and application of a bulky dressing. The wound is initially left open. Antibiotics should be given within 3 hours of arrival.
- For animal bites: Irrigation and débridement as for human bites. Small

wounds are closed. Prophylactic antibiotics are recommended for high-risk patients.
• Antibiotic therapy and tetanus and rabies prophylaxis as indicated.

PATIENT EDUCATION
• Take antibiotics as prescribed.
• Perform wound care and dressing changes as directed.
• Return for wound checks as directed. Return or call before scheduled follow-up for increased pain, fever, wound redness, swelling, heat, or drainage (pus).

Burn

See Chapter 22 for discussion of burn wounds.

Contusion

Formation of a hematoma beneath unbroken skin because of the rupture of small blood vessels. Caused by blunt trauma.

ASSESSMENT
• Assess for depth of hematoma and potential damage to underlying vascular, nerve, and bony structures. Test circulation, sensation, and motor function.
• Is the patient currently receiving anticoagulation therapy?
• Assess need for analgesia.

THERAPEUTIC INTERVENTIONS
• Apply ice pack to affected area.
• Elevate contused area or extremity.
• Observe progression of swelling and discoloration. Monitor circulation, sensation, and motor function.

PATIENT EDUCATION
• Take analgesia as prescribed. Avoid aspirin or aspirin-containing products.
• Keep affected area elevated, with ice pack to affected area (20 minutes on and 20 minutes off) as necessary for the first 24 hours.
• Return or call if affected area or limb becomes significantly more painful; normal function is affected from significant swelling; limbs become numb, cool, cyanotic, or insensate; fever develops; or hematoma becomes significantly larger and fluctuant. Tell the patient that hematomas take 2 to 3 weeks to resolve, but very large hematomas may need to be drained after a week or two for patient comfort, function, or to decrease the risk of infection.

Crush injury

Injury to multiple tissues, muscle, or bone in which there is a blunt, high-energy exchange, such as in a fall, pedestrian versus motor vehicle incident, or an industrial injury.

ASSESSMENT

- Assess for blood loss, tissues involved, wound depth, neurovascular status of the affected area.
- Assess need for analgesia.
- Assess tetanus prophylaxis status.
- Because the patient will likely require surgical intervention for further evaluation, irrigation and débridement, fasciotomy, amputation or fracture repair, prepare for operation (e.g., place intravenous line, assess time of last meal, and withhold fluids by mouth).

THERAPEUTIC INTERVENTIONS

- Control bleeding by direct pressure.
- Apply dry, sterile dressing (pressure dressing if bleeding).
- Elevate extremity.
- Administer pain medication as needed.
- Administer antibiotics as directed.
- Monitor for signs of compartment syndrome. These include pain, firmness of the muscle compartment, and paresthesia.
- Apply dressing type as determined by the injury and treatment plan.

PATIENT EDUCATION

- Take antibiotics as prescribed.
- Take pain medication as directed.
- Keep the affected extremity elevated above the level of the heart to decrease swelling and pain.
- Keep the wound and dressing clean and dry at all times.
- Change dressings daily as directed.
- Return sooner than scheduled follow-up if redness, swelling, increased pain, numbness, coolness, blue discoloration of fingers or toes, fever, or wound drainage (pus) develop.

Laceration

A cut or tear of the skin that may involve the epidermis and dermis (superficial) or deeper structures (deep); may be caused by blunt or sharp objects.

ASSESSMENT

- Assess age of wound, depth, degree/type of contamination, associated injuries, neurovascular status distal to wound.
- Assess need for analgesia.
- Assess tetanus prophylaxis status.

• Control bleeding with direct pressure.
• Apply local anesthetic as prescribed.
• Cleanse and irrigate thoroughly. Be certain to remove all debris and foreign bodies. May require physician exploration/débridement.
• Wound closure by suture, skin staples, or tape if indicated.
• Apply dressing/immobilization appropriate to wound type, location, and closure versus nonclosure treatment plan (see section on wound dressings). Assess need for home nursing services for wound care.
• Administer tetanus prophylaxis and systemic or topical antibiotics as prescribed.

• Apply topical antibiotic ointment twice daily as directed.
• Take analgesia as prescribed.
• Keep sutures clean and dry.
• Change dressings as directed.
• It is not necessary to cover sutured wounds after 24 hours.
• Return for wound check sooner than scheduled appointment if wound becomes reddened, hot, or swollen, or if drainage (pus) or fever develops.
• Return for suture removal in the prescribed number of days. Suture removal is determined by wound location (see section on suture material).
• Apply sunscreen to wound once it is completely healed or whenever area is exposed to the sun or wear protective clothing when in direct sunlight.
• Scars take 6 to 12 months to develop into their final cosmetic appearance.

Puncture

A wound created by a small-diameter sharp object that externally may not produce a large defect, but may penetrate superficial and/or deeper tissues.

• Assess for presence of foreign bodies/materials, impaled objects, depth of tissue penetration, underlying structural damage, type/degree of contamination, and need for analgesia.
• Assess tetanus prophylaxis status.

• Control bleeding by direct pressure.
• Secure any impaled objects.
• Administer local and/or systemic analgesia as necessary.
• Soak the wound in warm isotonic solution for several minutes.
• Remove any easily dislodged debris, necrotic tissue, or foreign bodies. This may require physician intervention and placement of drains.

- Cleanse and irrigate the wound as described (see section on wound cleansing).
- Apply appropriate dressing (may include loose packing).
- Administer systemic or topical antibiotics and tetanus prophylaxis as prescribed.

PATIENT EDUCATION

- Take antibiotics as directed.
- Take analgesia as directed.
- Keep wound clean and dry.
- Change dressings as directed.
- Assess need for home nursing services for wound care and checks.
- Observe for retained foreign bodies or material.
- Return before scheduled follow-up if wound becomes reddened, swollen, hot to touch, begins to drain pus, or if fever develops.

PREVENTION OF INFECTION

Antibiotic therapy in trauma

Prophylactic antibiotics are usually not indicated for minor, uncomplicated wounds with low contamination, or for those wounds in which there has been adequate and appropriate cleansing, débridement, and closure.

There are certain situations in which it is generally believed that antibiotics are indicated, considering that the morbidity of a wound or systemic infection can be significant or even life or limb threatening. These include[2]:

- Open joint, tendon, nerve, or fracture injuries (including teeth)
- Heavily contaminated wounds (i.e., soil, mammalian bites)
- Wounds with major soft tissue injury or losses (i.e., degloving injuries)
- Premorbid conditions such as valvular disease or replacement, immunosuppression, or diabetes
- Delays in wound management such as cleansing, débridement, and repair

Antibiotics must be present in adequate tissue levels before wound closure and during operative management to be effective; therefore the timing of administration in trauma is important. The specific antibiotic for a particular wound is determined by the age of the wound, as well as the type, location, and degree of contamination.

Tetanus prophylaxis in trauma

Clostridium tetani, the causative organism of the disease tetanus, exists in animal and human excreta and is found in soil and dust. It enters the human body through an open wound. Tetanus is easily prevented through appropriate vaccination, immunization, and wound care. Table 8-1 outlines current recommendations for tetanus prophylaxis.[3]

Table 8-1   Summary Guide to Tetanus Prophylaxis* in Routine Wound Management, United States

	Clean, minor wounds		All other wounds†	
	Td§	TIG¶	Td§	TIG
Uncertain or <3	Yes	No	Yes	Yes
>3**	No††	No	No§§	No

From Centers for Disease Control: Update on adult immunization: recommendations of the Immunization Practices Advisory Committee (ACIP), *MMWR* 40(RR-12):70, 1991.

*Refer also to text on specific vaccines or toxoids for contraindications, precautions, dosages, side effects, adverse reactions, and special considerations. Important details are in the text and in the ACIP recommendations on diphtheria, tetanus, and pertussis (DTP) (MMWR 1991: 40[RR-10]).

†Such as, but not limited to: wounds contaminated with dirt, feces, and saliva; puncture wounds; avulsions; and wounds resulting from missiles, crushing, burns, and frostbite.

§Td = Tetanus and diphtheria toxoids, adsorbed (for adult use). For children <7 years old, DTP (DT, if pertussis vaccine is contraindicated) is preferred to tetanus toxoid alone. For persons ≥7 years old, Td is preferred to tetanus toxoid alone.

¶TIG = Tetanus immune globulin.

**If only three doses of fluid toxoid have been received, a fourth dose of toxoid, preferably an adsorbed toxoid, should be given.

††Yes, >10 years since last dose.

§§Yes, >5 years since last dose. (More frequent boosters are not needed and can accentuate side effects.)

The need for immunization after injury depends on the condition of the wound and the patient's vaccination history. In addition to the most recent dose of tetanus toxoid, it is important to ascertain whether patients have ever received the full primary vaccination series of three doses. Patients with unknown or uncertain vaccination histories should be considered to have had no previous tetanus toxoid doses. Those who have served in U.S. military forces at any time since 1941 usually have received the complete primary series. Patients 60 years of age or older are most at risk of being unvaccinated or inadequately vaccinated.[3]

Rabies prophylaxis in trauma

Rabies, an extremely rare but fatal disease, is preventable through proper wound care and postexposure prophylaxis. Rabies is transmitted when the virus, carried by an infected animal, is introduced into open cuts or wounds in the victim's skin or mucous membranes. Over half of recent cases in the United States have been traced to bats. Other cases have been attributed to carnivorous wild animals, especially skunks, raccoons, and foxes; woodchucks; exotic pets; dogs and cats.[4,5]

The risk of rabies infection and the need for prophylaxis vary with the nature and extent of exposure. Wounds are categorized as bite

Table 8-2 Rabies Postexposure Prophylaxis Guide, United States, 1991

Animal type	Evaluation and disposition of animal	Postexposure prophylaxis recommendations
Dogs and cats	Healthy and available for 10 days' observation	Should not begin prophylaxis unless animal develops symptoms of rabies*
	Rabid or suspected rabid	Immediate vaccination
	Unknown (escaped)	Consult public health officials
Skunks, raccoons, bats, foxes, and most other carnivores; woodchucks	Regarded as rabid unless geographic area is known to be free of rabies or until animal proven negative by laboratory tests†	Immediate vaccination
Livestock, rodents, and lagomorphs (rabbits and hares)	Consider individually	Consult public health officials. Bites of squirrels, hamsters, guinea pigs, gerbils, chipmunks, rats, mice, other rodents, rabbits, and hares almost never require antirabies treatment

From Centers for Disease Control: Rabies prevention—United States, 1991: recommendations of the Immunization Practices Advisory Committee (ACIP), *MMWR* 40(RR-3):4, 1991.

*During the 10-day holding period, begin treatment at first sign of rabies in a dog or cat that has bitten someone. The symptomatic animal should be killed immediately and tested.

†The animal should be killed and tested as soon as possible. Holding for observation is not recommended. Discontinue vaccine if immunofluorescence test results of the animal are negative.

wounds or nonbite wounds. Nonbite exposures (scratches, abrasions, open wounds, or mucous membrane contacts) rarely cause rabies. Bat exposures are a special category: seemingly insignificant physical contact with bats may result in viral transmission. Therefore rabies postexposure prophylaxis should be considered in all situations in which there is reasonable probability of contact with a bat, unless the bat is tested and found negative. In addition to known bites, scratches, and mucous membrane contacts, examples of potential contact include a sleeping person awakening to find a bat in a room or a person finding a bat in a room with an unattended child or a mentally disabled or intoxicated person.[4,5]

Patient management begins with appropriate wound care. A decision should then be made concerning the need for postexposure prophylaxis (Table 8-2). If needed, rabies vaccine and rabies immune globulin are given

Table 8-3 Rabies Postexposure Prophylaxis Schedule, United States, 1991

Vaccination status	Treatment	Regimen*
Not previously vaccinated	Local wound cleansing	All postexposure treatment should begin with immediate thorough cleansing of all wounds with soap and water.
	HRIG	20 IU/kg body weight. If anatomically feasible, up to one-half the dose should be infiltrated around the wound(s) and the rest should be administered IM in the gluteal area. HRIG should not be administered in the same syringe or into the same anatomical site as vaccine. Because HRIG may partially suppress active production of antibody, no more than the recommended dose should be given.
	Vaccine	HDCV or RVA, 1.0 ml, IM (deltoid area†), one each on days 0, 3, 7, 14 and 28.
Previously vaccinated§	Local wound cleansing	All postexposure treatment should begin with immediate thorough cleansing of all wounds with soap and water.
	HRIG	HRIG should not be administered.
	Vaccine	HDCV or RVA, 1.0 ml, IM (deltoid area†), one each on days 0 and 3.

From Centers for Disease Control: Rabies prevention—United States, 1991: recommendations of the Immunization Practices Advisory Committee (ACIP), *MMWR* 40(RR-3):7, 1991.

HRIG, Human Rabies Immune Globulin; *HDCV,* Human Diploid Cell Vaccine; *RVA,* Rabies Vaccine Adsorbed.

*These regimens are applicable for all age groups, including children.

†The deltoid area is the only acceptable site of vaccination for adults and older children. For younger children, the outer aspect of the thigh may be used. Vaccine should never be administered in the gluteal area.

§Any person with a history of preexposure vaccination with HDCV or RVA, prior postexposure prophylaxis with HDCV or RVA, or previous vaccination with any other type of rabies vaccine and a documented history of antibody response to the prior vaccination.

according to a standard regimen (Table 8-3). State or local health departments should be consulted for additional advice regarding prophylaxis.[4,5]

REFERENCES

1. Wilson RF, Balakrishnan C: General principles of wound care. In Wilson RF, Walt AJ, editors: *Management of trauma: pitfalls and practice,* ed 2, Baltimore, 1996, Williams & Wilkins.
2. Stewart RM, Page CP: Wounds, bites, and stings. In Feliciano DV, Moore EE, Mattox KL, editors: *Trauma,* ed 3, Stamford, CT, 1996, Appleton & Lange.
3. Centers for Disease Control: Update on adult immunization: recommendations of the Immunization Practices Advisory Committee (ACIP), *MMWR* 40(RR-12):16-19, 1991.

4. Centers for Disease Control: Rabies prevention—United States, 1991: recommendations of the Immunization Practices Advisory Committee (ACIP), *MMWR* 40(RR-3):1-19, 1991.
5. Human rabies—Montana and Washington, 1997, *MMWR* 46:770, 1997.

SUGGESTED READINGS

Cardona VD, Hurn PD, Mason PJB, and others: *Trauma nursing from resuscitation through rehabilitation,* ed 2, Philadelphia, 1994, Saunders.
Herman ML, Newberry L: Wound management. In Emergency Nurses Association: *Sheehy's emergency nursing: principles and practice,* ed 4, St Louis, 1998, Mosby.

CHAPTER 9

Trauma Laboratory Tests

Patricia Brueske

When a trauma patient enters the Emergency Department, a predetermined set of laboratory tests known as *trauma labs* or *trauma lab panels* are often performed. Recent studies have begun to question the justification and cost effectiveness of these routine tests, as often they have no influence on clinical management.[1,2] Still, they remain part of the standard trauma patient treatment plan. In most institutions these panels consist of chemistry, hematologic, and coagulation profiles, or a combination of the following studies:

Type & screen or Type & crossmatch	(T&S/T&CM)
Kleihauer-Betke	
Arterial blood gases	(ABGs)
Complete blood count	(CBC)
Red blood cells & indices	(RBCs)
White blood cells & differential	(WBCs)
	(Diff)
Hematocrit	(Hct) ⎱ Known as *H & H*
Hemoglobin	(Hgb) ⎰
Platelets	
Coagulation studies	(Coags)
Prothrombin time	(PT)
Activated partial thromboplastin time	(APTT)
Fibrinogen	
D-dimer	
Chemistry profile	
Serum glucose	
Potassium	(K)
Sodium	(Na)
Chlorides	(Cl)
Carbon dioxide	(CO_2)
Blood urea nitrogen	(BUN)
Creatinine	(Creat)
Urine tests	
Urine analysis	(UA)
Urine toxicology	(Urine tox)
Urine and serum hCG (pregnancy)	

Serum alcohol   (ETOH)
Serum amylase
Serum lactate
Alanine aminotransferase   (ALT)
Aspartate aminotransferase   (AST)

TYPE & SCREEN OR TYPE & CROSSMATCH

The type and screen (T & S) or type and crossmatch (T & CM) blood serum test is one of the most important lab tests to be performed on the critically injured trauma patient. Often obtaining even one blood sample is difficult because of multiple injuries or the presence of shock. However, this test should be performed for the trauma patient requiring blood transfusions.

Type and screen tests are performed for the patient's own blood grouping antigen (A, B, AB, or O) and the presence (positive) or absence (negative) of the Rh antigen.

Type and crossmatch tests are performed for compatibility between a mixture of the patient's own blood and the donor's blood. Successful type and crossmatch occurs when no hemolysis or clumping occurs in the mixture.

General rule

O negative = universal donor
AB positive = universal recipient

Procedure

Collect 5 to 10 cc of blood in a red top evacuated specimen tube. Date and sign the sample. Send to the lab.

Kleihauer-Betke

The Kleihauer-Betke blood serum is occasionally ordered for the pregnant trauma patient who is Rh negative. For injured patients at risk for abruptio placenta or other pregnancy-related complications, this test is used to determine the amount of fetomaternal hemorrhage that has occurred in the mother and the amount of Rhlg (RhoGAM) to be given. RhoGAM prevents the Rh negative mother from producing antibodies against future pregnancies in which the fetus is Rh positive.

Procedure

Collect 7 cc of blood in a purple (EDTA) top specimen tube. Send immediately to the lab.

ARTERIAL BLOOD GASES

Arterial blood gases (ABGs) are obtained from arterial blood samples. The values help to evaluate the effectiveness of gases exchanged at the alveolar capillary cellular membrane level. They also assist in evaluating the efficiency of lung ventilation and perfusion and in determining the acid-base balance of the body.

Normal values

Pao_2	Measures the amount of oxygen in arterial blood available for combining with Hgb	80-100 mm Hg
O_2 saturation	Measures the quantity of O_2 that is actually combined to Hgb	94%-100%
pH	Measures the acidity or alkalinity of arterial blood; also an expression of hydrogen ion concentration	7.35-7.45
$Paco_2$	Measures the partial pressure of carbon dioxide (CO_2) in arterial blood to determine how well the lungs are maintaining acid-base balance. The lungs do this by "blowing off" or retaining CO_2 (acid).	35-45 mmHg (respiratory component of acid-base)
HCO_3	Measures the amount of bicarb (HCO_3) in arterial blood to determine how well the kidneys are maintaining acid-base balance. The kidneys do this by retaining or excreting HCO_3 (base).	22-26 mEq/L (metabolic component of acid-base)

NOTE: $Paco_2$ and HCO_3 are proportional to pH: $\uparrow Paco_2 = \downarrow pH$, $\downarrow Paco_2 = \uparrow pH$ $\uparrow HCO_3 = \uparrow pH$, $\downarrow HCO_3 = \downarrow pH$

Abnormal values		**Possible cause**
Pao_2	<50 mmHg	Hypoxia
pH	<7.35	Acidosis
	>7.45	Alkalosis
$Paco_2$ (resp acidosis)	>45 mmHg	Hypoventilation/$\uparrow CO_2$ retained by lungs
$Paco_2$ (resp alkalosis)	<35 mmHg	Hyperventilation/$\uparrow CO_2$ blown off by lungs
HCO_3 (metab acidosis)	<22 mEq/L	$\uparrow HCO_3$ excreted by kidneys
HCO_3 (metab alkalosis)	>26 mEq/L	$\uparrow HCO_3$ retained by kidneys

Common *traumatic* causes of abnormal blood gas values

Test	**Value:**	**Possible cause**
Pao_2	$\downarrow$	• hypovolemic shock
O_2 saturation	$\downarrow$	(hypoventilation and
pH	$\downarrow$ (late)	hypoperfusion)
$Paco_2$	$\uparrow$ (late)	
HCO_3	$\downarrow$	

NOTE: Hyperventilation in early shock may $\uparrow pH$ & $\downarrow Paco_2$.

Pao_2	↓	• airway obstruct/anoxia
O_2 saturation	↓	• chest trauma ↓ respira-
pH	↓	tions
$Paco_2$	↑	• head trauma/CNS
HCO_3	ok-↑ (mild)	injury with ↓ respira-
		tions

NOTE: Bicarb may be mildly ↑ to compensate resp acidosis.

Pao_2	↓	• simple pneumothorax
O_2 saturation	↓	
pH	ok	
$Paco_2$	ok	
HCO_3	ok	
Pao_2	ok	• hyperventilation may be
O_2 saturation	ok	because of CNS injury
pH	↑	or pain
$Paco_2$	↓ (mild)	
HCO_3	ok-↓ (mild)	

NOTE: Bicarb may be mildly ↓, compensating resp alkalosis.

Procedure

Collect 3 to 5 cc of arterial blood in a preheparinized syringe from the radial, brachial, or femoral artery. Write on the specimen the patient's temperature and the amount of oxygen being received at the time of the sample collection (including room air oxygen). Place the sample on ice and immediately send it to the lab.

COMPLETE BLOOD COUNT

A complete blood count (CBC) is obtained to identify the amount of red blood cells, blood cells with differentiation, hematocrit, hemoglobin, and platelets in whole blood.

Procedure

Collect 5 cc of blood serum in a purple (EDTA) top evacuated specimen tube. Avoid clotted specimen. Send to lab.

Red blood cells (erythrocytes)

Red blood cell (RBC) values will vary, depending on the age, sex, and geographic location (in relation to sea level) of the patient.

Normal values

Neonates (up to 2 months)	4.4-5.8 million/µl
Infants (>2 months)	3-3.8 million/µl
Children (>1 year)	4.6-4.8 million/µl

Adults	
Males	4.5-6.3 million/µl
Females	4.2-5.4 million/µl
Pregnant females	Decreased

Abnormal values	Possible cause
↑	• Dehydration
↓	• Hemorrhage
	• Fluid overload (dilutional)
	• Anemia (iron deficient)
	• Pregnancy

Red blood cell indices

The following lists RBC indices:
• Mean Corpuscular Volume (MCV)
• Mean Corpuscular Hemoglobin (MCH)
• Mean Corpuscular Hemoglobin Concentration (MCHC)
• Red Cell Size Distribution Width (RDW)

Red blood cell indices define the size, weight, and Hgb content of RBCs. They are routinely done as part of a CBC and are useful in identifying different types of anemia that may be present, including that of trauma patients.

Normal values

MCV	80-95 m
MCH	27-31pg
MCHC	32-36g/d
RDW	11%-14.5%

Abnormal values		Possible causes
MCV, MCHC	↓	Iron deficient anemia
MCV	↑	Alcoholism, ↓ Vitamin B$_{12}$ or Folic acid

White blood cells (leukocytes)

A white blood cell (WBC) count is obtained to identify the presence of an infection.

Normal values

4100-10,900/µl (may be elevated in pregnancy)

Abnormal value	Possible cause
>10,900/µl	• Infection/inflammation
	• Tissue necrosis
	• Immunocompromise

NOTE: Elderly patients may respond weakly to severe bacterial infection.

White blood cell differential

A white blood cell differential (diff) count is done in trauma patients to identify current infections and their severity and to determine the body's ability to resist and fight infection. Each component represents a relative percentage of the total WBC count.

Normal values

Neutrophils	55%-70%
Eosinophils	0%-3%
Basophils	0%-1%
Monocytes	3%-7%
Lymphocytes	25%-40%

Abnormal values		**Possible causes**
Neutrophils (pyogenic infect)	↑	• Bacterial infection • Stress response • Ischemic necrosis
	↓	• Viral infections
Eosinophils (allergic and parasite disorders)	↑	• Drug sensitivity • Allergic reaction
	↓	• Stress response • Shock • Burns
	↑	• Postsplenectomy (uncommon)
Basophils (parasite infection)	↓	• Stress
Monocytes (severe infection)	↑	• Chronic infection
	↓	• Prednisone treatment
Lymphocytes	↑	• Viral infection
	↓	• Renal failure • Steroid therapy

NOTE: Neutrophils are the most numerous and first in to fight infections. With overwhelming infections, there is a production of immature neuts (bands), reflecting a shift to the left on the CBC results.

Hematocrit

A hematocrit (Hct) value is obtained to determine the percentage of RBCs in whole blood. Hematocrit values parallel RBC values. Serial Hcts may be done at short intervals of time to detect hemorrhage.

Normal values

Neonate	55%-68%
7 day infant	47%-65%
1 month infant	37%-49%

3 month infant	30%-36%
1 year old	29%-41%
10 year old	36%-40%
Adult:	
Male	42%-54%
Female	35%-46%
Pregnancy/Elderly	Slightly ↓

Abnormal values in trauma

↓	• Hemodilution
	  From compensated hypovolemia
	  From excessive volume replacement
	• Anemia
	• Hemorrhage

↑	• Hemoconcentration • Burns • Dehydration

NOTE: When blood is lost acutely, the amount of hematocrit lost is in the same ratio as that of whole blood. Therefore, the percentage of hematocrit in a whole blood sample would remain normal. It is only after hemodilution occurs (from shock compensation or crystalloid replacement) that hematocrit will drop.

Hemoglobin

Hemoglobin (Hgb) value is obtained to measure the amount of hemoglobin in whole blood. The amount of hemoglobin determines the oxygen-carrying capacity of blood. Hemoglobin values closely reflect RBC values. Serial Hgbs may be done at short intervals of time to detect hemorrhage.

Normal values

Neonate	17-22 g/dl
1 week infant	15-20 g/dl
1 month infant	11-15 g/dl
Child	11-13 g/dl
Adult	
Male	14-18 g/dl
Female	12.4-14.9 g/dl
Pregnancy/ Elderly	Slightly ↓

Abnormal values in trauma

Possible cause

↑	• Hemo concentration • Severe burns • Dehydration
↓	• Hemorrhage • Anemia • Transfusions of incompatible blood

NOTE: When whole blood is lost acutely, the amount of hemoglobin that is lost is proportionate. It is only after hemodilution occurs (as a result of shock compensation or crystalloid volume replacement) that hemoglobin will drop.

Platelets (thrombocytes)

A platelet count is obtained to test the amount of platelet function. Platelets play an essential role in coagulation. Particularly in trauma, platelets are essential to hemostasis when vascular trauma occurs.

Normal values

130,000-370,000/mm^3

Abnormal values	Probable causes
↑	• Splenectomy
	• Injury
	• Infection
	• Hemorrhage
↓	• Disseminated intravascular coagulation (DIC)

COAGULATION STUDIES

Research has shown that within 1 to 4 hours after severe head trauma, patients can develop a disseminated intravascular coagulation (DIC) syndrome leading to more serious coagulopathy and then death.[3] In cases of significant head trauma, the collection of immediate coagulation studies has been recommended to provide early and effective treatment. Head injury coagulation studies may include PT/APTT, fibrinogen, platelets, and D-dimer.

Procedure

Collect 5 to 7 cc of blood in a blue (sodium citrate) top evacuated specimen tube. Do not underfill; an incorrect test result can occur from altered blood-to-anticoagulant ratio. For head injury coagulation studies, as many as three blue top specimens may be required. Send specimens to the lab.

Prothrombin time (protime)

A prothrombin time (PT) is evaluated in trauma patients to measure clotting time (caused by factors V, VII, and X; fibrinogen/factor I; and prothrombin/factor III). PT is important in determining the blood's ability to clot.

Normal values

PT	10-14 sec
Critical	>20 sec

Abnormal values	Possible cause
↑	Deficiency of factors V, VII, X, fibrin, or prothrombin; 2.5 × normal times means that there is an abnormal bleeding tendency

NOTE: There may be prolonged clotting times in the presence of liver disease, couma-rin ingestion, DIC, and massive blood transfusions.

Activated partial thromboplastin time

Activated partial thromboplastin time (APTT) is obtained to screen for prob-lems with intrinsic clotting factors (except factors VII and XIII). It can also be used to monitor the effectiveness of anticoagulation with heparin. This labo-ratory test measures the amount of time it takes for fibrin to form a clot. In the trauma patient, it is used to determine the patient's tendency to bleed.

Normal values

| APTT | 30-45 sec for clot to form after clinical reagent is added |
| Critical | >70 sec |

Abnormal values	Possible cause
↑	• DIC (after head injury)
	• Heparin therapy
↓	• Early DIC

Fibrinogen

Fibrinogen is a protein in the blood clotting network that rises sharply in re-sponse to acute phase injury or tissue necrosis. In trauma it is used to screen for DIC.

Procedure

Same as for PT/APTT

Normal value

| Fibrinogen | 200-400 mg/dl or 2-4 g/L |
| Critical | >100 |

Abnormal value	Possible cause
↑	• compensated DIC
	• various cerebral accidents
↓	• DIC
	• liver disease

D-dimer

D-dimers are fibrin degradation fragments that are produced through fibrino-lysis in conditions like DIC. Normal plasma does not contain them. The D-dimer is a specific test used for diagnosing DIC.

Procedure

Same as for PTT/APTT

Normal value

| D-dimer | 0 < 250mg/ml |

Abnormal value	Possible cause
↑	• DIC

CHEMISTRY PROFILE

In most institutions, a modified version of the complete chemistry panel (chem panel) exists. The most commonly ordered chemistries in this test include serum glucose, K, Na, Cl, CO_2, BUN, and creatinine.

Procedure

Collect 5 cc of blood in a red top or red/black "tiger" top evacuated specimen tube. Send to the lab. Serum glucose may be tested at a bedside glucose monitor.

Serum glucose

Serum glucose is produced from digestion of carbohydrates and from the liver when it converts glucagon. Serum glucose is necessary for cellular metabolism to occur. In trauma cases, this test rules out metabolic causes of decreased level of consciousness like hypoglycemia.

Normal values

Random blood glucose	70 mg/dl
Critical	<70 mg/dl

Abnormal values	Possible causes
↓	• Hypoglycemia
↑	• Hyperglycemia/DKA • Stress response

Potassium

The primary electrolyte in intracellular fluid is potassium (K) (90%). It is essential for the maintenance of cellular osmosis and plays a critical role in the electrical conduction of cardiac and skeletal muscle. Potassium is also important to acid-base balance and kidney function.

Normal values

Potassium	3.5-5.5 mEq/L
Critical	<2.5 mEq/l > 7mEq/L

Abnormal values	Possible causes
↑ (hyperkalemia)	• Major burns/cell damage • Renal failure • Major crush injuries
↓ (hypokalemia)	• Hypovolemia • IV fluid therapy without KCl supplement

NOTE: Hemolysis of the blood specimen will result in inaccurately high K levels.

Sodium

Sodium (Na) is one of the two major extracellular cations. It is the major cause of osmotic pressure in extracellular fluid. Sodium also plays a major part in both acid-base balance and neuromuscular function.

Normal value

Na	135-145 mEq/L
Critical	<120 mEq/L
	>160 mEq/L

Abnormal values	Possible causes
↑ (hypernatremia)	• Fluid intake/fluid loss
	• Sodium intake
↓ (hyponatremia)	• Sodium intake
	• Sodium loss
	• Severe burns
	• Excess fluid

Chlorides

Measurement of serum chlorides (Cl) is important for the assessment of acid-base status. Chloride is a major extracellular anion that plays a role in the maintenance of oncotic pressure and, thus, blood volume and arterial pressure. It is also important in the assessment of acid-base balance.

Normal value

Cl	100-108 mEq/L
Critical	<80 mEq/L
	>115 mEq/L

Abnormal values	Possible causes
↑ (hypochloremia)	• Dehydration
	• Renal failure
	• CNS trauma with central neurogenic breathing
	• Hyperventilation
↓ (hyperchloremia)	• Excess vomiting
	• Excess gastric suctioning
	• Overhydration
	• Burns

Carbon dioxide

Serum carbon dioxide (CO_2) is the end product of food metabolism and is controlled by the kidneys. CO_2 is measured to assist with acid-base balance determination. When CO_2 levels are excessive, CO_2 is released with blood and absorbed by plasma. When CO_2 is in blood, it combines with water (H_2O) to form carbonic acid (H_2CO_3). Carbonic acid breaks down into hydrogen (H) and bicarbonate (HCO_3).

Normal value

CO_2	22-34 mEq/L
Critical	<6 mEq/L

Abnormal values	Possible causes

	• Metabolic alkalosis
	  ↑ vomiting
	  ↑ gastric suctioning
	• Respiratory acidosis
	  ↓ ventilation

Blood urea nitrogen

A blood urea nitrogen (BUN) study evaluates renal function and determines the patient's hydration status. Urea is an end product of metabolism and is excreted in urine.

Normal values

BUN	8-20 mg/dl
Critical	>100 mg/dl

Abnormal values	Possible causes
↑	• Shock • Dehydration • Tissue necrosis
↓	• Overhydration

Creatinine

Creatinine (creat) is a by-product in the breakdown of muscle mass for energy metabolism. The creatinine study in trauma patients detects the amount of muscle damage that has occurred and tests kidney function. It is a more sensitive test than BUN.

Normal values

Creat	0.6-1.3 mg/dl
Critical	>4 mg/dl

Abnormal values	Possible causes
↑	• Shock • Dehydration

NOTE: Before using IV contrast in computed tomography scans, BUN and creat levels should be checked for normal kidney function.

URINE TESTS

Urine tests are indicated in trauma to test for injury (hematuria), toxicology, and pregnancy.

Procedure

Collect approximately 10 cc of urine in a red top specimen tube. Send it to the lab. Before collection, the following steps must be taken:

Avoid contamination of the voided sample by ensuring no external blood is on the patient's body or hands. For females on their menses, a catheterized sample should be obtained.

To prevent further injury to males with GU trauma, always look for blood at the meatus before catheterization. In addition, a rectal exam must be done to check for prostate position.

Normal values

Color	Yellow-straw
Appearance	Clear
Specific gravity	1.005-1.020
pH	4.5-8.0
Protein	Negative
Glucose	Negative
Ketones	Negative
Microscopic	
RBCs	0-3/hpf
WBCs	0-4/hpf
Epithelial cells	Few
Casts	0
Crystals	Few
Bacteria	0
Yeast	0
Parasites	0

Abnormal values

		Possible causes
Color	Dark or red	• Presence of blood
Appearance	Dark or red	• Presence of blood
Specific gravity	>1.020	• Shock
pH	Alkaline >8.0	• Alkalosis
	Acidic <4.5	• Acidosis
Glucose	Present	• Diabetes
		• Increased intracranial pressure
Protein	Present	• Renal failure
Ketone	Present	• Diabetes/DKA
		• Diarrhea/vomiting
Microscopic		
RBCs	3/hpf	• Kidney, ureteral, bladder trauma
WBCs	4/hpf	• UTI
Epithelial	↑	• Renal tubular necrosis
Casts	↑	• Glomerular capsule trauma
Bacteria/yeast/parasites	↑	• Infection

Urinalysis

Urinalysis (UA) in trauma checks for genitourinary trauma and specific disease states. The absence of hematuria can exclude a penetrating injury to the genitourinary tract with 90% confidence.[4]

Procedure

A gross visual exam of the urine color, concentration, and amount should be done first. The sample can then be tested quickly for the presence of blood or certain disease states at the patient's bedside using a dipstick reagent strip. Finally, a microscopic study can be carried out by the lab.

Urine toxicology

Urine tox screens on trauma patients determine possible causes for altered levels of consciousness. The most common urine drug tests include:

Amphetamines	Alcohol	Barbiturates
Benzodiazepines	Cocaine/Crack	Cyanide
Opiates	Marijuana	PCP
LSD	Analgesics	Sedatives
Major tranquilizers	Stimulants	Sympathomim

Normal/abnormal values

A normal value would detect no evidence of drugs. The presence of one or more of these is an abnormal finding.

Urine and serum hCG (pregnancy)

The urine pregnancy test determines if the female trauma patient who is within child-bearing years is pregnant. It is a qualitative test that measures for the presence or absence of human chorionic gonadotropin (hCG). The test is carried out by placing a few drops of the patient's urine on a urine hCG reagent strip at the bedside and waiting a few moments for the results: hCG Present = pregnant

---

NOTES:
- Obtain a catheterized specimen if urine is grossly bloody
- A blood serum hCG may also be sent to the lab to test for pregnancy (5 cc of blood in a red top evacuated tube).

SERUM ALCOHOL (ETHYL ALCOHOL)

Serum alcohol (ETOH) detects alcohol in trauma patients to determine possible causes for altered levels of consciousness. Serum is the preferred medium for testing ETOH levels because the concentration is more elevated.

Procedure

Collect 5 cc in a red top or gray (potassium oxalate) top evacuated specimen tube. Avoid cleaning the puncture site with alcohol. Send to the lab.

NOTE: Alcohol can also be tested in urine and using a breath analyzer.

Normal/abnormal values

Normal value is negative for the presence of blood alcohol.
Critical value >300 mg/dl

SERUM AMYLASE

Serum amylase is an enzyme that is secreted by the pancreas and is used for carbohydrate catabolism. This test is performed in trauma patients to detect acute pancreatic injuries.

Procedure

Collect 5 to 7 cc of blood in a red top evacuated specimen tube and send it to the lab.

Normal values

Serum amylase	60-180 Somogyi units/dl
Critical	>640 Somogyi units/dl

Abnormal values	Possible causes
↑	• Pancreatic injury
	• Aortic aneurysm rupture
	• ETOH toxicity
↓	• Severe burns

SERUM LACTATE

Serum lactate is an end product of carbohydrate metabolism. Excessive amounts of lactate may be produced when anaerobic metabolism occurs because of lack of oxygen.

Procedure

Collect 4 cc of arterial or venous blood in an evacuated tube and send immediately to the lab.

Normal values

Venous lactate	0.5-2.2 mEq/L
Arterial lactate	0.5-1.6 mEq/L

Abnormal values	Possible causes
↑	• Lactic acidosis
	• Hemorrhage/Shock
	• Cardiac/Respiratory failure
	• DKA

ALANINE AMINOTRANSFERASE (FORMERLY SGPT) AND ASPARTATE AMINOTRANSFERASE (FORMERLY SGOT)

Alanine aminotransferase (ALT) and aspartate aminotransferase (AST) are enzymes that exist in the liver, especially ALT. A transient rise in their levels will occur following trauma.

Procedure

Collect 5 cc of blood in a red top evacuated specimen tube and send it to the lab.

Normal values

ALT	10-30 U/L
AST	8-20 U/L

Abnormal values	Possible causes
↑ ALT	• Hepatic injury
	• Trauma to striated muscle
	• Shock/severe burns
↑ AST	• Skeletal/multiple trauma
	• Severe deep burns

REFERENCES

1. Chu UB, Clevenger FW, Imami ER, and others: The impact of selective laboratory evaluation on utilization of laboratory resources and patient care in a level-I trauma center, *Am J Surg* November 558-563, 1996.
2. Namius N, McKenney MG, Martin LC: Utility of admission chemistry and coagulation profiles in trauma patients: a reappraisal of traditional practice, *J Trauma* 41(1):21-25, 1996.
3. Hulka F, Mullins RJ, Frank EH: Blunt brain injury activates the coagulation process, *Arch Surg* September 923-928, 1996.
4. Wachtel TL: Critical care concepts in the management of abdominal trauma, *Crit Care Nurse Q* 17(2):34-50, 1994.
5. Frankel HL, Rozycki GC, Ochsner MG, and others: Minimizing admission laboratory testing in trauma patients: use of a microanalyzer, *J Trauma* 37(5):728-736, 1994.

SUGGESTED READINGS

Committee on Trauma, American College of Surgeons: *Advanced trauma life support instructor manual,* ed 5, Chicago, 1993, American College of Surgeons.

Emergency Nurses Association: *Trauma nursing core course instructor manual,* ed 4, Park Ridge, IL, Emergency Nurses Association.

Fischbach FF, editor: *A manual of laboratory and diagnostic tests,* ed 5, Philadelphia, 1996, Lippincott.

Flomenbaum N, Goldgran L, Jacobsen S, editors: *Emergency diagnostic testing,* ed 2, St Louis, 1995, Mosby.

McFarland MB, Grant NM: *Nursing implications of laboratory tests,* ed 3, Albany, NY, Delmar Publishers.

Miller DT, Lunde JR: Laboratory tests. In Sheehy SB: *Emergency nursing,* ed 4, St Louis, 1997, Mosby.

Pagana KD, Pagana TJ: *Mosby's diagnostic and laboratory test reference,* ed 3, St Louis, 1995, Mosby.

Ravel R: *Clinical laboratory medicine,* ed 6, St Louis, 1995, Mosby.

Selfridge-Thomas J: *Emergency nursing: an essential guide for patient care,* Philadelphia, 1997, Saunders.

CHAPTER 10

Crisis Intervention in Trauma

Gail E. Polli

> *"A crisis is an acutely time-limited state of disequilibrium resulting from situational, developmental, or societal sources of stress. A person in this state is temporarily unable to cope with or adapt to the stressor by using previous methods of problem solving."*[1]

Death, grief, loss of a body part, disfigurement, concerns about the cost of care, loss of property, and family relationships are all issues that can factor into crises experienced by patients, family, and staff during the emergency.

Whatever the cause, a crisis can threaten to overwhelm a person's emotional resources. Tyhurst defines three phases of crisis and potential reactions.[2]

PHASE 1: IMPACT

An impact reaction usually occurs in one of three forms. The impact will occur from minutes to hours after the incident.
- The person is cool and collected—aware of the situation, able to evaluate, plan, and implement action(s).
- The person is stunned and bewildered. Most commonly, span of attention is restricted, and the person acts on reflexes and lacks awareness of subjective feelings or emotions.
- The person is confused and experiences paralyzing anxiety with inappropriate responses.

PHASE 2: RECOIL

The time span for the recoil phase varies widely according to the individual and the incident.

- The immediate threat has passed, and the person is left with many continuing stresses.
- The person experiences a gradual return of self-consciousness and awareness of the immediate past.
- The person needs the opportunity to talk about the incident; to express fear, anger, and concerns.
- This is a time to begin to mobilize defenses—a *crucial time for intervention*. After a person passes through this phase, he may refuse to seek or accept help.

PHASE 3: POSTTRAUMATIC

Phase 3 is one of rehabilitation. It continues for the remainder of one's life.
- This is the period of first insight into full awareness of the incident and the loss.
- This is the period of readjustment.
- In this period the person often experiences fatigue, anxiety, anorexia, and mood swings, and has nightmares or dreams about the incident.

In crisis intervention one must define the crisis as the individual sees it, not as the caregivers see it. Crisis intervention is structured to assist the individual in dealing with the stress of the situation. The outcome of crisis intervention is mastery of the stress.

   This mastery of stress includes two types of behavior:
- Behavior that results in reducing the physiologic and psychologic manifestations of emotional arousal to tolerable limits during and shortly after the stressful event
- Behavior that mobilizes the person's internal and external resources to develop new capabilities that lead to changing his environment or his relationship to it to reduce the stress or find alternative sources of satisfaction

The balancing factors in crisis and crisis intervention are:
- Perception of event—realistic or unrealistic
- Situational support—family, friends, and staff
- Coping mechanisms—help the person to identify what he or she usually does to reduce stress

STEPS IN CRISIS INTERVENTION

Most crises resolve on their own. The changes experienced become integrated into a person's life over time. With this in mind, the goal of crisis intervention is to support the healing process, help the person utilize available resources, and facilitate ongoing treatment and/or access postcrisis when necessary.
- Assess the person in crisis.
   Identify the degree of impact defined by the behaviors exhibited, emotions expressed, and cognition of the response

- Assist the person to define the crisis.
  Give concrete information about the incident, the extent of injury or illness, and the cause, if known.
- Allow the person to express feelings about the incident.
  Help the person to focus on the crisis and steps that may lessen stress.
- Explain hospital procedures and why certain things must be done.
- Provide support.
  To the staff: both verbal and nonverbal.
  To the family and friends: help the family and friends to understand the crisis; give information and support those giving support.

COPING MECHANISMS

To assist a person in mobilizing coping mechanisms, do the following:
- Confront the crisis. This may need to be done in small doses.
- Identify feelings. Assist the person to talk about feelings. This takes time, patience, understanding, and the ability to be a good listener.
- Promote problem solving. Assist the person in setting tasks. The task must be manageable. The person must have support and encouragement. Help to reassess the situation and plan the next step.
- Assist the person to move from dependence to independence.

Identification of maladaptive coping mechanisms

When a person is not coping well, it is important to recognize signs and to redirect the process. The following are some signs of possible maladaptive coping:
- Excessive denial or withdrawal—uses fantasy to replace or merge with reality
- Impulsive behavior and scapegoats used to vent rage
- Denial of feelings—overcontrol of emotions
- Too much dependence or too much independence
- Inability to ask for or use help when it is offered/needed
- Ritualistic behavior

POSSIBLE SYMPTOMS OF A PERSON IN CRISIS

- Increased tension
- Increased anxiety
- Confusion
- Helplessness
- Narrow focus of attention
- Sense of urgency
- Impaired cognitive functioning
- Regression in managing interpersonal relationships

NURSING DIAGNOSES RELATED TO CRISIS INTERVENTION

Ineffective coping

Ineffective coping is seen when usual methods of coping with stressful life situations are insufficient to control anxiety, fear, or anger.

ASSESSMENT

- Expressed or unexpressed fear, anxiety, or anger
- Verbalization of inability to cope
- Inability to act on or solve problems
- Inability to make necessary decisions
- Inability to ask for help
- Inability to meet basic needs
- Inability to meet role expectations
- Acting-out behavior toward self and others

THERAPEUTIC INTERVENTIONS

- Assist the person to define the crisis; give needed information.
- Help the person to set a course of action; use small manageable activities that will lead to mastery and eventual return of coping skills.
- Be a receptive listener; assist in sorting out fact from fiction.

EVALUATION

- The person will be able to take charge of small tasks (such as calling a family member or friend).
- The person will begin to understand the scope of the crisis and be able to ask for and accept help.
- The person will be able to verbalize the details of the incident.
- The person will be able to verbalize feelings.

Anticipatory grieving

Grief reactions can occur over expectation of loss or significant disruption in familiar patterns or relationships (death, loss of significant other, loss of body part, disfigurement).

ASSESSMENT

- Potential of significant loss
- Verbal expression or anticipation of loss
- Anger
- Sadness
- Crying at frequent intervals
- Choked feeling; difficulty breathing
- Alteration in concentration or pursuit of a task

THERAPEUTIC INTERVENTIONS

- Allow and encourage the person to express concerns, anger, and sadness.
- Allow and encourage the person to cry.

- Help the person to differentiate reality from fiction.
- Give specific, correct, and truthful information in a kind and gentle way.

EVALUATION

- The person will feel supported in his or her grief.
- The person will have a clear understanding of the issues.

Spiritual distress

Spiritual distress is a disruption in life principles that pervades a person's entire being and integrates and transcends his or her biopsychosocial nature.

ASSESSMENT

- Expresses concern about the meaning of life, death, or spiritual beliefs
- Expresses anger toward God
- Questions meaning of suffering
- Verbalizes inner conflicts about spiritual beliefs
- Questions the meaning of existence
- Seeks spiritual assistance
- Questions the moral/ethical implications of therapeutic interventions
- Expresses *gallows humor*
- Displaces anger toward a religious representative

THERAPEUTIC INTERVENTIONS

- Allow person to express concerns. Do not try to reason or suggest that he or she should not feel the way he feels.
- Offer to call a religious representative of the person's faith if he or she so desires.

EVALUATION

- The person will feel supported by staff or religious representative.
- The person will express a desire for help or support.

Impaired verbal communication

Impaired verbal communication is an inability to verbalize as a result of a language barrier, a mechanical barrier (such as an endotracheal tube), or mental, emotional, or physical deficits.

ASSESSMENT

- Endotracheal tube in place
- Inability to understand or speak the language used by caregivers
- Inability to communicate because of:
    Expressive aphasia
    Receptive aphasia
    Hearing loss
    Absence of intelligible speech

THERAPEUTIC INTERVENTIONS

- For the patient with an endotracheal tube, ask questions that can be answered "yes" or "no." Assist the patient with communication devices (such as paper and pencil).
- For the patient with a language barrier, find an interpreter who can translate the individual's concerns, who also understands medical terminology and has had some training in crisis intervention.
- For the patient with mental, emotional, or physical deficits, find a close family member, friend, or caregiver who is familiar with the patient's communication problems and can help with communication.

EVALUATION

- An effective means of communication will be found to support the needs of the individual.

Ineffective family coping (compromised)

The supportive primary person (family member or friend) may provide insufficient, ineffective, or compromised support.

ASSESSMENT

- Supportive primary person is absent because of death, injury, or distance.
- Supportive primary person is preoccupied with personal reactions to the situation.
- Supportive primary person describes or confirms inadequate knowledge that interferes with effective assistance.
- Supportive primary person attempts assistive or supportive behavior with less than satisfactory results.
- Conflict exists between family members and the supportive primary person that prevents or limits communication.

THERAPEUTIC INTERVENTIONS

- When possible, assist the supportive primary person to be available in person or by phone.
- Assist the supportive primary person to:
  Deal with own feelings
  Understand the situation and medical therapies necessary for optimal care
  Deal effectively with others in supportive way
- Assist all members of the family to deal with conflicts, role expectations, and so on. This may require referral to a social worker, psychologist, psychiatrist, or psychiatric nurse, as appropriate.

EVALUATION

- The primary supportive person will be able to regain or maintain supportive relationships.

REFERENCES

1. Kneis LC, Riley E: *Psychiatric Nursing,* ed 5, Menlo Park, CA, 1996, Addison-Wesley.
2. Tyhurst JS: The role of transition states—including disasters—in mental illness. In *Proceedings of the symposium on preventative and social psychiatry,* Washington, DC, 1957, Walter Reed Army Institute.

SUGGESTED READINGS

Aguilera DC: *Crisis intervention: theory and methodology,* ed 7, St Louis, 1994, Mosby.
Blazyl S, Canavan MM: Managing the discharge crisis following catastrophic illness or injury, *Social Work Health Care* 11:19-32, 1986.
Lindemann E: Symptomatology: management of acute grief, *Am J Psychiatry* 101:101-148, 1944.
Lundin T: The treatment of acute trauma: post traumatic stress disorder prevention, *Psych Clin North Am* 17(2):385-391, 1994.
Townsend MC: *Nursing diagnoses in psychiatric nursing,* ed 2, Philadelphia, 1991, FA Davis.
Wilson HS, Kneiss LC: *Psychiatric nursing,* ed 5, Menlo Park, CA, 1996, Addison Wesley.

CHAPTER 11

Critical Incident Stress Management

William T. Briggs

Emergency care professionals treating trauma victims are constantly placed in stressful situations. The very nature of the job requires work in an environment that is uncontrolled and, at many times, dangerous. Physicians, nurses, paramedics, and emergency medical technicians (EMTs) do not know which patients they will be caring for, what illnesses or injuries will present, in what environments they will work, or how many patients they will see. In addition, the threat of physical violence is omnipresent. The specter of hepatitis, human immunodeficiency virus (HIV), tuberculosis (TB), and other infectious diseases has further complicated their work. Yet, they are required to perform highly technical work with compassion while often working long and erratic hours.

Stress takes its toll on many emergency caregivers. Some "burn out" and leave the profession. Others turn to drugs or alcohol. Suicide rates are high. Many emergency caregivers continue to function in a healthcare setting in a less than optimal capacity.[1]

Stress is defined as a state of physical and psychologic arousal that follows any demand placed on a person. Stress is a normal part of life and, in most cases, is adaptive. Stress motivates people to stay up late studying for exams, allows people to meet the demands of a busy shift, and gives people the strength to flee or fight when faced with an emergency. Beneficial stress is often referred to as *eustress;* detrimental stress is called *distress.*

The constant demands of caring for the sick and injured is one of the most stressful forms of human activity.[2] Cumulative stress refers to this going and building form of dystress. Frequently, emergency personnel were taught to ignore the stress, "keep a stiff upper lip," and show no emotion. Persons affected by stress were considered weak or unfit for duty.

A critical incident is any situation faced by emergency service personnel that causes them to experience unusually strong emotional reactions that have the potential to interfere with their ability to function during or after an event.[3] There are no specific criteria that determine a critical incident. This is

---

BOX 11-1

EXAMPLES OF CRITICAL INCIDENTS

Death occurring in the line of duty
Death or serious injury of a child
Serious injury or illness encountered in the line of duty
Providing care to a person you know or relate to (e.g., a co-worker)
Suicide of a co-worker
Prolonged situations with a negative outcome (e.g., resuscitation)
Multiple casualty situations
Incidents with high press coverage

---

affected by the individuals involved, their previous experience, their current emotional status, and their perception of the event. What is a critical incident for one may not be for another. For example, the death of a child may be a critical incident in a rural hospital where the child is known to many of the caregivers, but such an incident may not cause much stress in a large, urban children's hospital where the experience of the death of a child is more common.

Although there is not a standard list, certain events are considered high risk and should be evaluated for the probability of being a critical incident (Box 11-1). Often emergency caregivers will know an event has had a significant emotional impact by noting that "things seem different in this one" or "the staff just isn't snapping back." When in doubt, it is best to consult a critical incident stress management (CISM) team.

Critical incidents lead to critical incident stress (CIS), which is also known in the literature as *traumatic stress,* referring to psychologic trauma. The signs and symptoms of CIS vary greatly between individuals. Three individuals exposed to the same circumstances may have no reaction, a minimal reaction, or a severe reaction. The signs and symptoms can range from opposites of insomnia to sleeping 12 hours per day or from loss of appetite to overeating. Box 11-2 summarizes the signs and symptoms that have been observed in CIS. Some symptoms, such as chest pain or shortness of breath, should never be assumed to be symptoms of CIS until an organic cause has been ruled out.

The rate at which symptoms subside varies. Most people find the symptoms relieved or diminished within 4 to 6 weeks after an incident. If the symptoms persist after that time, a mental health consultation is necessary.

The most severe and debilitating reaction to a critical incident is post traumatic stress disorder (PTSD). This is a psychiatric disorder with the potential to incapacitate the individual. The diagnosis of PTSD requires ongoing symptoms of CIS lasting over a month and severely affecting the person's ability to function (Box 11-3). Although treatment for PTSD has greatly improved since the Vietnam War, it is still a devastating diagnosis.

BOX 11-2
SIGNS AND SYMPTOMS OF TRAUMATIC STRESS

Cognitive
Confusion
Difficulty making decisions
Loss of attention span
Lowered concentration
Problems with abstract thinking
Memory dysfunction
Lowering of all higher cognitive
    functions

Physical
Headaches
Fatigue
Excessive sweating
Chills
Dizzy spells
Lightheadedness
Globus hystericus
Thirst and hunger
Increased heart rate
Elevated blood pressure
Tachypnea
Chest pain
Difficulty breathing
Cardiac arrest

Emotional
Irritability
Emotional numbness
Anger
Grief
Depression
Feeling overwhelmed
Anxiety
Panic feelings
Loss of emotional control
Fear

Behavioral
Changes in ordinary behavior pat-
    terns
Changes in eating
Decreased personal hygiene
Increased or decreased association
    with fellow workers
Withdrawal from others
Loss of interest in work
Prolonged silences

From Everly GS: *A clinical guide to the treatment of the human stress response,* New York, 1989, Plenum.

Fortunately, a program of critical incident stress management has emerged and shown success in mitigating the effects of CIS and decreasing the possibility of developing PTSD. Although the effects of stress have been described in war since before Christ, work on stress in the emergency services didn't emerge until the 1960s when police psychologists started working with officers involved in shootings.[3] In the 1970s there were descriptions of early stress management programs in the prehospital and hospital environments.[4,5]

It was in 1976 that Jeffrey Mitchell, Ph.D., a firefighter-paramedic and psychologist published the first article on Critical Incident Stress Debriefing.[8] His concept was simple. If an individual is allowed to talk about an event and given the support and resources to deal with its effects, he or she will have a

---

BOX 11-3

CHARACTERISTICS OF POST TRAUMATIC STRESS DISORDER

1. The person is exposed to a traumatic event that involved actual or threatened death or serious injury or a threat to the physical integrity of self or others, **and** the person's response involved intense fear, helplessness, or horror.
2. The traumatic event is persistently reexperienced in one or more ways:
   • Recurrent and intrusive distressing recollections of the event including images, thoughts, or perceptions.
   • Recurrent distressing dreams of the event (nightmares).
   • Acting or feeling the event were recurring (including hallucinations, illusions, and flashbacks).
   • Intense distress at cues that symbolize or resemble the event.
   • Psychologic reactivity on exposure to these cues.
3. Persistent avoidance of stimuli associated with the trauma or event.
4. Persistent symptoms of increased arousal not present before the event (insomnia, irritability, difficulty concentrating, hypervigilance, etc.).
5. Duration of symptoms lasting greater than one month.
6. The disturbance causes clinically significant distress or impairment in social, occupational, or other areas of functioning.

From American Psychiatric Association: *Diagnosis and statistical manual of mental disorders (DSM-IV)*, ed 4, Washington, DC, 1994, American Psychiatric Association.

quicker and better recovery. This concept has been accepted throughout the United States and much of the world. Although CISM research is in its infancy, there is good anecdotal evidence of its success. Currently, there are over 300 CISM teams world wide utilizing the Mitchell model.

Critical Incident Stress Management has been realized in recent years to require more than just debriefing. It must be a carefully planned and managed effort. There must be a commitment by the employers to provide the resources necessary for CISM. Staff must be given time to participate as both a CISM team member and/or to attend a debriefing. There must be no retribution to the individual who seeks help.

COMPONENTS OF A COMPREHENSIVE CRITICAL INCIDENT STRESS MANAGEMENT PROGRAM

Preincident education

The institution of preincident education is the most essential part of a comprehensive CISM program. Emergency care providers need to know what CIS is, how to recognize the signs and symptoms, and how to get help. They also

---

BOX 11-4

TOPICS FOR STRESS EDUCATION

Definition of stress
Cumulative stress versus critical incident stress
Stressors in the emergency services environment
Developing a personal stress relief program
Critical incidents (definition and examples)
Effects of critical incident stress
Signs and symptoms
Effects of stress on the family
The role of the CISM team
How to contact the CISM team

---

need to know the effects of chronic stress and how to mitigate them. CISM training is becoming the standard in police and fire academies and EMT programs. Unfortunately, hospitals have been slower to recognize the benefits of CISM. A sample outline of a CISM education program is included in Box 11-4. Preincident education should be part of every emergency care provider's basic education and on-going training. Spouses, significant others, and families should also be included in education programs, since they can also be affected and often may be the first to recognize the symptoms of stress.

On-scene support

On-scene support, sometimes called midaction support, is utilized during large-scale or prolonged emergency situations. A CISM team member is available to provide support as needed, as well as to identify personnel that may need help. Actions by the team member are short-term emotional first aid. The team member can also ensure that personnel are receiving adequate breaks and that their physical needs are being met.

Defusing

Defusings are one of the most commonly used techniques. The sessions are a shortened version of a debriefing occurring within a few hours of an incident. Defusings are very cost-effective since they only last 20 to 45 minutes, can be conducted by one or two CISM team members, and can sometimes eliminate the need for a formal debriefing. A defusing most often occurs as a particular shift is going off duty. The process is a conversation consisting of an introductory discussion of the process, a discussion of the incident itself, and some helpful hints are given for managing the stress. After the defusing, the team determines if a formal debriefing is necessary.

Demobilization

Demobilizations are utilized in mass casualty incidents when emergency workers are required to return to the scene to provide additional aid. The participants are brought to a room and given a 10-minute talk about the possible effects of the stress. No one is asked to talk. Any questions are answered and then the participants are fed and given a rest period before returning to the scene.

Debriefing

A critical incident stress debriefing (CISD) is one of the most helpful, yet complex stress mitigation processes. It is reserved for especially traumatic events that affect multiple members of a group. Critical incident stress debriefing is a group process that is conducted by a specially trained team consisting of at least one mental health professional and several peers representing the group being debriefed. One member of the team acts as the team leader and the others support the leader and aid in the discussion. A debriefing typically lasts 2 to 3 hours and is conducted in a private location that is free of disturbances.

Ideally a CISD is held 24 to 72 hours after an incident. This allows time for the affected group members to handle physical matters and for the team to make the necessary preparation. In some circumstances, such as when the funeral of a co-worker is pending, it is better to wait till after the services. Although the maximum benefit is obtained during this window, a debriefing should never be declined because of time factors.

The debriefing should be open to all members of the emergency care team who are *directly involved in the incident.* An effort should be made to contact and invite all personnel. Peripheral personnel such as emergency medical services (EMS) dispatchers or social service workers are often deeply affected by an incident and inadvertently left off the debriefing list. In some cases, a department will chose to mandate attendance. This is best done by a preexisting policy, rather than at the time of the incident. Persons who were not involved in the incident, such as supervisors, observers, and the press should be excluded. Multidisciplinary debriefings bring together personnel from all aspects of an incident (e.g., police, firefighter, EMS, and hospital personnel). These are very successful in building respect and ongoing relationships between disciplines. In some cases, it may be necessary to limit the debriefing to one discipline.

Before the debriefing, the team members get together and plan the debriefing. At that time, they discuss what they know of the incident and any special circumstances involved. They assign roles for the debriefing, including a member to be available to anyone who leaves the room. The team sets up the room in an informal manner, usually a circle.

The debriefing is a guided discussion, not a therapy session, and follows a defined format. The process consists of the following seven phases as defined by Dr. Jeffrey Mitchell.[6]

- **Introductory Phase**   The leader creates a comfortable, nonthreatening environment. The process is explained, and a set of rules is established. At this time, it is important for every participant to maintain confidentiality and only speak for themselves. The debriefing is not an operational critique, and all rank is left behind.
- **Fact Phase**   Each participant is asked to introduce themselves and describe their role in the incident. The leader then guides the participants to reconstruct the incident and provide the entire group with a realistic, collective account of the event. This phase usually lasts the longest and is the most crucial to a successful debriefing.
- **Thought Phase**   Each participant is asked to share what their first or most prominent thought was after they came off of "auto-pilot."
- **Reaction Phase**   Participants discuss what was most stressful for them during the incident. Often, this is posed as an open-ended question, such as "What was the worst part of this for you?" As feelings are shared, the team members validate and support the participants. The mental health professional keeps the discussion from becoming a therapy session. This is the most emotionally powerful portion of the debriefing.
- **Symptom Phase**   A discussion of symptoms that the participants may have encountered since the incident occurs. This gives the team the opportunity to validate normal reactions and start the next phase.
- **Teaching Phase**   The team teaches participants techniques that will help mitigate the effects of the incident. Participants are also taught what symptoms are normal and which ones should trigger further action. Participants are also encouraged to ask questions and participate in discussion.
- **Reentry Phase**   This final phase is a time for any issues that were not previously discussed to be addressed. The team provides a summary of what occurred and reaffirms the standards of confidentiality. After the debriefing ends, refreshments may be served, and the team is available to any individual who may not have wanted to speak in the group or needs extra help.

After the debriefing, the team evaluates the process and discusses their own feelings. They also arrange for any follow-up action indicated, which may include checking with individual participants or the group as a whole or rarely, a second debriefing.

CRITICAL INCIDENT STRESS MANAGEMENT TEAM

The development of a CISM team in a city, county, or regional area can be an asset to many different organizations, and the sharing of one team generally improves the close cooperation of the agencies that work together in emergency care. Depending on the size of the institution and the frequency of occurrence of internal traumatic events, a hospital may elect to maintain its own CISM team. It must be remembered that an internal team may not be able to function when its own members have been affected by the incident. For the team to be proficient and effective, the members need to be adequately trained and have the opportunity to use and improve their skills. The cost effectiveness of the team must also be evaluated. Each organization needs to evaluate its own requirements.

The following is a list of considerations in forming a CISM team:

Need   Is there a need for a team in the area? Where is the closest team available to you? Can they provide you with all the services you need? Can you join their team? Is the perception of need shared with other agencies and/or within your own agency?

Funding   Do you have a source of funding? Are there agencies that will help?

Members   Do you have adequate potential members? Do you have committed mental health professionals? Do you have members willing to teach? Do you have support staff?

Other Resources   Clerical help? Pagers? Dispatching?

Once you have identified the need and the resources, you are ready to start a team. The first step is to identify leadership through officers or a steering committee. From there you need to develop a plan to start the team. Contact other CISM teams for examples of their bylaws and standard operating procedures. The International Critical Incident Stress Management Foundation in Baltimore is an excellent source of materials and advice. Box 11-5 provides you with a checklist of actions that will ensure the success of the team.

Generally teams are either associated with one lead agency such as a hospital or fire department or are a community team. In either case, you need a strong organization. A community may represent a single town or a broad geographic area. It is important to determine the geographic area or agencies that you will serve.

The team has to establish and abide by a budget. The budget consists of income and expenses. Since CISM teams generally are staffed by volunteers who do not charge for their services, it is necessary to determine sources of income. In some cases the lead agency provides all the income, but many teams need to raise funds. A lawyer will be able to help you obtain tax-exempt status to obtain charitable contributions. Other sources of income include dues, fund raising events, such as bake sales, car washes, or raffles, and providing continuing education programs. The expenses of the team may include office supplies, answering service, beepers, printing, and training.

A volunteer team should enlist a variety of talented members. Some members may be best suited for debriefings, whereas others may be better at providing support services. A job description or list of qualifications for member roles should be established. Members who are providing direct services should have a minimum two-day basic CISM training and an interview with the CISM team's clinical director. Mental health professionals such as psychologists, social workers, and psychiatric nurses should be selected for their experience in traumatic stress management. One of these professionals should be selected as the team's clinical director.

BOX 11-5

CHECKLIST FOR FORMING A SUCCESSFUL CISM TEAM

Organization and Structure
Establish constitution and by-laws
Elect leaders
Obtain legal counsel
Seek incorporation and tax-exempt
  status as appropriate
Budget

Standard Operating Procedures
Area of service
Policies and procedures
How the team is activated and dis-
  patched

Membership
Qualifications for membership
Qualifications for debriefer and
  team leaders
Qualifications for mental health pro-
  fessionals
Qualifications for trainers
Selection and interviewing process

Training and Quality Improvement
Initial CISM training for debriefers
  and mental health
Advanced CISM programs
Continuing education for team
  members
Regular team meetings and case
  reviews

Outreach
Fliers, brochures
Visiting agencies
Preincident education
Family education

Record Keeping
Records of activities to support
  funding and grant applications
Financial and tax records

Fund Raising
Set up a fund raising committee or
  team
Agency budget
Dues
Donations or grants
Events (raffles, bake sales, etc.) or
  continuing education seminars

The team needs written policies and procedures to guide them. One of the most important aspects is to determine how the team is going to be contacted and dispatched. An answering service or an existing emergency service dispatcher can handle the initial calls and contact an on-call team member by telephone or beeper. This member screens the call and determines what services are needed. He or she in turn notifies the other team members.

Once the team is established and organized, the next step is to provide outreach to the agencies served. A brochure and telephone stickers are good first steps. Meetings with the leadership of the agencies you serve is critical to your success. The best outreach may be providing preincident education to the agency personnel.

REFERENCES

1. Mitchell JT, Bray GP: *Emergency services stress: guidelines for preserving the health and careers of emergency personnel,* Englewood Cliffs, NJ, 1990, Prentice Hall.
2. Patrick PK: *Health care worker burnout, what it is, what to do about it,* Chicago, 1981, Inquiry Books (Blue Cross/Blue Shield Association).
3. Reese JT, Horn JM, Dunning C: *Critical incident stress in policing—revised,* Washington, DC, 1991, US Government Printing Office.
4. Graham NK: Done in, fed up, burned out: too much attrition in EMS, *J Emer Med Serv* 6(1):24-29, 1981.
5. Epperson-Sebour M: *Role stressors and supports for emergency workers,* Washington, DC, 1985, Center for Mental Health Studies of Emergencies, US Department of Health and Human Services.
6. Mitchell JT: Rescue crisis intervention, *EMS News* 4(3):4, 1976.

SUGGESTED READINGS

Mitchell JT: Comprehensive traumatic stress management in the emergency department, leadership and management in emergency nursing, *Emergency Nurses Association Monograph Series* 1(8):1992.

CHAPTER 12

Nursing Diagnosis in Trauma

Luann Loughlin

Although nursing diagnosis is not new to nursing, standard nursing diagnoses for rapid, individualized care planning are being used more frequently. The patient care plan ensures safe, efficient care and justifies the need for nursing care. In an emergency setting, little or no time is available for an individual plan for each patient. This does not mean that nurses work without a plan; rather, the plan is frequently not written. Because emergency care must be given rapidly, nurses often work with very specific protocols (standardized care plans) that experienced nurses have committed to memory. These protocols have usually been developed by nurses and physicians and have been adapted to fit the role that the nurse must perform in cooperation with the trauma team. These protocols do not necessarily delineate all the patient's nursing needs. For that reason, protocols that can be easily modified for a specific patient can facilitate rapid, efficient care delivery.

The following nursing diagnosis care plans were developed around common injuries sustained by trauma patients. Under each topic is a specific care plan. Many nursing diagnoses can be applied to a number of trauma patients. For example, *infection; risk for;* or *comfort, altered: pain* may appear under various types of trauma. These diagnoses have been more fully developed for some than for others because the problem may be more acute in one type of injury than in another. Frequently, to reduce repetition, a note refers the reader to another injury topic for a more complete care plan. The reader may use these diagnoses to help develop standardized care plans (in checklist or computerized format) for patients with specific types of injury.

NURSING DIAGNOSES FOR PATIENT WITH FLUID LOSS AND SHOCK

Fluid volume deficit, actual

Defining Characteristics

- Excess loss of intravascular fluid
- Hemorrhage

NURSING INTERVENTIONS

- Monitor vital signs: pulse, blood pressure, respirations
- Monitor level of consciousness
- Monitor intake and output
- Monitor skin for temperature, color, turgor, and moisture
- Maintain IV fluid flow rates as prescribed to restore normal vital signs
- Draw blood type and crossmatch as indicated; ensure that adequate amounts of blood are available for patient
- Administer blood according to protocol to ensure safety
- Administer warm fluids and blood to prevent hypothermia

OUTCOMES

- Vital signs will be restored to normal and will be maintained
- Blood will be given safely without undue risk to patient
- Hypothermia will be prevented or corrected

Cardiac output, decreased: risk for

Defining Characteristics

- Fluid volume deficit because of hemorrhage or loss of intravascular volume
- Cardiac disease or injury compromising the pumping action of the heart
- Neurogenic shock caused by loss of vascular tone

NURSING INTERVENTIONS

- Assess skin color, turgor, and temperature
- Assess for external hemorrhage; apply pressure above or directly over the area of hemorrhage
- Monitor vital signs: temperature, pulse, blood pressure
- Monitor changes in mental status
- Place ECG leads on patient and monitor rhythm
- Monitor intake and output closely
- Monitor laboratory values (hematocrit, white blood count [WBC], coagulation parameters, electrolytes, and arterial blood gases)
- Test urine and emesis or stool for blood
- Place patient flat or with head slightly elevated (no more than 15 degrees)
- Administer IV fluids and blood as prescribed
- Prepare and assist with diagnostic or therapeutic procedures such as pericardiocentesis, peritoneal lavage, and thoracotomy

NURSING DIAGNOSES FOR PATIENT WITH HEAD INJURY

Although many nursing diagnoses may be applied to the patient with a head injury, the following diagnoses apply to most of these patients. As indicated, some of these are thoroughly discussed under other injury topics so that only important differences are noted here.

Fluid volume deficit, actual or risk for

This diagnosis is thoroughly discussed under *fluid volume deficit: actual*, p. 126. The important factors to note in these patients include the following:
- Fluid volume deficit may be caused by injuries unrelated to head trauma
- With head trauma, a high incidence of spinal cord injury and the potential for spinal shock exists
- If intracranial bleeding occurs, hypovolemia is not usually the cause

Nursing interventions and evaluation for this diagnosis are discussed on p. 126.

Breathing pattern, ineffective

Although ineffective breathing pattern is discussed under several different areas, the etiologic factors are somewhat different in the patient with a head injury. Because respiratory rate, depth, and patterns are mainly controlled by the respiratory center of the brain, injury to the brain may cause the following changes in breathing patterns:

Central neurogenic
Ataxia
Biot's sign
Apneustic

Nursing intervention and evaluation are discussed on p. 135.

Comfort, altered: pain

- Pain management in the patient with a known or suspected head injury is complicated by the possibility of masking changes in level of consciousness. Therefore narcotics, especially long-acting ones, usually are not given.
- When pain management is necessary, such as for painful procedures in setting fractures, either short-acting drugs or brief administration of analgesic doses of anesthetics may be used.
- Severe agitation in patients with head injury may be caused by the injury itself or by anoxia or pain. If anoxia is ruled out, the possible causes of pain should be sought and corrected. Pain may result from a distended bladder or dressings or casts applied too tightly. If agitation is not relieved by removing the cause, medications may be administered.

Further discussion of nursing interventions and evaluation of pain management may be found on p. 142.

Tissue perfusion, altered: cerebral

DEFINING CHARACTERISTICS

- Direct injury to brain tissue
- Intracranial edema
- Decreased tissue perfusion related to low-flow states or hypoxia
- Herniation syndrome

NURSING INTERVENTIONS

- Monitor the following assessment parameters every 5 to 15 minutes or as indicated. Note any changes in any of the following, and notify the physician:
  - Level of consciousness using the Glasgow Coma Scale or DERM
  - Pupillary response
  - Blood pressure, pulse, respiratory rate, and respiratory pattern
  - Temperature
  - pO_2, pCO_2, and ICP, if available
  - Motor and sensory changes
- If patient is hyperthermic, administer antipyretics or use hypothermia blanket
- Administer diuretics or steroids as prescribed
- Prepare patient for possible emergency surgery

OUTCOMES

- Changes in neurologic status will be noted rapidly
- Surgical intervention, if necessary, will be carried out with appropriate speed to prevent further deterioration
- Temperature will remain within normal limits

Infection, risk for

DEFINING CHARACTERISTICS

- Scalp lacerations
- Wounds penetrating into brain tissue

NURSING INTERVENTIONS

- Cleanse wound with gentle irrigation and débride as indicated
- Protect exposed brain tissue with moist, sterile dressing covered by dry, sterile dressing
- Administer systemic antibiotics as prescribed
- Administer tetanus prophylaxis as indicated
- Assist with wound repairs while maintaining aseptic technique

OUTCOMES

- Wound will be appropriately cleansed, débrided, and dressed to protect exposed tissue
- Wounds will be protected from additional injury and contamination

Injury, risk for

DEFINING CHARACTERISTICS

- Seizure activity
- Altered sensorium

NURSING INTERVENTIONS

- If patient is experiencing seizure activity, the nurse should
  - Administer anticonvulsants as prescribed
  - Pad side rails of bed or stretcher
- Restrain for protection, as indicated
- Protect cervical spine with appropriate immobilization device until cervical spine injury is ruled out
- Administer analgesics or sedatives, as prescribed

OUTCOMES

- Patient will be free from seizures or seizures will be controlled rapidly
- Patient will remain free from injury
- Cervical spine will remain in neutral alignment

NURSING DIAGNOSES FOR PATIENT WITH SPINAL CORD INJURY

Injury, unintentional, risk for

DEFINING CHARACTERISTICS

- Fracture or dislocation of vertebrae
- Impalement of fragments into spinal cord

NURSING INTERVENTIONS

- Place patient with suspected injury in rigid cervical collar
- Use immobilization devices to prevent movement
- When necessary to turn patient, use log-roll technique or turn entire backboard (with patient secured to prevent movement)
- During procedures that require removal of rigid collar, maintain head/neck immobilization manually

OUTCOMES

- Patient will show no further progression of signs of spinal cord injury, such as decrease in movement or sensation

Fluid volume deficit, risk for

In patients with spinal cord injuries, a relative fluid volume deficit exists that is caused by reduced vascular tone secondary to spinal cord injury (i.e., neurogenic shock).

DEFINING CHARACTERISTICS

- Hypotension; bradycardia; warm, dry, flushed skin; and loss of thermoregulation

NURSING INTERVENTIONS

- Monitor vital signs (i.e., blood pressure, pulse, respirations, and temperature)
- Carefully monitor fluid intake and urinary output
- Keep patient flat
- Keep patient warm
- Administer fluids and vasoactive drugs, as prescribed
- Administer steroids, as prescribed

OUTCOMES

- Patient's vital signs will be returned to and maintained within normal limits
- Patient will have urinary output of 1 ml/kg/hr
- Patient's skin color will be normal, and skin will be warm and dry

Skin integrity, impaired, risk for
DEFINING CHARACTERISTICS

- Patients with paraplegia or quadriplegia will be unable to feel pressure or move to relieve that pressure

NURSING INTERVENTIONS

- Bony prominences should be padded to relieve pressure and prevent pressure sores from forming
- Skin over bony prominences should be inspected frequently
- Areas of pressure should be massaged to improve circulation
- Removal of backboard as soon as appropriate x-ray films have been taken and removal has been approved

OUTCOMES

- Skin will remain intact without evidence of undue pressure such as redness, discoloration, or breakdown

Aspiration, risk for
DEFINING CHARACTERISTICS

- Depressed cough and gag reflex
- Spinal immobilization devices and/or paralysis

NURSING INTERVENTIONS

- Maintain patency of airway by frequent, cautious suctioning, if indicated
- Insert gastric tube to prevent gastric distention

• If unable to maintain airway, be prepared to assist with endotracheal intubation

OUTCOMES

• Patient's airway and lungs will remain clear

The following nursing diagnoses may be present in the patient with spinal cord injury and are discussed in more depth in other sections.

Breathing pattern, ineffective

DEFINING CHARACTERISTICS

• Breathing may be partially or totally compromised, depending on level of spinal cord injury
    See Chest, pp. 134 and 135.

NURSING INTERVENTIONS

See Chest, p. 135.

OUTCOMES

See Chest, p. 135.

Communication, impaired verbal and nonverbal

DEFINING CHARACTERISTICS

• Depending on level of cord damage, patient may have little or no ability to speak
• Because of necessity of intubation, patient may also have impaired communication
• Because of decreased muscle activity of upper extremities, patient may not be able to communicate with his or her hands

NURSING INTERVENTIONS

See Crisis, p. 145.

OUTCOMES

See Crisis, p. 145.

Ineffective individual coping

See Crisis, p. 143.

Anticipatory grieving

See Crisis, pp. 143 and 144.

NURSING DIAGNOSES FOR THE PATIENT WITH FACIAL/EENT TRAUMA

Airway clearance, ineffective

DEFINING CHARACTERISTICS

- Facial trauma with airway obstruction secondary to edema
- Blood clots from injury to nose or face, obstructing airway
- Airway obstruction by foreign objects such as teeth

NURSING INTERVENTIONS

- Monitor respiratory rate and pattern
- Monitor increasing hoarseness or respiratory stridor as sign of airway occlusion by edema or air (subcutaneous emphysema); patient may require intubation.
- Suction airway to remove clots and foreign bodies (suction via oral route if there is suspicion of cranial fractures or cerebrospinal fluid [CSF] leak)
- Maintain cervical spine immobilization until cervical spine x-rays have ruled out fracture or dislocation
- Prepare patient for intubation, if necessary
- Instruct patient in system of communication if intubation required

OUTCOMES

- Airway patency will be maintained
- Blood clots and foreign bodies will be removed, if necessary

Pain

DEFINING CHARACTERISTICS

- Injury to eye, ear, or nose
- All facial structures are highly sensitive, and patients with injuries in these areas will have significant pain

NURSING INTERVENTIONS

- Assess patient's reaction to pain: verbal and nonverbal
- Administer anesthetics, narcotics, and sedatives, as prescribed
- Apply cold packs initially
- With eye injury, patch both eyes to decrease motion and pain
- Instruct patient in distraction techniques
- Instruct patient in relaxation techniques

OUTCOMES

- Patient will exhibit less verbal and nonverbal expression of pain
- Patient will verbalize adequacy of pain relief measures

Body image, disturbance of

DEFINING CHARACTERISTICS ▰▰▰▰▰▰▰▰▰▰▰▰▰▰▰▰▰▰

- Major changes in self-concept or body image associated with injury to face, especially if injury is result of domestic violence, in which case injured party may also suffer from low self-esteem
- Verbalized actual or potential change in appearance of bodily function
- Verbalized fear of rejection or reaction to others
- Verbalized negative feelings about outcome of injury

NURSING INTERVENTIONS ▰▰▰▰▰▰▰▰▰▰▰▰▰▰▰▰▰

- Encourage patient to verbalize fears and concerns
- If patient is intubated, explain injuries and verbalize perceived feelings
- Be careful not to overemphasize feelings that may not be true for individual patient
- Explain injuries, treatment, and any major complication or defect that may occur
- Encourage patient to seek help if he or she continues to have concerns about appearance or emotions.

OUTCOMES ▰▰▰▰▰▰▰▰▰▰▰▰▰▰▰▰▰

- Patient will understand significance of injury in realistic terms
- Patient will know how or from whom to seek additional help for physical and emotional problems related to injury

The following nursing diagnoses may be present in the patient with facial/EENT trauma and are discussed in more depth in other sections:

Trauma syndrome

See Crisis, p. 146.

Violence, risk for

See Crisis, p. 147.

Infection, risk for

See Wound, pp. 142 and 143.

NURSING DIAGNOSES FOR PATIENTS WITH CHEST TRAUMA

Airway clearance, ineffective

DEFINING CHARACTERISTICS ▰▰▰▰▰▰▰▰▰▰▰▰▰▰▰

- Decreased air movement
- Abnormal breathing sounds (rales, crackles, rhonchi, wheezes)
- Ineffective cough
- Change in rate or depth of respiration

- Dyspnea
- Cyanosis
- Alterations in blood gases
- Subcutaneous emphysema

NURSING INTERVENTIONS

- Remove obstruction, if possible
- Suction, if necessary
- Administer oxygen
- Control airway; surgical airway may be needed
- Monitor vital signs and adequacy of air movement

OUTCOMES

- Patient will be able to maintain adequate ventilation without assistance
- Patient will maintain adequate oxygenation via mechanical airway and ventilator

Breathing pattern, ineffective

ETIOLOGY

- Flail chest
- Pneumothorax
- Hemothorax
- Tension pneumothorax
- Diaphragmatic rupture

DEFINING CHARACTERISTICS

- Dyspnea
- Paradoxic chest wall movement
- Use of accessory muscles
- Presence of stridor
- Epigastric or supraclavicular retractions
- Absence of bilateral breath sounds
- Presence of bowel sounds in chest
- Tachypnea
- Changes in depth of respiration
- Cyanosis
- Distended jugular veins
- Air fluid levels seen on chest x-ray
- Alterations in arterial blood oxygenation

NURSING INTERVENTIONS

- Administer oxygen
- If pneumothorax or hemothorax suspected, prepare patient for decompression needle or chest tube

- Set up chest drainage/chest suction equipment
- If flail chest suspected, respirations should be assisted by intubation and positive pressure ventilation
- If open pneumothorax present, cover wound with nonporous dressing taped on three sides
- Administer medication to relieve pain
- Continue to monitor vital signs and assess for other problems
- Measure oxygen saturations
- Draw or redraw blood gases to determine adequacy of oxygenation
- Insert orogastric tube to decompress stomach and reduce pressure within thoracic cavity

OUTCOMES

- Patient will be able to maintain adequate oxygenation with or without intubation and mechanical ventilation
- Vital signs will return to normal

Gas exchange, impaired

ETIOLOGY

- Impaired ventilation because of injury to lung and/or inadequate perfusion (shock)
- Cardiac tamponade

DEFINING CHARACTERISTICS

- Dyspnea
- Agitation
- Confusion
- Somnolence
- Increased respiratory rate
- Cyanosis
- Increased pulse rate
- Decreased blood pressure
- Alterations in blood gases

NURSING INTERVENTIONS

- Administer oxygen
- Suction airway
- Intubate and ventilate, as needed
- Correct hypovolemia by IV fluid replacement
- If cardiac tamponade suspected, prepare patient for pericardiocentesis
- Insert orogastric tube to relieve gastric distention and pressure on diaphragm

OUTCOMES

- Patient will maintain adequate oxygenation with or without mechanical intubation and ventilation
- Vital signs will return to normal

Cardiac output, altered: decreased

ETIOLOGY

- Tension pneumothorax
- Cardiac tamponade
- Hypovolemic shock

DEFINING CHARACTERISTICS

- Increased pulse rate
- Decreased blood pressure
- Narrowed pulse pressure
- Flat or distended neck veins
- Agitation
- Confusion
- Cold, clammy skin
- Cyanosis
- Muffled heart sounds
- Tracheal deviation
- Decreased breathing sounds unilaterally or bilaterally

NURSING INTERVENTIONS

- Restore effective breathing pattern as under gas exchange, impaired
- Monitor vital signs
- If cardiac tamponade present, prepare patient for pericardiocentesis
- Monitor for dysrhythmias and possible cardiogenic shock from myocardial infarction
- Patient should be prepared immediately for necessary surgical intervention

OUTCOMES

- Hemodynamic, cardiac, and respiratory parameters will return to normal

Other nursing diagnoses that may be operant but are discussed in detail elsewhere include:
- Fluid volume deficit, actual or risk for
- Comfort, altered: pain
- Anxiety, anticipatory (mild, moderate, severe)
- Fear

NURSING DIAGNOSES FOR PATIENT WITH ABDOMINAL TRAUMA

Fluid volume deficit: actual or potential

See Shock, p. 126.

Cardiac output, decreased: actual or risk

See Shock, p. 126.

Infection, risk for

DEFINING CHARACTERISTICS

- Bowel injury
- Multiple invasive procedures

NURSING INTERVENTIONS

- Administer antibiotics promptly, as prescribed
- Administer tetanus toxoid, if indicated
- Ensure use of gloves and sterile technique for all invasive procedures
- Cover exposed tissue with sterile, moist dressing

OUTCOMES

- All invasive procedures will be carried out in aseptic manner
- All precautions will be taken to prevent infection, including adequate fluid resuscitation, administration of antibiotics, and appropriate wound care
- Patient will have vital signs restored to normal levels and maintained at these levels

NURSING DIAGNOSES FOR PATIENT WITH EXTREMITY/ VASCULAR TRAUMA

Tissue perfusion, impaired peripheral, risk for

DEFINING CHARACTERISTICS

- Dressing or cast applied too tightly
- Immobilization
- Extremity injuries with excessive swelling

NURSING INTERVENTIONS

- Monitor extremities for neurovascular compromise
- Notify physician promptly if patient develops any of following signs and symptoms:
  - Pain
  - Pallor
  - Pulselessness
  - Paresthesia
  - Paralysis

- Elevate extremity above level of heart unless compartment syndrome is suspected
- If patient demonstrates signs and symptoms of compartment syndrome, keep extremity level but not dependent
- Protect extremities with decreased circulation and neurologic compromise from additional injuries
- Avoid pressure from constricting bed linen or restraints

OUTCOMES

- Signs of decreased tissue perfusion will be prevented or diagnosed quickly
- Additional tissue loss will be prevented (See discussion under Burn injury, p. 141)

Impaired physical mobility

DEFINING CHARACTERISTICS

- Imposed restrictions of movements (e.g., casts, braces, traction)
- Limited range of motion
- Decreased muscle strength or control
- Impaired coordination

NURSING INTERVENTIONS

- Teach mobility restrictions to patient and family
  - What movements patient can and cannot do
  - Expected duration of restrictions
  - Activities patient and family can perform to maintain strength and functionality in extremity while mobility is limited
- Teach patient and family how to regain maximum mobility
  - Use of assistive devices (e.g., bed trapeze, crutches, walkers, canes, wheelchairs) for moving in bed, transferring, or ambulating
  - Use of medically ordered therapeutic devices (e.g., braces, casts, splints, traction) to maintain good alignment, treat and prevent injury, and promote healing
- Medicate patient if pain is experienced with motion
- Discuss risk of injury and/or falls with impaired mobility
- Teach patient and family methods that reduce risks
- Consult with physical or occupational therapist if additional assistance needed

OUTCOMES

- Patient will experience return of independent physical mobility
- Patient will safely and correctly use assistive or therapeutic devices

The following nursing diagnoses may be present in the patient with extremity trauma but are discussed further in other sections:

Infection, risk for

See discussion under Wound, pp. 142 and 143.

Fluid volume deficit, risk for

See discussion under Shock and Fluid Replacement, p. 126.

Comfort, altered: pain

See discussion under Burn injuries, p. 142.

NURSING DIAGNOSES FOR PATIENT WITH BURN INJURY

Fluid volume deficit, actual

DEFINING CHARACTERISTICS

- Increased pulse
- Decreased blood pressure
- Increased respirations
- Central venous pressure (CVP) below 3 cm H_2O
- Decreased urine output
- Hematocrit level >50 mg/dl
- Diminished capillary refill
- Restlessness or confusion
- Nausea or vomiting
- Paralytic ileus

NURSING INTERVENTIONS

- Ascertain extent and severity of burns
- Monitor vital signs, CVP, level of consciousness
- Initiate IV therapy according to institutional protocol
- Adjust flow rates or administer fluids to maintain vital signs
- Maintain accurate intake and output record
- Notify physician if assessment parameters cannot be maintained without increase of more than 20% of ordered flow rates or quantities of fluid
- Secure all IV lines to prevent dislodgment

OUTCOMES

- Assessment parameters will be maintained within normal limits
- Patient will receive prescribed or needed volume of fluid over appropriate time period

Gas exchange, impaired, risk for

DEFINING CHARACTERISTICS

See list under Chest trauma, p. 135. In addition:
- Increased carbon monoxide level of carboxyhemoglobin measurement
- Hoarseness

- Edema and redness of posterior pharynx
- Carbonaceous sputum
- Full thickness, circumferential burns of chest wall

NURSING INTERVENTIONS ▬▬▬▬▬▬▬▬▬

- Recognize risk factors (possible smoke inhalation or chest wall burns)
- Monitor respiratory parameters:
  - Rate and character of breathing
  - Increasing hoarseness
  - Difficulty in handling secretion
  - Difficulty with chest wall expansion
- Monitor patient for signs of airway obstruction
- Observe for carbonaceous sputum
- If appropriate, draw blood gases and evaluate pO_2, pCO_2, and pH
- If patient is intubated, secure tube to prevent extubation
- Maintain ventilator settings for appropriate function
- Explain procedure to allay patient's fears
- Provide patient with method to communicate needs
- Suction as necessary to assist with elimination of secretions
- Administer sedatives or pain medication as appropriate to allay anxiety and help patient get used to ventilator

OUTCOMES ▬▬▬▬▬▬▬▬▬

- Impending respiratory problems will be recognized promptly and corrected
- Assessment parameters will be returned to normal limits
- Patients requiring intubation will be managed safely
- Fear and anxiety will be diminished

Infection, prevention of
DEFINING CHARACTERISTICS ▬▬▬▬▬▬▬▬▬

- Presence of burn wound
- Need for invasive procedures

NURSING INTERVENTIONS ▬▬▬▬▬▬▬▬▬

- Provide aseptic environment
- Cleanse wound
- Apply topical antibacterial therapy according to protocol
- Cleanse nonburned areas
- Administer tetanus prophylaxis and systemic antibiotics, as prescribed
- Provide aseptic management of all invasive lines and procedures

OUTCOMES ▬▬▬▬▬▬▬▬▬

- Patient's wounds and environment will be managed aseptically
- Topical and systemic antibiotics will be administered in timely, safe manner to prevent infection

Tissue perfusion, impaired, peripheral, risk for

DEFINING CHARACTERISTICS

- Edema of extremities
- Full thickness, circumferential burns of extremities
- Electrical injuries

NURSING INTERVENTIONS

- Recognize potential risk factors in patients (full-thickness circumferential burns, electrical injury, other muscle trauma, or low-flow states)
- Monitor extremities for:
    - Capillary refill
    - Pulses distal to area of injury
    - Pain or paresthesias
    - Decreased nerve and muscle function
    - Cyanosis of unburned distal areas
- Elevate extremities slightly to reduce edema unless compartment syndrome is suspected; arms and legs elevated more than 30 to 40 degrees may lead to increased edema formation.
- If compartment syndrome suspected, keep extremities level but not dependent
- If escharotomies or fasciotomies needed, prepare patient:
    - Explain procedure
    - Administer pain medication or sedatives, as prescribed
    - Prepare sterile equipment and assist with procedure
    - Prepare patient for surgery, if patient is to go to operating room for fasciotomy
    - Protect extremities with decreased circulation and neurologic functions from additional injury (avoid pressure from constricting bed linens or restraints)

OUTCOMES

- Signs of decreased tissue perfusion will be prevented or diagnosed and treated quickly
- Additional tissue loss will be prevented
- If escharotomies are required, these will be accomplished under aseptic conditions with the least discomfort possible

Comfort, altered: pain

DEFINING CHARACTERISTICS

- Patient complaining of pain
- Nonverbal expression of pain
- Agitation

NURSING INTERVENTIONS

- Observe for and record objective and subjective data consistently
- Administer medications as prescribed and as requested
- Assist patient and family to understand various pharmacologic and non-pharmacologic therapies that may help to relieve pain

OUTCOMES

- Objective signs and subjective complaints of pain will diminish
- Patient will feel that he or she has control over pain management

The following nursing diagnoses may be present in the patient with burn injury but are discussed further in other sections:

Fear

See Crisis, p. 146.

Anticipatory grieving

See Crisis, pp. 143 and 144.

Spiritual distress

See Crisis, p. 144.

NURSING DIAGNOSES FOR PATIENT WITH WOUND

Infection, risk for

DEFINING CHARACTERISTICS

- Infection-prone wound (e.g., dirt in wound, human or animal bite; old, untreated wound)
- Redness, pain, warmth, swelling around area of wound
- Purulent material draining from wound
- Fever, chills, malaise

NURSING INTERVENTIONS

- Administer tetanus toxoid, if indicated
- Administer antibiotics, as prescribed
- Teach patient how to care for wound aseptically to prevent infection
- Encourage slight elevation of body part for at least 72 hours

OUTCOMES

- Wound will remain free of infection, or infection will resolve over time

Comfort, altered: pain

See discussion under Burn injuries, p. 142.

NURSING DIAGNOSES RELATED TO CRISIS INTERVENTION

Coping, ineffective individual

DEFINING CHARACTERISTICS

- Usual methods of coping with stressful life situations are insufficient to control anxiety, fear, or anger
- Specific assessment data:
  - Expressed or unexpressed fear, anxiety, or anger
  - Verbalization of inability to cope
  - Inability to act on or solve problems
  - Inability to make necessary decisions
  - Inability to ask for help
  - Inability to meet basic needs
  - Inability to meet role expectations
  - Verbal manipulation
  - Acting out behavior toward self and others

NURSING INTERVENTIONS

- Assist patient to define crises; give needed information
- Help patient to set a course of action: small, manageable activities that will lead to mastery and eventual return of coping skills
- Be receptive listener and assist person in sorting out reality from fiction

OUTCOMES

- Patient will be able to take charge of small tasks (e.g., call family member or friend, find coffee shop)
- Patient will be able to verbalize details of accident
- Patient will be able to verbalize feelings
- Patient will begin to understand meaning of incident and be able to ask for and accept help

Grieving, anticipatory

DEFINING CHARACTERISTICS

- Potential of significant loss
- Verbal expression or anticipation of significant loss
- Anger
- Sadness
- Crying at frequent intervals
- Choked feeling
- Alteration in concentration or pursuit of task

NURSING INTERVENTIONS

- Allow and encourage patient to express concerns, anger, and sadness
- Allow and encourage patient to cry
- Help patient distinguish reality from fiction
- Give specific, correct information

OUTCOMES

- Patient will feel supported in his or her grief
- Patient will have clear understanding of potential problems.

Spiritual distress

DEFINING CHARACTERISTICS

- Concern with meaning of life, death, or belief systems
- Anger toward God
- Questioning of meaning of suffering
- Verbalizing of inner conflicts about beliefs
- Seeking of spiritual assistance
- Questioning of moral and ethical implications of therapeutic regimen
- Gallows humor
- Displacement of anger toward religious representative

NURSING INTERVENTIONS

- Allow patient to express concerns
- Do not try to reason with patient or suggest that he or she should not feel that way
- Offer to call religious representative of patient's faith, if desired

OUTCOMES

- Patient will feel supported by staff or religious representative
- Patient will express desire for help or support

Communication, impaired verbal

DEFINING CHARACTERISTICS

- Endotracheal tube in place
- Inability to speak dominant language
- Inability to communicate because of
    - Difficulty forming words
    - Difficulty expressing thoughts verbally
    - Loss of hearing
    - Absence of intelligible speech

NURSING INTERVENTIONS

- For patient with endotracheal tube, express thoughts for patient that can be answered yes or no
- Help patient to use communication devices or systems to communicate needs
- For patient with language barrier, find interpreter who can interpret patient's concerns and who understands medical terms well enough to interpret these, as well
- For patient with mental, emotional, or physical deficits, find close family member, friend, or caregiver who is familiar with communication problems of patient

- Effective means of communication will be found to support person's needs

Coping, ineffective family, compromised

Usually the supportive primary person (family member or friend) provides insufficient, ineffective, or compromised support.

- Supportive primary person is absent because of death, injury, or distance
- Supportive primary person is preoccupied with personal reaction
- Supportive primary person describes or confirms inadequate knowledge that interferes with effective assistance
- Supportive primary person attempts assistive or supportive behavior with less than satisfactory results
- Conflict between family members and supportive primary person prevents or limits communication

- When possible, assist supportive primary person to be available in person or by phone
- Assist supportive primary person to
  - Deal with own feelings
  - Understand situation and medical therapies necessary for optimal care
  - Deal effectively with others in supportive way
- Assist all members of family to deal with conflicts, role expectations, and other situations appropriate to coping, which may require referral to social worker or psychologist, as appropriate

- Primary supportive person will be able to regain or maintain supportive relationships

Fear

Fear in trauma patients may be related to factors such as body image change or the potential loss of life or livelihood.

- Verbalization of fear of loss of life, disfigurement, or other losses
- Restlessness
- Increased muscle tension
- Increased verbalization
- Increased information seeking

NURSING INTERVENTIONS

• Encourage patient to discuss fears or anxiety
• Maintain accepting but hopeful outlook as patient discusses problems or lashes out at staff members
• Encourage family and friends to maintain close contact with patient

OUTCOMES

• Patient will be able to talk freely about fears and anxiety
• Patient and family will feel supported by staff members

Trauma syndrome

DEFINING CHARACTERISTICS

• Domestic violence
• Fear of additional injury or death
• Anger
• Embarrassment
• Fear of identifying perpetrator of injury
• Revenge
• Self-blame

NURSING INTERVENTIONS

• Encourage patient to express fear, anger, and concerns
• In cases of domestic violence, encourage patient to seek help and protection through social and law enforcement agencies

OUTCOMES

• Patient will understand that he or she is not to blame for abuse
• Patient will identify how to seek help and protection when he or she is ready

Violence, risk for

DEFINING CHARACTERISTICS

• Expression of anger
• Abusive language
• Threatening language or behavior
• Overt and aggressive acts
• Increased motor activity
• Destruction of objects in environment
• Evidence of intoxication
• History of alcohol or drug abuse
• History of psychosis

NURSING INTERVENTIONS

• Prevent physical harm to self or others; may be necessary to restrain patient
• Provide safe environment for patient

- Isolate patient from other patients
- Set limits for patient behavior
- Do not respond defensively to anger
- Assist patient to identify causes of anger
- Assist patient to identify constructive action to deal with anger
- Reinforce efforts to express anger in positive manner
- Encourage staff members and family to support and understand patient's appropriate expression of anger

OUTCOMES

- Patient will not injure self or others during hospitalization
- Patient will demonstrate absence of signs and symptoms of violent behavior

SUGGESTED READINGS

Emergency Nurses Association: *Trauma nursing core course instructor manual,* ed 4, Park Ridge, IL, 1995, Emergency Nurses Association.

Gordon M: *Manual of nursing diagnoses,* New York, 1982, McGraw-Hill.

North American Nursing Diagnosis Association: *Nursing diagnoses: definitions and classifications, 1997-1998,* Philadelphia, 1997, North American Nursing Diagnosis Association.

Sheehy SB: *Electronic nursing care plans,* Albany, NY, 1998, Delmar Publishers.

CHAPTER 13

Organ and Tissue Donation

Michael J. Pineau

Across the United States, the name of a new patient is added to the national waiting list for organs every 18 minutes. As of July 1997, more than 50,000 patients were registered on waiting lists for organs from one of 281 transplant centers across the country.[1] Each patient is dependent on the generosity of others who make organ donations. The ideal organ donor is a person in good health who has been declared brain dead, often as a result of traumatic injury, and whose organs are being maintained by artificial life support.

Because most trauma patients enter the hospital system through the Emergency Department, emergency care personnel are frequently involved in requesting the donation of organs and tissues. Emergency care personnel should be familiar with the process of organ donation and should be able to offer the patient's next of kin the opportunity for organ or tissue donation. They should check whether the patient has an organ donor card or has made any wishes known to his or her family regarding organ and tissue donation.

Whenever a patient dies or is near death, that patient should be considered for tissue and/or organ donation. With the exception of patients with massive systemic infections, almost all other patients are potential organ or tissue donors. Although family members are grieving, they have the right to be offered the possibility of donation.

Organ donation should be considered when the patient experiences a fatal assault to the brain, such as
- Major head injury from trauma
- Nontraumatic event such as severe stroke or ruptured aneurysm
- Secondary brain injury from an anoxic event such as near-drowning, with the patient maintained by mechanical ventilation and pharmacologic agents

Tissue donation can be considered in almost any patient, even after asystole has occurred. Organ donation usually cannot be considered if asystole has occurred; however, some transplant centers are beginning to consider the use of organs from asystolic patients to increase the number of available donors.

For organ donation to be considered, the patient must be maintained on mechanical ventilation; and blood pressure, fluid and electrolyte balance, and arterial blood gases must be maintained within normal ranges. Therefore pharmacologic agents may be required. Brain death must be declared before organ donation can occur.

HISTORY OF ORGAN AND TISSUE DONATION

In 1968 the Uniform Anatomical Gift Act was passed and enacted in all 50 states. This law allowed people to choose to be organ or tissue donors. Persons who are 18 years of age or older may signify their intent by including donation provisions in their living will, making advanced directives, carrying a donor card (signed by two witnesses), or placing an identifying sticker or stamp on their driver's license. There are legal criteria for each of these methods of donation.

In the 1980s, Vice President and former Senator Albert Gore (D, Tennessee) led an inquiry to determine problems with the organ transplantation process. From this, the Organ Transplantation Act (Public Law 98-507) became law. This law provides for a request from next of kin and has increased the numbers of organs and the amount of tissue available. A task force was formed to review issues surrounding organ and tissue donation and transplantation, including legal, ethical, medical, and economic issues.

The report of this task force was published in 1986.[2] According to this report, families were not offered donation possibilities consistently, and healthcare workers were hesitant to ask families to consider donation. Authors of the report requested that states enact legislation mandating hospitals to develop and implement organ request and donation policies. The authors also encouraged states to support health professional and public education about donation and transplantation and encouraged states to enact the Uniform Determination of Death Act. Federal rules currently require each state to have "required request" legislation, which require hospitals to maintain a protocol for asking family members for permission to donate a deceased relative's organs and tissues. In addition, the task force mandated that the Department of Health and Human Services establish a single network to act as a clearinghouse for the identification and distribution of tissues and organs to be transplanted. Thus the Organ Procurement and Transplantation Network was created. A private agency, the United Network for Organ Sharing (UNOS), was contracted to carry out this task.

The Consolidated Omnibus Budget Reconciliation Act (COBRA) includes a provision that provides for Medicare funding for hospitals to (1) develop policies for informing families of their rights to choose or deny organ or tissue donation and (2) ensure that a designated organ procurement agency be notified when a potential organ donor exists. These organ procurement agencies have formed a regional network throughout the United States (Fig. 13-1). To make a referral for donation, an emergency care provider should contact the

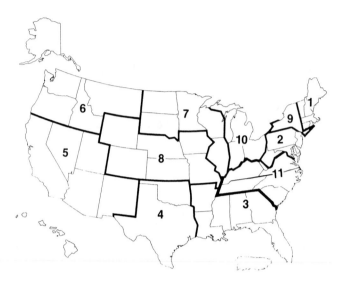

Fig. 13-1   UNOS regional map.

regional organ procurement agency for their locality and for information on donation.

   In addition to donor cards and license stickers, it is important for the patient's next of kin to be aware of the patient's wishes, because they will have the ultimate decision about donation. Next of kin are given the following authorization priority: (1) spouse, (2) adult child, (3) parent, (4) brother or sister, (5) legal guardian. Any next of kin must be at least 18 years of age to make the decision for donation. Although giving permission for donation is the ultimate responsibility of one person, the actual decision is usually made by many of the patient's family members.

DONATION

For donation to take place, the following must be documented:
   • Determination of death by protocol
   • Pronouncement of death
   • Consent for donation from next of kin
   • Approval by the state medical examiner in accordance with state law
Determination of death is made by one of two criteria:
   • Cessation of circulatory and respiratory function
         Made by clinical examination
         Irreversibility (persistent cessation of functions during observed period of time)
   • Cessation of all brain and brain stem functions
         Absence of brain functions for observed time period
         Absence of brain stem functions for observed time period

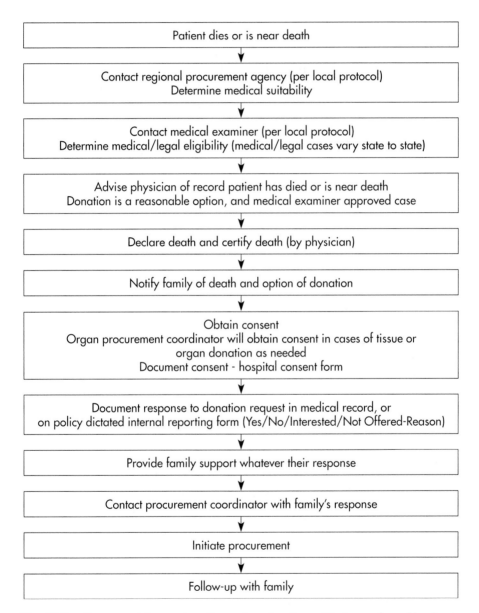

Fig. 13-2   Organ and tissue donation referral pattern. (Redrawn from Newberry L, editor: Sheehy's *Emergency Nursing,* ed 4, St Louis, 1998, Mosby.)

Identified cause of coma that can cause loss of brain functions

No possibility of recovery

When brain death has been declared, it must be documented in the patient's medical record. Because criteria for organ and tissue donation change frequently, early contact with the regional organ procurement agency is essential. Historically a patient would not be considered for organ or tissue donation because of a septic condition, the presence of a communicable disease, or the high risk for HIV. These criteria should no longer preclude the patient from consideration as a donor because selected organs and tissues may still be suitable for transplant or use in research.

Permission must be granted by the medical examiner in certain types of cases. These may include, but are not limited to, accidental deaths, possible homicides, suicides, small children (under age 3 years), patients who die unexpectedly within 24 hours of hospital admission, and patients who are admitted to the hospital in a coma and later die. Criteria for requiring medical examiner permission varies from state to state, so emergency care providers must be familiar with their local requirements.

Consent of next of kin must be documented in the patient's medical record. This documentation should also name which tissues or organs may and may not be taken. A standard hospital form or a specific form designed for donation may be used.

A typical referral pattern for initiating organ or tissue donation is outlined in Fig. 13-2. Each institution must identify who is responsible for each step of the process. The process varies from institution to institution. Frequently, if the organ donor coordinator is contacted early, he or she becomes involved before the patient's death. This early involvement is essential in helping determine whether the patient is a potential donor and to work with and support the patient's family through the difficult decision-making process of donation. The organ donor coordinator also provides support and education to staff members who may not have experienced the process of requesting a donation from family members.

REQUESTING ORGAN OR TISSUE DONATION

On many occasions, the emergency care provider is in an ideal position to request organ/tissue donation from the patient's next of kin, because he or she has established a rapport with the patient's family. It is important for the person who does the requesting to be prepared to do so and to be relatively comfortable with the process. The family should be given some time to process the fact that their loved one has died or is about to die. Clinical personnel must be mindful that although families must be given some time to make their decision, organs and tissues will begin to deteriorate over time even with aggressive mechanical life support measures. Thus a family may lose the opportunity to donate a loved one's organs. When death is imminent because of a severe head injury, the patient may be transferred to the intensive care unit, where diagnostic tests will be performed to confirm brain death. Diagnostic tests for brain death include apnea testing, evaluation for the absence of reflexes and eye movement, and the use of cold-calorics testing. Additionally, EEG and radiologic evaluation of cerebral blood flow may also be used to assist in the determination of brain death. Because the patient is being maintained by mechanical ventilation and possibly by pharmacologic agents, the family can then be informed of the diagnostic findings and will have time to process information about organ donation. This death may be especially difficult for families, because they see that their loved one is "breathing" and still warm.

In the Emergency Department, when a patient dies from any condition, but the terminal event is asystole, the family can see that the patient is truly dead. However, this family has less time to consider a request for tissue donation.

Clinical personnel must find out what the patient's family has been told and whether the possibility of organ/tissue donation has been discussed. Families must understand that their loved one is dead before they can begin to contemplate organ/tissue donation. Good judgment and common sense will guide the caregiver or organ donor coordinator when the time is appropriate to ask for donation.

If the next of kin is not present and telephone contact must be made, permission for organ donation can be obtained by telephone. It is then essential to have two witnesses sign documentation that permission was obtained.

If internal organs are being donated, a person from the local organ procurement agency will usually be present to work with the family of the patient and the staff caring for the patient. In addition, the agency representative will ensure that protocols are carried out to maintain the patient's hemodynamic status until organ removal can take place.

PROCUREMENT OF TISSUES AND ORGANS

For tissue donation, a person representing the local organ procurement agency, perhaps a nurse or physician's assistant from the hospital who is specially trained in tissue retrieval, will assist in the process. Corneas, heart for valve replacement, skin, and bone may be removed in the morgue. A heart that is to be used for valve replacement may be recovered 6 to 10 hours following asystole. Bones may be recovered up to 10 hours, corneas and skin up to 24 hours following asystole.

Solid organs are retrieved by surgical specialists in the operating room. They can be retrieved only if the next of kin has given permission to retrieve that specific organ or organs. A representative from the local organ procurement agency will be present to work with the family and to assist the staff in maintaining the patient in a hemodynamically acceptable state for organ donation. For organs to be retrievable, the patient's systolic blood pressure must be maintained at or above 100 mmHg, Po_2 must be maintained at 100 or greater, and hematocrit at 30 or greater for the adult donor. Pediatric parameters are based on the size of the child.

After a patient is deemed acceptable for organ donation, his or her organs are assigned to waiting patients. The organ procurement teams coordinate their efforts to choose a time for retrieval that will fit all schedules. Often teams may travel great distances to perform organ retrieval. The patient continues to be hemodynamically maintained throughout surgical removal of the organs. The heart, heart and lungs, and single lungs must be transplanted within 6 hours of removal. The kidneys may be transplanted up to 24 hours after removal. Elapsed time for a pancreas or liver to be transplanted will vary depending on the institution doing the transplant.

COST OF ORGAN AND TISSUE DONATION

The donor's family should not be responsible for any costs associated with the organ and tissue retrieval process. Questions about cost should be referred to the local organ procurement agency. The cost of transplant is high and varies significantly depending on the type of transplant being performed and the resources needed to provide care for the transplant recipient.

SUMMARY

Emergency care workers must have knowledge about the organ requesting, procurement, and donation processes. Because many patients who become candidates for tissue and organ donation enter the hospital system through the Emergency Department, emergency care workers must be prepared to meet this enormous challenge. Any patient who dies or is about to die is a potential donor, and emergency care providers are obligated to provide every family of a potential donor the opportunity to give the gift of organs and tissues.

REFERENCES

1. United Network for Organ Sharing: *United States Waiting List Statistics*, Richmond, VA, 1997, United Network for Organ Sharing.
2. Department of Health and Human Services: *Organ Transplantation: issues and recommendations. Report of the Task Force on Organ Transplantation*, Washington, DC, 1986, US Department of Health and Human Services.

SUGGESTED READINGS

Albert PL: Overview of the organ donation process, *Crit Care Nurs Clin N Am* 6(3):553-565, 1994.
American Hospital Association, American Medical Association, and United Network for Organ Sharing: *Required request legislation: a guide for hospitals on organ and tissue donation*, Chicago, 1988, American Hospital Association, American Medical Association and the United Network for Organ Sharing.

President's Commission for the Study of Ethical Problems in Medicine and Biomedical Research: *Defining death: medical, legal and ethical issues in the determination of death,* Washington, DC, 1981, President's Commission for the Study of Ethical Problems in Medicine and Biomedical Research.

Emergency Nurses Association: *Role of the emergency nurse in organ procurement: ENA position statement,* Chicago, 1987, Emergency Nurses Association.

Laudicina SS: *Medicaid coverage and payment policies for organ transplants: findings of a national survey,* George Washington University, 1988, U.S. Department of Health and Human Services.

McNally-Pedersen ME: Organ and tissue transplantation. In Sheehy SB, editor: *Emergency nursing,* ed 3, St Louis, 1992, Mosby.

National Kidney Foundation: *For those who give and grieve: a booklet for donor families,* New York, 1990, The National Kidney Foundation.

Wisner DH, Lo B: The feasibility of organ salvage from non-heart-beating trauma donors, *Arch Surg* 131(9):929-934, 1996.

CHAPTER 14

Injury Prevention

IMPACT OF TRAUMA ON THE COMMUNITY

Barbara A. Foley

TRAUMA STATISTICS

Trauma has become the scourge of modern society. This is true not only for the United States and Canada but also for most industrialized nations. In the United States trauma is the largest killer of persons between ages 1 and 44, the most productive years of their lives. Every year, more than 59 million Americans are injured and more than 150,000 deaths result. In 1995 6% of all deaths were caused by an injury. In addition, 8% of all hospital discharges had a primary diagnosis of injury, and 37% of all Emergency Department (ED) visits were for injuries (Fig. 14-1). For each person who died from trauma in 1995, 18 were hospitalized, 251 received treatment in the ED, and 40 received some kind of medical care (including telephone advice) for their injury.[1] Estimates suggest that annually 99,000 Americans receive brain injuries severe enough to produce long-term disabilities.[2] In addition, each year more than 7600 trauma victims sustain spinal cord injuries that produce paraplegia or quadriplegia.[3] Trauma has been estimated to result in the loss of more than 4 million years of future work life per year, compared with 2.1 million resulting from heart disease and 1.7 million resulting from cancer.[4]

In the United States trauma is one of the most costly health problems, taking an economic toll greater than heart disease and cancer combined. In 1995 trauma cost the American public $434.8 billion including lost wages and productivity, medical expenses, administrative costs, and employer expenses. Lost quality of life from trauma incidents would add an estimated $775.8 billion, totaling $1210.6 billion in comprehensive costs in 1995.[5]

The indirect economic costs are even greater than the direct healthcare costs of these patients (Table 14-1).

Automobile crashes remain the number one single source of trauma deaths and nonfatal injuries (Box 14-1). In 1995 41,798 people were killed in motor vehicle accidents, and 3,386,000 people were injured; an average of 115

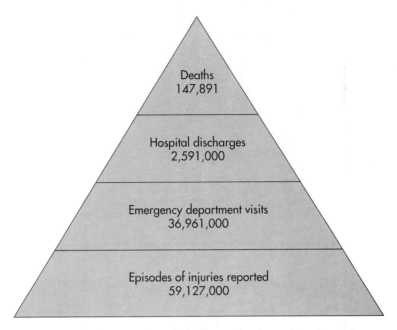

Deaths
147,891

Hospital discharges
2,591,000

Emergency department visits
36,961,000

Episodes of injuries reported
59,127,000

Notes: Injury deaths in 1995 excluded 2918 deaths resulting from adverse
events. Emergency department visits in 1995 excluded 262,000
visits for no specific injury identifier.

Fig. 14-1   Burden of injury: United States, 1995. (From Centers for Disease Control and Prevention, National Center for Health Statistics, National Vital Statistics System, National Hospital Discharge Survey, National Hospital Ambulatory Medical Care Survey, National Health Interview Survey)

persons died each day in motor vehicle accidents; that is, 1 person every 13 minutes. The leading cause of death for people 5 to 27 years old results from motor vehicle accidents. The age group with the highest incidence of death was between 15 and 24 years old, and males were involved twice as often as females.[6]

Alcohol abuse is a major contributor to automobile crash fatalities, and the blood alcohol level in at least one driver or nonoccupant of fatal crashes in 1995 was over 0.10% in approximately one third of instances. More than two thirds of the 13,564 people killed in such crashes were themselves intoxicated. The rate of alcohol involvement in fatal crashes is three and one-third times as high at night as during the day (i.e., 62.2% versus 18.8%). About 2 in every 5 Americans are involved in an alcohol-related crash at some time in their lives.[7] This information is invaluable in identifying target groups for education and in writing legislation that can aid in trauma prevention. Although alcohol continues to be a significant element in injuries associated with automobile crashes, the numbers have diminished slightly in the past 10

Table 14-1 Summary of Costs for All Motor Vehicle Injuries

Cost category	Cost, all injuries (million $)
Property damage	52,119
Medical costs	17,026
Productivity	54,748
Services	
Emergency	1,724
Legal	5,857
Administrative	18,995
Total	150,459

From National Highway Traffic Safety Administration: The economic cost of MVC's, Washington, DC, 1994 National Highway Traffic Safety Administration.

BOX 14-1

FATAL INJURY DEATH BY CAUSE, ALL AGE GROUPS, 1995

Motor vehicle crash	29%
Suicide	21%
Homicides	15%
Falls	7%
Poisonings	6%
Drowning	3%
Fire/flame	2%
Other	17%

From National Center for Health Statistics, Centers for Disease Control and Prevention 1995, Atlanta, Centers for Disease Control.

---

years with increasing penalties for impaired drivers. The problem remains large, but it is encouraging to see results of preventive efforts through education, legislation, and enforcement.

The Centers for Disease Control and Prevention (CDC) has identified priority health-risk behaviors that contribute to the leading causes of mortality, morbidity, and social problems among youth and adults that are often established during youth and extend into adulthood.[8] In 1996 CDC reported the results of their national survey based on their *Youth Risk Behavior Surveillance System*. They reported 72% of all deaths among school-age youth and young adults resulted from motor vehicle crashes, other unintentional injuries, homicide, and suicide. The study suggests that many high school students practice behaviors that may increase their likelihood of death, such as noncompliance with seat belt laws, driving while impaired or riding in a car with a driver whom they know is impaired, carrying a weapon, and frequent drug or alcohol use. The potential impact of altering high-risk behavior at an early age through local and community educational programs may result in decreasing trauma morbidity and mortality statistics.

In the United States an additional element of trauma epidemiology is the increasing numbers of intentional, violent injuries. The number of criminal injuries in the United States is disproportionately higher than in other developed countries. Handguns remain the weapon most used, and legislation for handgun control in this country is lacking. The issue of handgun regulation remains inconclusive, with many organizations supporting both sides of the debate. The specter of injury caused by intentional violence extends beyond urban trauma centers and has a serious, negative impact on community trauma centers.[9] Although there is a disproportionately higher incidence of intentional, violent injuries in males, 26% of injury-related deaths in women are classified as intentional.[10]

PREVENTION OF INJURIES

Given what we know about the incidence of injury and contributing social factors, the emphasis for reducing the dramatic figures must be on prevention of injuries and their severity. High-risk lifestyles that have become commonplace in technical and industrial countries are being recognized as significant contributors to the numbers of casualties associated with high-speed vehicles, sophisticated high-energy industrial machines, and the growing number of chemicals and toxins used in industry and everyday living.

In recent years an awareness of the preventability of injuries has been recognized, both by healthcare personnel and industrial leaders, but consumers need a great amount of education. The use of automobile restraints has dramatically decreased the severity of injuries incurred from automobile crashes, and the continuing improvement in automobile safety design, seat belts, air bags, and child restraint car seats creates a hopeful picture. Although legislation by many states requires the use of automobile passenger restraints, compliance continues to be a problem, and community education to emphasize the importance of these devices has become an essential part of a complete trauma program. Helmet use for motorcycles is mandated in many states, but only a few states consider bicycle helmet use a legislative problem, in spite of the dramatic number of adults and children who suffer significant head injury and death from bicycle incidents every year. A natural focus for community injury prevention programs is on children in the formative years when safe behavior can be integrated into daily living. The results of these programs are difficult to measure initially, but it is hoped that their effectiveness will be reflected in declining numbers of traumatic deaths and injuries in the future. Organized trauma systems that collect data of injuries include information on the mechanism of injury and the use of safety devices and will be invaluable in measuring the effectiveness of prevention efforts in local, state, and federal programs.

An area in which prevention programs have been particularly effective is burn injury prevention. In the past 20 years there has been a significant decline in home fire injuries, following a major effort in the 1970s by the American Burn Association to educate families about home burn risks and following widespread use of smoke alarms. The effectiveness of this effort is dramatic and encouraging as we look to other areas of behavior that education and technologic advances for safer living can affect.

There are several aspects of prevention that we as healthcare providers should consider. *Patient education* is the natural first approach, with the opportunity to speak one-on-one with patients and families about the behavior that brought them to the hospital for their current visit.

Community education through school programs and presentations to youth and philanthropic groups can be very effective. Graphic visual aids and handouts that are appropriate to the activities of the age group being addressed are very helpful and can be inexpensively obtained through state injury prevention organizations, local fire and rescue groups, and many manufacturers of protective devices and sports equipment. Coordination of a community-wide injury prevention program with other public services, such as law enforcement agencies, fire departments, and bicycle clubs, can be crucial to a comprehensive approach to educating consumers.

As trauma prevention education becomes more common, an increasing number of options for community education are becoming available. Local grants from industries can often be obtained to fund prevention projects, and generally when such programs are presented to community service groups, enthusiasm for these efforts builds. Injury is a potential risk to all age and social groups; it is therefore not difficult to generate enthusiasm when the need for financial support is presented in an organized and informative fashion.

Another major area of trauma prevention in which the trauma team can be involved is *safety legislation.* Legislators need to hear from professionals to support legislation that mandates safe behavior. When laws such as those enforcing stringent penalties for driving under the influence of drugs or alcohol and enforcing mandatory helmet use are being introduced or revised, it is an opportunity to both educate legislators and demonstrate support for these issues. Interest in these issues can be organized through state Emergency Medical Service (EMS) and Trauma Divisions, local EMS councils and trauma programs, professional organizations such as the Emergency Nurses Association (ENA), Society of Trauma Nurses (STN), the American Trauma Society (ATS), and district legislators' offices (Fig. 14-2).

An additional area of influence for decreasing the number and severity of injuries is improving the environmental and technical development of consumer products. Again, this area may be most effectively managed by legislation, because it is frequently difficult to influence a manufacturer to change or add features to a product that will increase cost. Public demand for safer automobiles, home appliances, and toys for children should be part of educa-

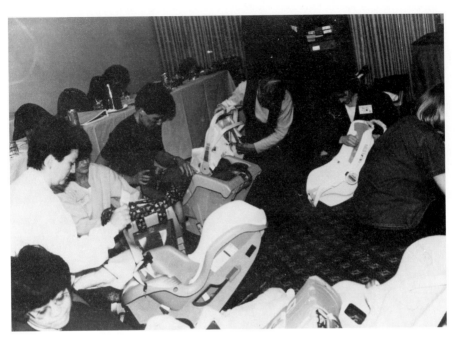

Fig. 14-2 Emergency Nurses during a 4-day child passenger safety technical training course that will enable the nurses to educate their patients and the community on the proper use of child passenger restraints. The course was a collaborative effort between ENA, ENCARE, and NHTSA. (Courtesy of Barbara Foley, RN, BS, Associate Executive Director, Emergency Nurses Care.)

tion presentations to consumers to broaden consumer demands and to put pressure on manufacturers to improve the safety of their products.

Awareness of the preventability of injuries needs to start with the professionals who witness the devastating effects of trauma every day. As part of our responsibility as caregivers, it is important to be informed of advances in trauma prevention, to support legislative and community efforts for safer living, and to share our knowledge with other citizens in the community.

REFERENCES

1. National Center for Health Statistics: *Health, United States, 1996-97 and injury chartbook,* 1997, Hyattsville, MD, National Center for Health Statistics.
2. Kraus J, Sorenson S: Epidemiology. In Silver J, Yudofsky S, Hales R, editors: *Neuropsychiatry of traumatic brain injury,* Washington, DC, 1994, American Psychiatric Press.
3. National Spinal Cord Injury Statistical Center: *Spinal cord injury: facts and figures at a glance,* 1996, Birmingham, AL, National Spinal Cord Injury Statistical Center.
4. Rice DP, MacKenzie EJ, and others: *Cost of injury in the United States: a report to Congress,* San Francisco and Baltimore, 1989, University of California and Johns Hopkins University.
5. National Safety Council: *Accident facts,* 1996, Itasca, IL, National Society Council.

6. National Highway Safety Traffic Administration, National Center for Statistics and Analysis: *Traffic safety facts 1995: overview,* Washington, DC, National Highway Safety Traffic Administration.
7. National Highway Safety Traffic Administration, National Center for Statistics and Analysis: *Traffic safety facts 1995: alcohol,* Washington, DC, National Highway Safety Traffic Administration.
8. Kunn L and others: *MMWR CDC Surveill Summ* 45(4):1-84, 1996.
9. Clancy TV and others: *J Trauma* 37(1):1-4, 1994.
10. Dannenberg AL, Baker SP, Li G: *Ann Epidem* 4(2):133-134, 1994.

PART III

Clinical Practice

CHAPTER 15

Trauma Initial Assessment

Mary M. Cushman

The primary and secondary trauma survey has been designed to provide an organized format for rapid assessment of the trauma patient. This process assures that any life-threatening conditions are identified, injuries are prioritized, and appropriate interventions occur in a systematic and orderly fashion. The primary survey should take approximately 2 minutes to complete. If problems are identified as life-threatening at any time during the survey, therapeutic interventions should be started immediately. Rapid assessment and appropriate therapeutic interventions must be provided without delay.

THE PRIMARY SURVEY: THE ABCs

Assessment of the patient's airway is the first step in the primary trauma survey. Assessment of the airway should be a reflex reaction on the part of the caregiver. It should be based on patient findings and should include the following:

A = AIRWAY

Airway patency
Assess the airway for signs of obstruction; to include facial, mandibular, or tracheal/pharyngeal fractures; or foreign bodies.[1]

Oxygen
All multiple trauma patients should receive supplemental oxygen by either nonrebreather mask, if the patient has adequate spontaneous respirations, or by airway adjuncts.

Head/neck position
Clinical personnel must assume that the patient has a cervical spine injury until it can be ruled out by x-rays or computed tomography (CT) scan, and

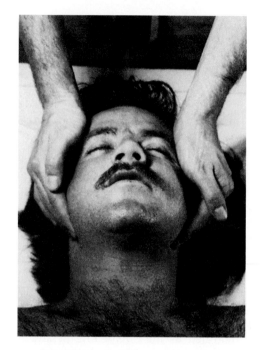

Fig. 15-1 Jaw-thrust maneuver.

clinical evaluation. All trauma patients should have a cervical collar in place to maintain the neck in a neutral, immobilized position. Head position becomes essential in management of the airway. The neck should not be hyperextended, hyperflexed, or rotated to establish and maintain a patent airway. The chin lift and jaw thrust maneuver (Fig. 15-1) are two interventions that can be used to open the patient's airway.

Airway adjuncts

The use of airway adjuncts may be essential to the management of the patient's airway. Familiarity with the various types of adjuncts available, including their indications and contraindications, is essential.

Oropharyngeal airway

The oropharyngeal airway should be used only in *patients who are unconscious and without a gag reflex* (Fig. 15-2). Even if the patient is endotracheally intubated, the oropharyngeal airway may be used as a bite block to prevent the patient from biting the endotracheal tube.

Nasopharyngeal airway

The nasopharyngeal airway may be used on patients who are conscious and have an intact gag reflex (Fig. 15-3). It is contraindicated in patients with se-

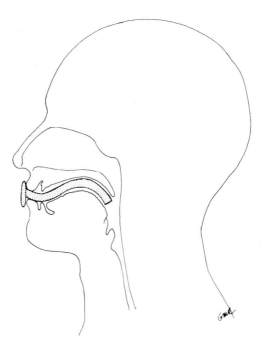

Fig. 15-2 Oropharyngeal airway in place.

vere facial fractures. It is better tolerated by the responsive patient and is less likely to induce vomiting.

Endotracheal tube

An endotracheal tube should be considered when total airway management is essential (Fig. 15-4). In the trauma patient, absolute care must be taken to avoid hyperextension of the neck at all times (before ruling out a cervical spine injury), especially when intubating.

Orotracheal intubation

Orotracheal intubation may be instituted in the unconscious patient in need of a definitive airway. In-line manual cervical spine immobilization must be maintained during the intubation process.

Nasotracheal intubation

Nasotracheal intubation is not commonly used in the trauma patient. It is contraindicated in those patients with severe midface fractures or basilar skull fractures or patients with no respiratory effort.

Cricothyroidotomy

Cricothyroidotomy is a technique that should only be used when airway management by another means cannot be accomplished (Fig. 15-5). This tech-

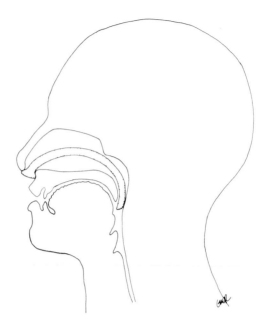

Fig. 15-3 Nasopharyngeal airway in place.

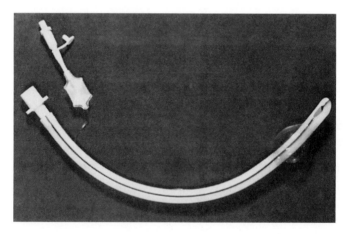

Fig. 15-4 Endotracheal tube.

nique provides oxygen to a patient in an emergent situation. It is considered a temporary airway until a definitive one can be established. Cricothyroidotomy may be carried out by:

• Needle placement and transtracheal jet insufflation

With this method, carbon dioxide (CO_2) rapidly accumulates, usually within 30 minutes. Therefore a definitive airway must be established quickly.

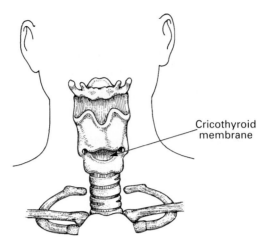

Fig. 15-5 Cricothyroidotomy.

- Small surgical incision and tracheal tube placement
  A surgical cricothyroidotomy should be converted to a formal tracheostomy as soon as the patient's clinical condition allows.

Appropriate equipment
Suction
Clinical personnel should assure that adequate suction is readily available. This includes the suction power of the unit, a container to hold the secretions, extra connecting tubing, and appropriate suction catheters. A backup system must be available if the first suction system malfunctions.

End Tidal Carbon Dioxide Detector
An end tidal CO_2 detector confirms placement of the endotracheal tube by indicating the presence of CO_2 in the exhaled gases.

Pulse Oximeter
A pulse oximeter is a noninvasive method to continuously measure oxygen saturation of arterial blood (SpO_2).[2]

B = BREATHING

The function of breathing and ventilation is the transportation of oxygen to the alveoli and diffusion across the alveoli to the vascular system, then diffusion of carbon dioxide from blood to the alveoli, where it is exhaled. With the trauma patient, as with any patient, clinical personnel must assure adequate oxygenation. If oxygenation is not being adequately accomplished by the patient, personnel must provide assistance to optimize oxygenation and gas diffusion. The effectiveness of ventilation can be evaluated by arterial blood gas

---

BOX 15-1

FACTORS THAT CONTRIBUTE TO TISSUE HYPOXIA IN THE TRAUMA PATIENT[3]

- Shifts to the left of the oxyhemoglobin dissociation curve (can be secondary to infusion of large volumes of banked blood, hypocarbia or alkalosis, or hypothermia)
- Reduced hemoglobin (secondary to hemorrhage)
- Reduced cardiac output (in presence of cardiovascular insults)
- Impaired cellular oxygen consumption (associated with metabolic alterations of sepsis)
- Increased metabolic demands (associated with stress response to injury)

(From Johnson KL: Critical care of the trauma patient. In Neff JA, Kidd PS, editors: *Trauma nursing: the art and science,* St Louis, 1993, Mosby.)

measurement (Box 15-1). Following are several methods of providing assisted ventilation:

- **Mouth-to-face mask** (one-person technique)   The mouth-to-face mask method provides a *barrier* between rescuer and victim. The advantages of this device are that it prevents exposure of the rescuer to communicable disease and that supplemental oxygen may be added. In accordance with universal precautions, ensure that the face mask has a one-way valve to prevent the backflow of air or secretions.
- **Bag-valve-face mask** (two-person technique)   With supplemental oxygen and tubing attached to add a dead space or with use of an added anesthesia bag, the bag-valve-face mask can deliver up to 95% oxygen. Clinical personnel will be able to sense lung compliance when they compress the bag.
- **Ventilators**   Appropriate equipment and skilled persons need to be available to accomplish optimal ventilation.

C = CIRCULATION

To assess circulatory status, begin by checking the carotid or femoral pulse. Peripheral pulses may be absent because of direct injury or of stimulation of the sympathetic nervous system, which causes peripheral vasoconstriction. Clinical personnel should assess vital signs, including pulse, respiration, blood pressure, temperature, and skin color, temperature, and moisture.

Delayed capillary refill (more than 2 seconds) at the nail bed or at the thenar eminence possibly indicates shock. Delayed capillary refill, together with cool, clammy distal extremities and an altered mental status, suggests shock *until proven otherwise.** A person who is hypothermic may demonstrate delayed capillary refill and *not* be in shock. A third trimester pregnant woman may be in shock and not demonstrate delayed capillary refill because of increased blood volume during pregnancy.

Hypovolemic shock

Hypovolemic shock is the most common type of shock that occurs in the trauma patient.[1] It results from the decrease in the amount of circulating blood volume and causes inadequate oxygen and nutrient delivery at the cellular level.

The average 70 kg (154 pound) person has a blood volume of approximately 5 liters.

- Class I—hemorrhage is up to a 15% blood loss (up to 750 ml)
- Class II—hemorrhage is a 15% to 30% blood loss (750 to 150 ml)
- Class III—hemorrhage is a 30% to 40% blood loss (1500 to 2000 ml)
- Class IV—hemorrhage is >40% blood loss (>2000 ml)

Recognition of hypovolemic shock

- Restless and anxious
- Cool and clammy skin
- Cool and clammy distal extremities
- Delayed capillary refill (>2 seconds)
- Weak and rapid pulse (>100 beats per minute)
- Decrease in blood pressure (<90 mmHg systolic†)
- Rapid and shallow (>29) or depressed (<10) respirations
- Decrease in level of consciousness (Glasgow Coma Scale <13)[1]

If the patient is conscious:

- Complains of being cold
- Complains of being thirsty

Compensatory mechanisms in shock

Sympathetic stimulation

Sympathetic stimulation causes the release of catecholamines (epinephrine and norepinephrine), providing α and β stimulation, which increases heart rate and peripheral resistance.

Activation of this compensatory mechanism will cause peripheral vasoconstriction, which causes the patient to have cool, clammy skin and cool distal extremities. The patient may complain of being cold.

Activation of renin-angiotensin mechanism

When blood flow through the renal system decreases, renin is released. Angiotensin I is then released, it is converted into angiotensin II, resulting

---

*Hypothermia patients with vascular insufficiencies may demonstrate these signs without the presence of shock.
†As defined by the American College of Surgeons (ACS).

in the secretion of aldosterone. Aldosterone causes the kidneys to retain sodium and thereby conserve water. As a result the compensatory mechanism, urinary output will decrease.[4] Urine output is a good indicator of adequate resuscitation in a patient with normal renal function (0.5 cc to 1 cc/kg).

Antidiuretic hormone

In hypovolemic shock, antidiuretic hormone (ADH) is secreted by the posterior pituitary gland, causing the kidneys to retain water at the collecting tubule. This compensatory mechanism results in an increased circulating intravascular volume and a decreased urinary output.

Jugular veins

If a patient is in shock, the jugular veins should be assessed.
* Vein distension may indicate that blood is unable to return to the right side of the heart. Clinical personnel should consider the possibility of a pericardial tamponade or a tension pneumothorax and treat accordingly.
* Jugular veins may be collapsed as a result of hypovolemia and therefore are an unreliable indicator of intravascular volume status.

Therapeutic interventions for trauma patient in shock
Intravenous lines
* Start two IV lines using crystalloid solution such as warmed Ringer's lactate
* Use large-bore, short cannulas (14 gauge or 7.5 Fr)
* Start in antecubital space, jugular veins, or any other large veins, such as femoral vein (upper extremity peripheral lines are preferred)
* Run solution at rate to maintain systolic pressure above 100 mmHg on an adult; consider rapid infusor devices
* Send blood specimen for type and crossmatch early in trauma resuscitation phase.
* Administer type-specific blood as indicated; uncrossmatched, low titer type O or O negative blood may be used when clinical situation warrants.[1]
* Warm all intravenous fluids.
* Send blood specimen for baseline hematologic studies; include serum pregnancy test for females of childbearing age.

100% oxygen
* Take extreme caution if positive pressure is utilized because of possibility of tension pneumothorax.
* Assure that patent airway exists (refer to Airway section, p. 166, for defined modalities).
* Administer supplemental oxygen.

Prevention of hypothermia

- Prevent heat loss in the patient by increasing the ambient air/room temperature.
- Removal of all clothing and wet dressings.
- Use blanket warmers.
- Warm all infused material.

Electrocardiographic (ECG) monitoring

- All patients should be continuously monitored to assess for dysrhythmias, pulseless electrical activity (PEA), or tachy or brady arrhythmias.

Pneumatic antishock garment

Use of the pneumatic antishock garment (PASG) is controversial in hospitals and in urban and rural areas. In general, PASG is thought to
- Increase peripheral vascular resistance
- *Possibly* increase venous return to the right side of the heart
- Tamponade bleeding (particularly as seen with pelvic fractures) and intraabdominal trauma
- Splint fractures

PASG is contraindicated when the patient is in pulmonary edema, when it is known that the patient has a diaphragmatic rupture, or when hemorrhage is occurring in a location not covered by the PASG, such as the scalp, face, upper extremities, or chest. Clinical personnel should be particularly cautious not to delay rapid transport or crystalloid or blood product replacement while the PASG is being placed.

Control of external bleeding

- Use direct pressure whenever possible
- Personnel should prepare for surgery if bleeding cannot be controlled or if internal hemorrhage is suspected

LIFE-THREATENING CONDITIONS IDENTIFIED IN PRIMARY SURVEY

Five types of chest injuries should be ruled out in the primary survey. If any of these five conditions are detected, it is imperative that immediate therapeutic intervention(s) are accomplished, because any of these conditions may be immediately life-threatening. In-depth discussion of these five types of chest injuries is found in Chapter 19.

Tension pneumothorax

ASSESSMENT

- Dyspnea
- Tachycardia
- Decreasing blood pressure
- Deviated trachea (away from tension)

- Diminished or absent breath sounds on affected side
- Distended jugular veins (if not in hypovolemic shock)
- Cyanosis (late sign)

THERAPEUTIC INTERVENTIONS

- Needle thoracentesis or chest tube placement

Open pneumothorax (open chest wound/sucking chest wound)

ASSESSMENT

- Dyspnea, tachypnea
- Diminished or absent breath sounds on the affected side
- Open, sucking wound with inspiratory effort
- Rapid pulse
- Decreased blood pressure
- Possible signs of tension pneumothorax

THERAPEUTIC INTERVENTIONS

- Cover defect with occlusive dressing taped on three sides
- Provide oxygen
- Consider endotracheal intubation and positive pressure
- Observe for signs and symptoms of tension pneumothorax; remove dressing if signs of tension pneumothorax appear
- Prepare for chest tube placement
- Prepare for operative intervention, if indicated

Massive hemothorax (>1500 ml blood)

ASSESSMENT

- Same as that for severe shock (see Chapters 7 and 19).

THERAPEUTIC INTERVENTIONS

- Same as that for severe shock (see Chapters 7 and 19)
- Oxygen
- IV lines/rapid blood replacement
- Chest tube(s) (large-bore: 36 Fr)
- Consider autotransfusion
- After tube insertion, obtain chest x-ray examination
- Prepare for surgery

Flail chest

ASSESSMENT

- Dyspnea
- Possible paradoxic movement of chest wall
- Pain
- Crepitus of rib fracture
- Cyanosis (late sign)

THERAPEUTIC INTERVENTIONS

- Selective endotracheal intubation (respiratory rate <24, PaO_2 < 60 on 50% O_2, tidal volume 5 ml/kg)
- 100% humidified O_2 under positive pressure
- Judicious fluid administration
- Analgesia
- Prevent hypoxia

Pericardial tamponade

ASSESSMENT

- Dyspnea
- Cyanosis (periorbital and peripheral)
- Beck's triad
  - Decreased blood pressure
  - Muffled heart sounds
  - Distended jugular veins (may be absent in presence of hypovolemic shock)
- Signs and symptoms of hypovolemic shock

THERAPEUTIC INTERVENTIONS

- High-flow oxygen
- High Fowler's position
- IV lines
- Pericardiocentesis or pericardial window
- Thoracotomy

ASSESSMENT OF LEVEL OF CONSCIOUSNESS

Initial assessment of neurologic status includes the Glasgow Coma Scale (Fig. 15-6).

Glasgow Coma Scale[6]

Best motor response	Points
Obeys simple commands	6
Localizes noxious stimulus	5
Flexion withdrawal	4
Abnormal flexion	3
Abnormal extension	2
No motor response	1

Best verbal response	
Oriented	5
Confused (imprecise)	4
Verbalizes/exclamatory, disorganized	3
Moans/groans (incomprehensible)	2
No vocalization	1

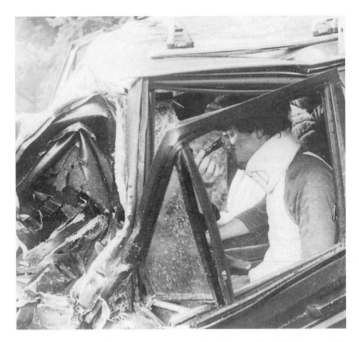

Fig. 15-6 Assess level of consciousness; check pupils. (Courtesy Tacoma Fire Department.)

Eye opening

Spontaneous	4
To speech (automatically, usually not conscious control)	3
To pain	2
No eye opening	1

A score of 11 or less indicates that the patient most likely has a severe injury. *Coma* is defined as no response and no eye opening or as a score of 7 or less.[5] The Glasgow Coma Scale may not be useful in patients who are severely hypovolemic or intoxicated or in infants and small children.

Pediatric Coma Scale*

The Pediatric Coma Scale should be used for infants and small children.

Eye opening	**Points**
Spontaneous	4
To speech	3
To pain	2
No response	1

*From Beyda, DH, Director, Pediatric Intensive Care, Phoenix Children's Hospital.

Best motor response

Spontaneous	6
Localizes pain	5
Withdraws to pain	4
Flexion to pain (decorticate)	3
Extension to pain (decerebrate)	2
No response	1

Best verbal response (age >2 yr)*

Oriented	5
Confused	4
Inappropriate	3
Incomprehensible	2
No response	1

Best response to auditory/visual stimulus (age <2 yr)*

Social smile, orients to sound, follows objects	5
Cries, consolable	4
Inappropriate, persistent cry	3
Agitated/restless	2
No response	1
TOTAL	3-15

A score of 11 or less indicates that the patient most likely has a severe injury. *Coma* is defined as no response and no eye opening or a score of 7 or less.[5]

SECONDARY SURVEY

After the primary survey has been completed and appropriate therapeutic interventions have been accomplished, clinical personnel should continue on to the secondary survey, examining the patient very carefully and methodically from head to toe, checking for obvious injuries, deformities, impaled objects, bruises, bleeding, and complaints of pain. Ongoing monitoring of vital signs is imperative.

To perform an adequate assessment, the patient should be undressed. The patient should be kept warm with blankets or a heating shield or other heating device during the physical assessment and therapeutic/diagnostic interventions. A complete neurologic evaluation (including GCS) should be performed.[6]

Patient history

• Obtain prehospital history of scene, events, conditions, mechanism of injury, field physical assessment, and clinical data.
• Obtain list of prehospital treatments and interventions.
• Obtain past medical history, past surgical history, comorbidities, medications, allergies, and transfusion history.

---

*From Beyda, DH, Director, Pediatric Intensive Care, Phoenix Children's Hospital.

Head

• Observe for bruises, lacerations, and deformities.
• Palpate for deformities.

Face

• Observe for bruises, lacerations, deformities, asymmetry.
• Palpate for deformities and "step-offs."

Eyes

• Observe for injuries, foreign bodies, periorbital ecchymosis, hemorrhage, contact lenses, enucleation, extraocular movement.
• Check pupil size and reaction to light.
• Check visual acuity, if appropriate.
• Palpate orbital rims.

Nose

• Observe for injuries, foreign bodies, epistaxis, cerebrospinal fluid (CSF) rhinorrhea.
• Palpate for deformities.

Mouth

• Observe for injuries, foreign bodies, hemorrhage, missing or broken teeth, malocclusion of teeth.
• Palpate for foreign bodies, malocclusion of teeth.

Ears

• Observe for injuries, foreign bodies, CSF otorrhea, Battle's sign, hemotympanum.

Neck

• Observe for penetrating or soft tissue injuries, ecchymoses, distended jugular veins, deviated trachea.
• Palpate for deviated trachea, subcutaneous emphysema, cervical vertebrae deformity, pain response.
• Auscultate for bruits.

Chest

• Observe for injuries, impaled objects, ecchymoses, chest wall bruising, chest expansion, respiratory rate, rhythm and depth, use of accessory muscles of respiration, and work of breathing.
• Palpate for pain response, subcutaneous emphysema, deformities (sternum, clavicles, ribs).
• Auscultate for breath sounds, heart sounds.

Abdomen

- Observe for injuries, impaled objects, ecchymoses, evisceration, distention, scars.
- Auscultate for bowel sounds.
- Palpate for pain response, guarding, rigidity.

Pelvis and genitalia

- Observe for injuries, bleeding, priapism.
- Palpate for pelvic instability.
- Check rectal sphincter tone.
- Note pain and/or urge to void but inability to complete act.

Table 15-1   Trauma Score

	Points
Respiratory rate	
10-24/min	4
25-35/min	3
36/min or greater	2
1-9/min	1
0	0
Respiratory effort	
Normal	1
Shallow, retracted, none	0
Blood pressure (systolic)	
≥90 mmHg	4
70-89 mmHg	3
50-69 mmHg	2
1-49 mmHg	1
0	0
Capillary refill	
<2 sec Normal	2
Delayed	1
None	0
Glasgow Coma Scale (Score)	
14-15	5
11-13	4
8-10	3
5-7	2
3-4	1
TOTAL =	

Table 15-2 Revised Trauma Score

Area of measurement	Coded value
Systolic blood pressure (mmHg)	
>89	4
76-89	3
50-75	2
1-49	1
0	0
Respiratory rate (spontaneous inspirations/minute)*	
10-29	4
>29	3
6-9	2
1-5	1
0	0
Glasgow Coma Scale Score	
13-15	4
9-12	3
6-8	2
4-5	1
3	0
Total possible points	**0-12**

The probabilities of survival for patients with various revised trauma scores are the following:

Score	Survivors (percent)
12	99.5%
11	96.9%
10	87.9%
9	76.6%
8	66.7%
7	63.6%
6	63.0%
5	45.5%
3–4	33.3%
2	28.6%
1	25.0%
0	3.7%

*Patient initiated, not artificial ventilations.

Lower extremities

- Observe for injuries, open wounds, deformities, edema, angulation.
- Palpate for crepitus, pain response, deformities, discolorations, pulses distal to injury, skin temperature, motor and sensory function, capillary refill.

Upper extremities

• Observe for injuries, open wounds, deformities, edema, angulation.
• Palpate for crepitus, pain response, deformities, discolorations, pulses distal to injury, skin temperature, motor and sensory function, capillary refill.

Posterior

• Patient's back must be inspected; patient should be logrolled, maintaining spinal alignment.
• Observe back, thorax, buttocks, and posterior legs for injuries, bruises, deformities, impaled objects, bleeding.
• Palpate for pain response, deformities.

It is important to assess and reassess the parameters of the primary survey throughout the secondary survey. After a secondary survey has been completed, the Trauma Score (Table 15-1) should be calculated and all findings documented. The revised Trauma Score measures the patient's physiologic response to injuries and includes the GCS, systolic blood pressure, and respiratory rate (Table 15-2).

REFERENCES

1. American College of Surgeons Committee on Trauma: *Advanced trauma life support instructor manual,* Chicago, 1993, American College of Surgeons.
2. Emergency Nurses Association: *Trauma nursing care course instructor manual,* Chicago, 1995, Emergency Nurses Association.
3. Johnson KL: Critical care of the trauma patient. In Neff JA, Kidd PS, editors: *Trauma nursing: the art and science,* St Louis, 1993, Mosby.
4. Thelan L and others: *Critical care nursing: diagnosis and management,* St Louis, 1994, Mosby.
5. Teasdale G, Jennett B: Assessment of coma and impaired consciousness, *Lancet ii* 81-84, 1974.
6. Champion HR, Sacco WJ, Copes WS, and others: A revision of the trauma score, *J Trauma* 29:623-629, 1989.

CHAPTER 16

Head Trauma

Nicki Gilboy

Head trauma is responsible for approximately half of all trauma-related deaths. In the United States, the incidence of head injury is approximately 200 per 100,000 people each year. The highest injury rate occurs in males between the ages of 15 and 30. Each year, approximately 120,000 head injuries are classified as severe (i.e., Glasgow Coma Score [GCS] of 9 or less); half of these individuals die before reaching a hospital. The three most common mechanisms of injury are motor vehicle crashes, falls, and assaults.[1] Penetrating head trauma, usually caused by an assault, is a significant problem in the United States. The incidence is currently 12 per 100,000.[2]

ANATOMY OF HEAD

The brain is well protected by the hair, scalp, skull, meninges, and cerebrospinal fluid (Fig. 16-1).

The scalp itself is composed of five layers of tissue: skin, connective tissue, aponeurosa, ligaments, and periosteum.

The skull is a bony structure whose main purpose is to protect the brain. It is divided into four main areas: the frontal area, the parietal area, the occipital area, and the temporal areas. The skull is also divided into two major sections: the calvarium or cranial vault (which houses the brain) and the base (which provides an opening for the spinal cord to enter the cervical area).

Three meningeal layers provide protection (or padding) for both the brain and the spinal cord. From the surface of the brain outward, the layers are the pia mater, the arachnoid, and the dura mater. The pia mater is thin and mucuslike and adheres to the cortex of the brain. The arachnoid layer is thin, vascular, and spiderlike (hence the term *arachnoid*). The dura mater (Latin words translating as "tough mother") adheres to the inner surface of the skull. In the area where the dura mater forms the tentorial notch, the tissue is knifelike and can cause severe damage to the brain when there is anterior-posterior movement of the brain.

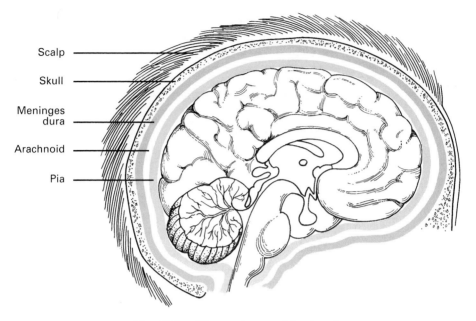

Fig. 16-1   The anatomy of the head.

The meningeal arteries are between the internal surface of the skull and the dura mater in an area known as the epidural (above the dura) space.

Cerebrospinal fluid

Cerebrospinal fluid (CSF) is produced in the ventricles of the brain and can be found in the subarachnoid space. CSF provides a cushion for both the brain and the spinal cord.

Brain

The body of the brain is a fluid-filled collection of very delicate tissues (Fig. 16-2) and water, which composes 80% to 85% of the cranial mass. The bulk of the brain is the cerebrum, which is divided into the right and left hemispheres. Each hemisphere is subdivided into four lobes: frontal, parietal, occipital, and temporal, named the same as the skull sections that are overlying.

The function of the frontal lobe is to conceptualize, think abstractly, and form judgments. When this lobe of the brain is injured, judgment and reasoning may become impaired and the patient may begin to shout out obscene and foul language. This is known as being *frontal lobish.*

The parietal lobe is the area in which the highest integration and coordination of perception and interpretation of sensory phenomena occur. Injury to this area of the brain may cause the patient to have difficulty with receptive communication.

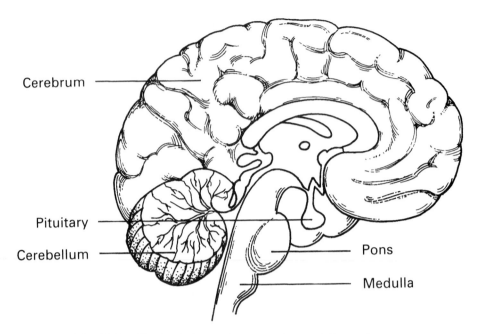

Fig. 16-2 The brain is a collection of very delicate tissues.

The occipital lobe is the area of the brain that is responsible for vision. Injury to this area of the brain may cause blurred vision, diplopia (double vision), or even blindness.

The temporal lobes (one is located on each side of the brain) resemble the thumbs of a boxing glove. These lobes are frequently injured because they are enclosed in relatively bony chambers. Injury to the temporal lobe or lobes may cause temporary or permanent memory loss.

The brain stem contains the reticular activating system and is responsible for consciousness. The medulla, which is the lower part of the brain stem, contains the cardiorespiratory centers.

The cerebellum is located next to the brain stem, under the cerebrum. It is responsible for movement and coordination. The area where the cerebrum and midbrain meet is the tentorial notch. The tentorial notch is formed by a separation of the dura mater and has extremely sharp edges; sudden contact with the brain may cause severe damage to the brain. This is also an area where there may be brain herniation.

Cranial nerves

There are 12 pairs of cranial nerves (Fig. 16-3).

Olfactory (I)

The olfactory nerve is responsible for the sense of smell. To test this nerve, the patient is instructed to close both eyes, occlude one nostril, and identify the

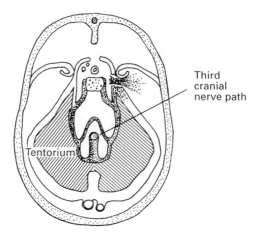

Fig. 16-3   The third cranial nerve path passes through the tentorium. Herniation of the brain through the tentorium will cause pressure on the nerve and a resulting fixed, dilated pupil, usually on the same side as the herniation.

odor from a common substance that has been placed under the open nostril. This procedure is repeated with the opposite nostril.

Optic (II)

The optic nerve controls visual acuity and the visual fields. Gross visual acuity is measured by instructing the patient to cover one eye and identify the number of fingers held up by the examiner. The procedure is repeated with the other eye.

Oculomotor (III), trochlear (IV), and abducens (VI)

The third, fourth, and sixth cranial nerves have much to do with the function and movement of the eye. They are tested by checking pupil size, shape, and reactivity to light. Extraocular movement can also be assessed by having the patient follow a moving finger with his or her eyes without moving the head: up, down, to the right, and to the left. The third cranial nerve (oculomotor) passes through the tentorial notch. Brain stem herniation causes pressure to be placed on this nerve and will cause pupil dilation on the ipsilateral (same) side as the herniation. Clinical personnel should be aware that a difference of 1 millimeter in pupil size may be a significant finding.

NOTE: Personnel should be sure that flashlight batteries are good and that the light used to test pupillary response is bright.

Trigeminal (V)

The trigeminal nerve controls facial sensation and jaw movement. It is tested by checking for facial sensation, strength of mastication muscles, and movement of the jaw.

Facial (VII)

The facial nerve controls facial expression and taste in the anterior two thirds of the tongue. It is tested by having the patient raise the eyebrows, close the eyelids tightly to resistance, show the teeth, smile, frown, and puff up the cheeks. If there is peripheral ipsilateral injury, both the upper and lower face will be involved. If there is a central injury, the brow of the contralateral (opposite side) will be spared.

Acoustic/auditory (VIII)

The eighth nerve is divided into two branches. The acoustic branch controls balance; it is tested by cold-water calorics. The auditory branch controls hearing; it is tested by acertaining the patient's response to a loud noise, such as a clap.

Glossopharyngeal (IX), vagus (X)

The glossopharyngeal and vagus nerves are usually evaluated together because of their close anatomic and functional relationships. The glossopharyngeal nerve controls taste in the posterior two thirds of the tongue and sensation in the nostrils and pharynx. The vagus nerve controls the soft palate, the pharynx and larynx muscles, the heart, the lungs, and the stomach. Both are tested by checking for the presence of a gag and a swallow reflex and by assessing the patient's ability to distinguish between salty and sweet tastes.

Accessory (XI)

The accessory nerve controls movement of the sternocleidomastoid and trapezius muscles. It is tested by asking the patient to turn his or her head against resistance or to shrug the shoulders.

NOTE: Before testing the accessory nerve, spinal cord injury or the potential for it must be ruled out.

Hypoglossal (XII)

The hypoglossal nerve controls movement of the tongue. It is tested by asking the patient to stick out the tongue. If the tongue is in midline, the nerve is considered to be intact.

RAPID NEUROLOGIC ASSESSMENT

When evaluating a patient with a head injury, the extent of the neurologic examination depends on the patient's level of consciousness. Patients who are awake, alert, and cooperative can have a detailed assessment performed; patients with a decreased level of consciousness will have a limited examination that includes GCS, pupils, reflexes, and vital signs. Reassessment should be performed at regular intervals.

Table 16-1   Glasgow Coma Scale (GCS)

Finding	Score
Eye opening	
Spontaneous	4
To voice	3
To pain	2
None	1
Best Verbal Response	
Oriented	5
Confused	4
Inappropriate words	3
Incomprehensible sounds	2
None	1
Best motor response	
Obeys commands	6
Purposeful movement (pain)	5
Withdraw (pain)	4
Flexion (pain)	3
Extension (pain)	2
None	1
POSSIBLE TOTAL SCORE	3-15

It is important to obtain a detailed history from the patient, bystanders, and prehospital personnel regarding the cause and mechanism of injury. Information about loss of consciousness, level of consciousness, and other events is the key.

Glasgow Coma Scale

The GCS has become a standard for objectively measuring the severity of a head injury (Table 16-1). Patients are assessed in three areas: eye opening, motor response, and verbal response. Clinical personnel should always use the patient's best score in each component. When testing motor response, the unaffected side of the body should be used if hemiplegia is present and the head or face if a spinal cord injury is present. A baseline score should be obtained before administering any medications. A neurologically intact patient would score the maximum possible score of 15. A patient with a score between 13 and 15 is classified as having no injury to having a mild head injury. A score between 9 and 12 indicates a moderate head injury. With a score of 8 or less, a severe injury is indicated. The lowest achievable score is 3 (i.e., one point in each area). The validity of the score depends on the absence of systemic abnormalities such as hypotension, hypoxia, hypothermia, hypoglycemia, and drugs that affect neurologic function.

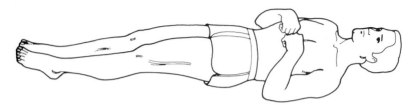

Fig. 16-4   Abnormal flexion (decorticate position).

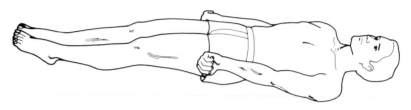

Fig. 16-5   Abnormal extension (decerebrate position).

DERM mneumonic

Components of the DERM mneumonic should be checked initially and then frequently thereafter (Table 16-2).

D = Depth of coma

• Give stimulus and note response.
    Verbal stimuli/painful stimuli
• Observe for flexion or extension.
    Abnormal flexion (decorticate posturing; Fig. 16-4): elbows are flexed, hands are pulled up toward the core; the lesion is higher in the brain stem, above the midbrain.
    Abnormal extension (decerebrate posturing; Fig. 16-5): elbows are in extension, wrists pointing downward, with hands clenched, rotating outward. The lesion is at the level of the brain stem, below the midbrain.

E = Eyes

• Check pupils for size in millimeters, accommodation, reactivity to light
    Check the eyes for any extraocular movement. Note that up to 20% of the population may have minor differences in pupil size (anisocoria) but that both pupils react to light.
• Normally, pupils constrict to light; if pupils are fixed and pinpoint, consider possible opiate use or pontine herniation.
• A pupil that is dilated and fixed unilaterally may indicate an early involvement of the third cranial nerve (Fig. 16-6). Be sure to rule out direct eye trauma, cataracts, or use of medications that can cause pupillary dilation.

Table 16-2 Assessing Brain Stem Function Using DERM Mnemonic

Brain stem	Herniation levels	D = Depth of coma	E = Eyes	R = Respirations	M = Motor function	Posturing
	None	Aware, alert, oriented	Equal and reactive	Eupnea	Normal	None
	Thalamus	Painful stimulus causes non-purposeful response	Small; reaction to light	Cheyne-Stokes respirations	Hyperactive deep tendon reflexes	Abnormal flexion (decorticate)
	Midbrain	Painful stimulus causes non-purposeful response	Midpoint to dilated; fixed; no reaction to light	Central neurogenic breathing	Decreased deep tendon reflexes	Abnormal extension (decerebrate)
	Pons and cerebellum	Painful stimulus causes no response	Pinpoint; fixed; no reaction to light	Biot's respirations	Flaccid	No tone
	Medulla	Painful stimulus causes no response	Midpoint to dilated; fixed; no reaction to light	Ataxia; apneusis	Flaccid	No tone

(From Budassi SA, Barber J: *Mosby's manual of emergency care*, ed 3, St Louis, 1989, Mosby)

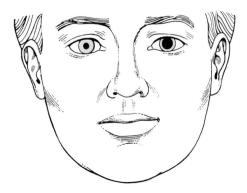

Fig. 16-6   Unilateral fixed, dilated pupil suggests early third nerve involvement.

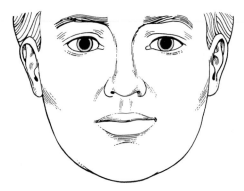

Fig. 16-7   Bilateral fixed, dilated pupils indicate complete third nerve involvement.

- Bilateral fixed dilated pupils are indicative of complete third cranial nerve involvement (Fig. 16-7).
- Ptosis is also indicative of third cranial nerve involvement. Horner's syndrome is a neurologic condition in which the patient demonstrates ptosis, miosis, and facial anhydrosis (Fig. 16-8).

R = Respirations

Pay close attention to respiratory rate, rhythm, and depth. (See Table 16-2 for types of respiratory rhythms.)

M = Motor/movement

- Assess each limb individually by major muscle groups, grading from 0 to 5:
  - 0 = no motor function
  - 1 = slight motion/flicker
  - 2 = moves if gravity is neutralized

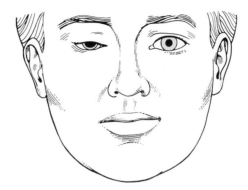

Fig. 16-8   Ptosis also indicates third nerve involvement.

3 = moves against gravity
4 = strength diminished
5 = normal function
• Note any abnormal position of the limbs at rest.
    If reflexes are hypoactive or there are none, there is a possibility of cerebellar involvement or peripheral nerve or horn cell disease.
    An upper extremity drift is a sensitive test of subtle proximal weakness.

Brain herniation

Herniation occurs when the brain protrudes through the tentorial notch and/or the foramen magnum, causing severe, permanent, neurologic deficits and alteration in cardiorespiratory function. Brain herniation is a result of increased intracranial pressure from an expanding hematoma or cerebral edema pushing the brain tissue toward the path of least resistance. There are two types of herniation:

Transtentorial (uncal) herniation

A transtentorial herniation occurs when pressure on the lateral middle fossa or the temporal lobe causes the inner edge (basal edge) of the uncus and hippocampal gyrus to be pushed toward the midline and into the lateral edge of the tentorial notch. This movement causes pressure to build at the tentorial notch and pushes the midbrain into the opposite side of the tentorial notch. As a result, the third cranial nerve (oculomotor nerve) and the posterior cerebral artery may become caught between the part of the uncus that has herniated and the edge of the tentorial notch.
    Early signs of transtentorial herniation are:
D = Depth of coma/decreased level of consciousness
E = Eyes/ipsilateral dilated pupil
R = Respirations/Cheyne-Stokes respirations
M = Motor and movement/contralateral hemiparesis and positive Babinski's reflex

Late signs of transtentorial herniation are:
D = Depth of coma/severely decreased level of consciousness
E = Eyes/midpoint and fixed pupils bilaterally
R = Respirations/central neurogenic breathing
M = Motor and movement/abnormal extension (decerebrate)

Central herniation (rostral-caudal deterioration)

When intracranial pressure is extremely high and uniformly distributed throughout the brain, the brain is forced downward and the cerebellar tonsils herniate through the foramen magnum. As this occurs, the medulla is compressed.

Early signs of central herniation are:
D = Depth of coma/restlessness to lethargy
E = Eyes/pupils equal and reactive but constricted
R = Respirations/Cheyne-Stokes breathing with yawns and sighs that deteriorate to central neurogenic breathing
M = Motor and movement/contralateral hemiparesis
Late signs and symptoms of central herniation are:
D = Depth of coma/severely altered level of consciousness
E = Eyes/nonreactive, midposition pupils
R = Respirations/central neurogenic breathing deteriorating to ataxic breathing
M = Motor and movement/posturing that deteriorates from abnormal flexion (decorticate) to abnormal extension (decerebrate)

REFLEXES

Pupil reflex

The pupils are compared to one another for size and reactivity. Normal pupils will constrict when the eyes are exposed to a bright light. Light that is shone into one pupil will cause the other pupil to constrict. If pupils are fixed and pinpoint size, opiate use or pons involvement is indicated. A unilateral, fixed, dilated pupil is indicative of early third cranial nerve involvement. Bilateral, fixed, dilated pupils usually indicate complete third cranial nerve involvement. Ptosis may also indicate third cranial nerve involvement.

Corneal reflex

When the cornea is stimulated by lightly brushing a piece of cotton across it, the normal response is to blink. No response indicates abnormality. Testing the corneal reflex provides information on the functioning of cranial nerves V and VII.

Gag reflex

The gag reflex is normally intact when stimulated. Loss of this reflex indicates abnormality (cranial nerves IX and X).

Deep tendon reflexes

Hypoactive or absence of deep tendon reflexes indicates that there may be cerebellar involvement, peripheral nerve disease, or anterior horn cell disease. Hyperactivity indicates pyramidal tract lesions or psychogenic disorders.

Deep tendon reflexes are scored from 0 to 4:

0 = absent
1 = decreased
2 = normal
3 = increased
4 = hyperactive

Babinski's sign or reflex

Babinski's sign or reflex is elicited by performing a cutaneous stimulation of the plantar surface of the foot. Normally, the toes flex. An abnormal response *positive Babinski,* occurs when the great toe points cephalad (toward the head, to where the problem is) and the other toes fan out.

DIAGNOSTIC TESTS

Many diagnostic tests can be employed when assessing the patient with a head injury. The more commonly used ones are presented in the following paragraphs. Clinical personnel should remember that some are more beneficial than others.

Computed tomography

Computed tomography (CT) can accurately detect 98% of intracranial injuries. It should be considered early when the patient has an altered level of consciousness, hemiparesis, or any type of aphasia.

Skull x-rays

Skull x-rays are no longer used as a routine diagnostic test, although they may be useful in evaluating penetrating injuries, intracranial foreign bodies, and the presence of old fractures.

Angiography

Angiography is used when a vascular injury is suspected. Radiopaque contrast is injected and serial images are obtained to visualize the blood vessels and cerebral circulation.

Nuclear magnetic resonance imaging

Nuclear magnetic resonance imaging (MRI) is not very useful in acute trauma situations because the procedure is time-consuming, the patient must be absolutely still, and access to the patient is limited during the procedure. MRI may, however, be useful in nonacute stages of trauma. MRI is particularly good at identifying soft tissue injuries, such as diffuse axonal injuries (shear injuries).

HEAD INJURIES

The concept of primary and secondary brain injury has become well accepted. The primary injury results from the initial insult. The secondary brain injury occurs after the primary injury and may lead to further tissue damage. Secondary injuries are a result of physiologic events like hypoxia, hypotension, cerebral edema, and increased intracranial pressure. Optimal initial management of the head-injured patient will decrease the chance of secondary brain injury and therefore decrease morbidity and mortality.

Primary head injuries can be broken down into scalp lacerations, skull fractures, and focal and diffuse brain injuries. With focal injuries, the damage is limited to a well-defined area and is the direct result of trauma to the tissues. Diffuse injuries produce damage throughout the brain resulting from widespread shearing and rotational forces. A general summary of therapeutic interventions is contained on pp. 207-208. Specific interventions are discussed with each injury.

Scalp laceration

The most frequently seen type of head injury is a scalp laceration. It is a common injury in children because their heads are large in relation to their bodies, they are relatively clumsy, and they have high activity levels. A scalp laceration can be caused by any blunt or penetrating force to the head. The scalp is extremely vascular, and a significant amount of blood can be lost from a scalp laceration.

ASSESSMENT

- Observe for profuse bleeding.
- Carefully examine the scalp with a gloved hand. Sometimes scalp lacerations are missed if hair is thick and bleeding is minimal.
- Check for concurrent neurologic injury.
- Check for other associated injuries.

DIAGNOSIS

- Observation of the laceration

THERAPEUTIC INTERVENTIONS

- Control bleeding.
  Direct pressure
  Ice
- Clip hair around laceration for better visualization, but do not shave

- Irrigate the wound with sterile normal saline.
- Inspect and palpate the wound.
- Devitalized tissue should be débrided. If bone fragments are present, a neurosurgical consultation is needed.
- The scalp should be sutured in layers. Closure of galea first with 2-0 or 3-0 absorbable suture; nylon or Prolene suture for the skin; skin staples may also be considered.
- Wound may be left open to air or covered with a small sterile dressing, depending on practitioner preference.
- Assure tetanus prophylaxis.
- Provide the patient with verbal and written discharge instructions for wound care and closed head injury.

Skull fracture

Skull fracture is a common injury. The diagnosis of skull fracture may be made by physical findings or x-rays. If a skull fracture is present, neurosurgical consultation should occur.

The patient's skull should be examined for bumps, defects, lacerations of the scalp, and bruises. In addition, neurologic status should be monitored. If the injury overlies the sinuses, profuse bleeding may occur. Also, the possibility of associated cervical spine injury and facial fractures should always be suspected and appropriate precautions taken.

Although large forces are necessary to produce a skull fracture, the extent of underlying brain injury varies. Because a skull fracture indicates significant trauma, a thorough assessment is necessary. Patients with a basilar skull fracture should also be observed for the presence of a CSF leak.

Linear/nondisplaced skull fracture

A linear/nondisplaced fracture is a fracture line in the skull that passes through its entire thickness. These fractures are not usually significant unless there are associated focal signs indicating underlying structural damage. These fractures are usually caused by a significant blow to the skull.

ASSESSMENT
- Difficult to palpate these fractures
- Seen on skull x-rays (if obtained)

THERAPEUTIC INTERVENTIONS
- Usually no specific therapeutic intervention is required.
- Discharge instructions should include observation for signs and symptoms of a more severe head injury.
- If the fracture is across a vascular groove or a suture line, consider observation for 24 hours and neurosurgical consultation.

Depressed skull fracture

A depressed skull fracture is an actual depression of a fragment or fragments of the skull. Great care should be taken for close observation of the presence or formation of an intracranial injury.

ASSESSMENT

- Patient may be unconscious, unresponsive, and not breathing adequately.
- Palpate the skull depression gently.
- Verify the depressed fracture on x-ray or CT scan.

THERAPEUTIC INTERVENTIONS

For closed depression:
- Neurosurgical consultation
- Hospital admission for close observation
- For depression greater than 5 mm, surgical intervention to elevate depressed segment

For open injury:
- Sterile wet-to-dry dressing over wound
- Neurosurgical consultation
- Surgical intervention to débride and elevate depressed segment
- Antibiotics
- Tetanus prophylaxis

Basilar skull fracture

A basilar skull fracture is a fracture at the base of the skull that may be difficult to diagnose because it is not readily visible on routine skull x-rays. This fracture could cause a CSF leak, which will usually close spontaneously.

ASSESSMENT

- Presence of intracranial air or opaque sphenoid sinuses
- Possibly seen on a Waters' view (open-mouth) x-ray
- Possibly seen on CT
- Patient may complain of severe headache
- Periorbital ecchymosis (Fig. 16-9), also known as *raccoon eyes* or *owl eyes;* this type of intraorbital bleeding usually seen with cribriform plate fracture or intraorbital root fracture
- Battle's sign (Fig. 16-10), an ecchymosis behind ear in mastoid region that usually occurs 12 to 24 hours after injury
- Hemotympanum (blood behind the tympanic membrane), usually caused by fracture of temporal bone
- Patient complaint of salty taste at back of throat (CSF leak)
- Possible CSF otorrhea or CSF rhinorrhea

    To test for this condition, drop some of the CSF drainage onto a filter paper. It may produce a finding known as a *ring sign,* a *halo,* or a *target sign,*

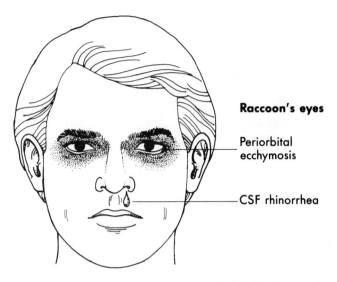

Raccoon's eyes

Periorbital
ecchymosis

CSF rhinorrhea

Fig. 16-9   Basilar skull fracture: periorbital ecchymosis.

where blood forms a central circle and CSF dissipates outward, forming a ring around the blood (Fig. 16-11). This drainage may also be tested for the presence of glucose. The CSF glucose level is approximately 25 mg.

THERAPEUTIC INTERVENTIONS ▐▬▬▬▬▬▬▬▬▬▬▬▬▬▬▬▬▬▬

- Admit patient for close observation.
- Avoid straining, which might exacerbate drainage (coughing, blowing nose, etc.).
- Monitor drainage.
- Assure tetanus prophylaxis.
- Consider antibiotics.

FOCAL INJURIES

Focal injuries account for about half of all head injuries. With this type of injury there is damage to a specific, well-defined area.

Contusion

A contusion is a bruise on the cortex of the brain, causing tissue alteration and neurologic deficit without hematoma formation (Fig. 16-12). There is a significant alteration in consciousness without localizing signs. Contusion is usually caused by a severe acceleration/deceleration force or a severe blunt trauma to the head.

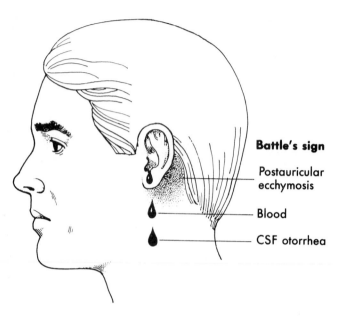

Battle's sign

Postauricular
ecchymosis

Blood

CSF otorrhea

Fig. 16-10   Basilar skull fracture: battle's sign.

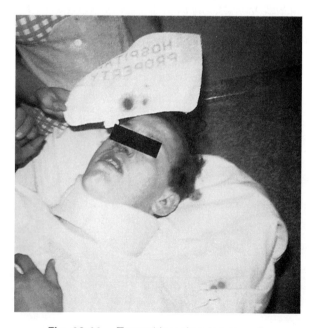

Fig. 16-11   Target/ring sign (on towel).

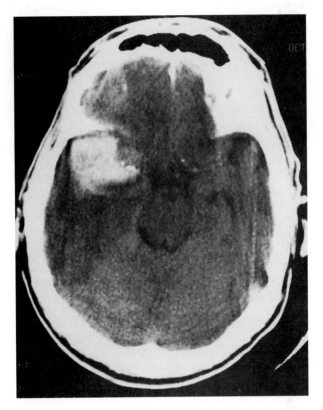

Fig. 16-12   CT: Contusion. (Courtesy of Laurence Cromwell, MD, Department of Radiology, Dartmouth-Hitchcock Medical Center.)

ASSESSMENT

- Decreased level of consciousness
- Loss of consciousness longer than 5 minutes
- Nausea and vomiting
- Hemiparesis
- Confusion or restlessness
- Speech difficulties
- Seizures

DIAGNOSIS

- History for event
- Clinical observation
- CT scan

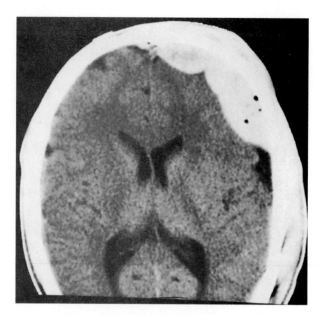

Fig. 16-13   CT: Acute epidural hematoma. (Courtesy of Laurence Cromwell, MD, Department of Radiology, Dartmouth-Hitchcock Medical Center.)

THERAPEUTIC INTERVENTIONS ▬▬▬▬▬▬▬▬▬▬▬▬▬▬▬▬▬▬▬▬▬▬▬

• Admit for close observation.
• Administer antiemetics as prescribed.
• Administer IV fluids judiciously, to avoid fluid overload.

Intracranial hemorrhage/hematoma

An intracranial hemorrhage is bleeding between the skull and the meningeal layers or within the brain tissue itself. In all cases of head trauma, clinical personnel should observe the patient carefully for associated injuries.

Acute epidural hematoma

An epidural hematoma (below the skull and above the dura mater in the epidural space) is usually arterial in origin (Fig. 16-13). Epidural bleeding is a rare type of intracranial hemorrhage that occurs in about 1% to 2% of all people with head injuries. It usually results from rupture of the middle meningeal artery or from a tear of the dural sinus. Death may be rapid because of the nature of the bleeding (arterial) causing an uncal herniation. It may be seen with a skull fracture in the temporal or parietal region near the middle meningeal artery. Many patients, however, will have no evidence of a skull fracture. The mortality is 25% to 50%; there is an equally high rate of morbidity.

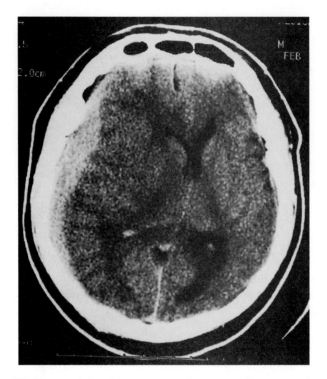

Fig. 16-14 CT: Acute subdural hematoma. (Courtesy of Laurence Cromwell, MD, Department of Radiology, Dartmouth-Hitchcock Medical Center.)

ASSESSMENT

- Possibly loss of consciousness, followed by lucid interval, followed by another period of unconsciousness
- In conscious patient, complaint of severe headache or contralateral hemiparesis
- Possibly fixed, dilated pupil on ipsilateral side as hemorrhage
- Seizures
- Bradycardia
- Systolic hypertension

Acute subdural hematoma

A subdural hematoma results from bleeding between the dura and the arachnoid layers of the meninges, usually caused by a torn bridging vein or cortical artery (Fig. 16-14). It is usually venous and may be life-threatening. It is the most frequently seen type of intracranial bleeding. It may occur instantly (acute) or may develop over a period of days to weeks (subacute or chronic), and it usually results from a severe trauma to the head. Bleeding will usually be gradual, because the nature of the bleeding is venous. The brain is often extensively injured. If an acute subdural hemorrhage is detected in a child under 1 year of age, clinical personnel should suspect that the cause was severe shaking associated with child abuse. Elderly patients, chronic alcoholics, and those on anticoagulant therapy are at high risk, even with a minor injury.

The prognosis for a patient with acute subdural hematoma is poor, with a 60% to 80% mortality rate. Mortality usually results from the severe underlying brain injury and extensive cerebral edema. If this condition is not rapidly treated, it will result in transtentorial herniation and death. If bleeding is bilateral, a ventricular shift may not be evidenced on CT.

ASSESSMENT

- Decreased level of consciousness
- Hypertension, bradycardia
- Fixed, dilated pupil or pupils
- Decreased motor function
- Hemiparesis
- Hyperreflexia
- Positive Babinski's reflex
- Possibly febrile

DIAGNOSIS

- CT scan

THERAPEUTIC INTERVENTIONS

- Surgical evacuation
- See summary on pp. 207-208.

Subarachnoid hemorrhage

A hemorrhage between the arachnoid and pia meningeal layers is known as a subarachnoid hemorrhage (Fig. 16-15). It may be the result of severe head trauma, severe hypertension, or a ruptured aneurysm. In head trauma, subarachnoid hemorrhage is often an incidental finding associated with other injuries. CSF will be bloody, and the patient will demonstrate signs of meningeal irritation.

ASSESSMENT

- Grand mal seizures
- Unconsciousness or restlessness
- Headache

DIAGNOSIS

- CT scan

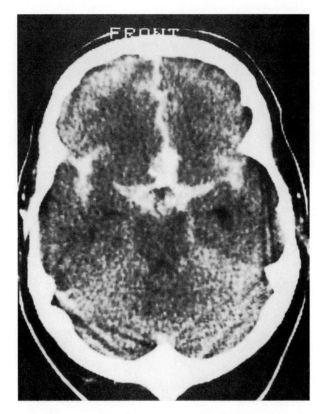

Fig. 16-15 CT: Subarachnoid hemorrhage. (Courtesy of Laurence Cromwell, MD, Department of Radiology, Dartmouth-Hitchcock Medical Center.)

THERAPEUTIC INTERVENTIONS

• See summary on pp. 207-208.

Intracerebral (brain) hemorrhage

An intracerebral hemorrhage is a hemorrhage in the brain tissue itself (Fig. 16-16). It may occur at any location in the brain. It may result from a penetrating injury and may be a result of a laceration, especially in the basilar area where the skull has bony prominences, or may be a diffuse injury. With a closed head injury, it is usually frontal or temporally located. Besides hemorrhage, there is usually an area of edema. Signs, symptoms, and prognosis will depend on the size and location of the hemorrhage.

ASSESSMENT

• Hemiparesis
• Visual disturbances

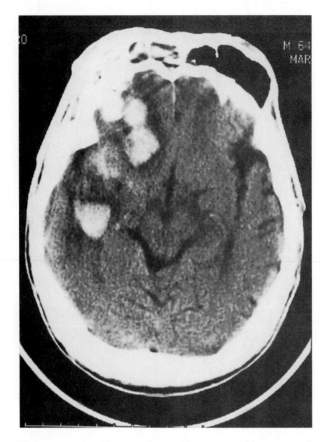

Fig. 16-16   CT: Intracerebral hemorrhage. (Courtesy of Laurence Cromwell, MD, Department of Radiology, Dartmouth-Hitchcock Medical Center.)

- Unconsciousness
- Other neurologic findings

DIAGNOSIS

- CT scan

THERAPEUTIC INTERVENTIONS

- Minimize cerebral edema
- See summary on pp. 207-208.

DIFFUSE INJURIES

Concussion

A concussion is a temporary disruption of the reticular activating system without structural defect and with possible microscopic bruising of the brain

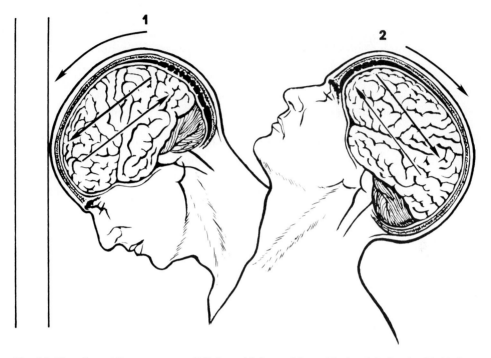

Fig. 16-17 Coup(1)-contre coup(2)injury. (Adapted from Thelan LA, Davie JK, Urden, LD: *Textbook of critical care nursing: diagnosis and management,* St Louis, 1990, Mosby.)

tissue (Fig. 16-17). The mechanism of injury is an acceleration/deceleration force or a direct blow, usually resulting from blunt trauma. Temporary loss of consciousness results from the disruption of the reticular activating system. The patient with a concussion will usually give a history of unconsciousness or memory loss for the event, followed by consciousness. The period of unconsciousness is usually short.

ASSESSMENT

- History of head trauma
- Temporary amnesia for the event
- Complaint of headache
- Dizziness
- Nausea and vomiting
- Other neurologic deficits
- Identification of associated injuries

DIAGNOSIS

- History of event
- Clinical observation
- CT scan to rule out more serious injury

- Admit for observation if the loss of consciousness is more than 5 minutes or if the patient is less than 12 years old. Otherwise, the patient may be sent home with careful aftercare instructions if there is someone reliable who can stay with the patient.
- Administer antiemetics, as required and prescribed
- Administer nonnarcotic/nonaspirin analgesics, as prescribed

Diffuse axonal injury (shear injury)

Diffuse axonal injury, also known as shear injury, is a tearing or shearing of axonal nerve fibers that results in diffuse brain damage. Coma usually occurs immediately and lasts for a prolonged period. The coma results from extensive damage to the white matter of the brain. Diffuse axonal injury has a high mortality rate, and the majority of survivors have major residual disabilities.[3]

ASSESSMENT

- History of head trauma with immediate decrease in level of consciousness
- Decerebrate/decorticate posturing
- Hypertension
- Hyperthermia
- Excessive sweating

DIAGNOSIS

- History
- Clinical observation
- MRI

THERAPEUTIC INTERVENTIONS

- Assure airway, breathing, and circulation
- Prevent secondary injury
- See summary on pp. 207-208.

PENETRATING HEAD INJURIES

The incidence of penetrating head injuries is increasing. An impaled object, knife, or missile projected into the skull and cranial vault may or may not cause severe injury, depending on the type and velocity of the object causing the injury. The most common types of missile wounds are caused by guns and bullets. These wounds are particularly devastating because the structural brain damage is extensive. The amount of damage will depend on the site of the wound and the caliber, velocity, and angle of yaw of the missile. Lacerations, contusions, and destruction of tissue may occur from the missile itself or as a result of the energy dissipated by the missile.

ASSESSMENT

- ABCs
- Neurologic survey
- Examination for entrance and exit wounds
- Observation for associated injuries

DIAGNOSIS

- Observation
- X-rays
- CT scan

THERAPEUTIC INTERVENTIONS

- Maintain cervical spine alignment.
- Prevent movement.
- Do not remove the impaled object!
- Secure the impaled object.
- Control bleeding.
- Anticipate a neurosurgical consultation.
- Assure tetanus prophylaxis.
- Administer antibiotics, as prescribed.

SUMMARY OF THERAPEUTIC INTERVENTIONS FOR ALL PATIENTS WITH SEVERE HEAD INJURIES

The goal of therapeutic intervention is to adequately resuscitate the patient and prevent secondary injury resulting from hypoxia and hypovolemia. The initial priority, as in all trauma patients, is stabilization of airway, breathing, and circulation.

- Secure the airway and assure cervical spine immobilization.
- Endotracheal intubation using rapid sequence technique is indicated in any patient with a GCS less than 9.[4]

  This is the safest method of managing the airway for these patients. The drugs used for intubation should not adversely affect intracranial pressure or cerebral perfusion pressure. Induction agents that meet these criteria include thiopental, etomidate, and fentanyl. For paralysis, succinylcholine is frequently used, preceded by a dose of a nondepolarizing agent to prevent muscle fasciculations. Lidocaine 1.5 to 2.0 mg/kg IV push may be given 2 to 3 minutes before the succinylcholine to prevent an intracranial pressure surge during intubation.[4] Patients with a GCS over 9 should receive oxygen via a nonrebreather mask and be monitored for early signs of hypoxemia and hypoventilation.

- Obtain IV access and initiate fluid replacement to correct or prevent hypotension, maintaining mean arterial pressure greater than 90 mmHg.

  The goal is to maintain adequate cerebral perfusion pressure. IV fluids should be normal saline, lactated Ringer's, or packed red cells, and not D5W solution.

- Monitor neurologic status frequently; includes GCS, pupillary response, depth of coma, and vital signs.
- The use of prophylactic hyperventilation (pCO_2 <35 mmHg) is no longer recommended.

  In fact, it should be avoided during the first 24 hours after injury.[5] Hyperventilation decreases intracranial pressure by causing cerebral vasoconstriction and subsequent decrease in cerebral blood flow. Cerebral blood flow during the first day postinjury is less than half that of normal individuals; thus routine hyperventilation can further compromise cerebral perfusion and risk causing cerebral ischemia. Hyperventilation may be necessary for brief periods when there are signs of increased intracranial pressure and mannitol is unavailable, contraindicated (hypovolemia), or ineffective.[5]
- Mannitol, an osmotic diuretic, is recommended to reduce intracranial pressure.

  Mannitol has a plasma-expanding effect that decreases hematocrit, decreases blood viscosity, and increases cerebral blood flow and cerebral oxygen delivery. The maximum effect occurs 30 to 60 minutes after administration. It is more effective if administered in repeated boluses of 0.25 to 1.0 gm/kg. Loop diuretics such as furosemide (Lasix) have been used as an adjunct to mannitol; however, there is little research to support this use.[4] Also, steroids are no longer recommended for severe head injury.[5]
- Insert a urinary catheter and record intake and output.
- Maintain the patient's head in a midline position to assure unobstructed jugular venous return. Elevate the head of the stretcher 15 to 30 degrees if possible, to facilitate CSF drainage.
- Prevent agitation and combativeness, which may lead to increased intracranial pressure.

  Provide a quiet, low-stimulating environment. Consider intravenous sedation and/or pain medication. Short-acting neuromuscular blocking agents may also be needed to prevent uncontrolled movement and straining.
- Control seizure activity.

  For active seizures, diazepam (Valium) 2.5 to 5 mg or lorazepam (Ativan) 2 to 4 mg may be given intravenously and titrated to effect. Phenytoin (Dilantin) 18 mg/kg is administered for acute prophylaxis. Fosphenytoin (Cerebyx) may be used instead. Prophylactic use of anticonvulsants is not recommended for the prevention of late posttraumatic seizures.[5]
- For patients with signs of increasing intracranial pressure, intracranial pressure monitoring will be needed and may be initiated in some Emergency Departments.

  The ventricular catheter is the recommended monitoring modality. For the patient with increased intracranial pressure and a ventricular catheter, drainage of CSF should be employed as the first treatment option.[5]
- Antibiotics are given to reduce the risk of infection in patients with open injuries.
- Consider transfer to a facility that can provide more definitive care.

REFERENCES

1. Olshaker JS, Whye DW: Head trauma, *Emerg Med Clin North Am* 11(1):165-186, 1993.
2. Ward DJ, Chisholm AH, Prince VT, and others: Penetrating head injury, *Crit Care Nurs Q* 17(1):78-89, 1994.
3. Hilton G: Diffuse axonal injury, *J Trauma Nurs* 2(1):7-14, 1995.
4. Zink BJ: Traumatic brain injury, *Emerg Med Clin North Am* 14(1):115-150, 1996.
5. *Guidelines for the management of severe head injury,* New York, 1995, Brain Trauma Foundation.

SUGGESTED READINGS

American College of Surgeons Committee on Trauma: *Advanced trauma life support instructor manual,* Chicago, 1993, American College of Surgeons.

Emergency Nurses Association: *Trauma nursing core course instructor manual,* Park Ridge Il, 1995, Emergency Nurses Association.

Howard PK: Head trauma. In Newberry L, editor: *Sheehy's emergency nursing principles and practice,* ed 4, St Louis, 1998, Mosby.

Mitchell PH: Central nervous system I: closed head injuries. In Cardona VD, Hurn PD, Mason PJB, and others: *Trauma nursing from resuscitation through rehabilitation,* ed 2, Philadelphia, 1994, Saunders.

Teasdale G, Jennett B: Assessment of coma and impaired consciousness: a practical scale, *Lancet* 2(81):1974.

Tintinalli J, and others: *Emergency medicine: a comprehensive study guide,* New York, 1996, McGraw Hill.

CHAPTER 17

Spine and Spinal Cord Trauma

Janet L. Orf

Spine and spinal cord injuries are serious. A spinal cord injury (SCI) with the resultant neurologic deficit is a catastrophic injury leading to enormous physical, psychologic, social, and economic challenges for the patient, the affected family, and society. Although, in comparison to other injuries, the incidence of spinal cord trauma is relatively low, it is estimated that approximately 10,000 people are injured in the United States each year. Spinal cord injuries occur most often in males (80%) with the majority of injuries (60%) happening between the ages of 16 and 30. Most SCI is associated with motor vehicle crashes. Falls, sports injuries, and assaults account for the remaining cases.[1]

Morbidity and mortality rates continue to improve for SCI patients. Factors that affect survival include the level of the spinal cord lesion, the extent of the paralysis, the age of the patient at the time of injury, and the ability to survive the first few months after injury. Although mortality continues to decrease, a recent study determined that the 1-year survival rate for a group of ventilator-dependent SCI individuals was only 25.4%.[2] The leading cause of death after SCI injury continues to be respiratory complications, particularly pneumonia. Quadriplegic patients face a lifetime of complications, primarily those related to infection, respiratory compromise, and complications from decreased mobility. Despite its low incidence, SCI remains a high-cost disability, with aggregate U.S. costs for 1 year exceeding $5.6 billion.[3]

ANATOMIC CONSIDERATIONS

The function of the spinal column is to protect the spinal cord and provide vertical stability for walking. The spinal column is made up of 7 cervical, 12 thoracic, 5 lumbar, 5 fused sacral, and 4 fused coccygeal vertebrae (Fig. 17-1). Although most of the vertebrae have similar structures, the first two are unique. The atlas, or C1, is a ringlike structure that articulates with the

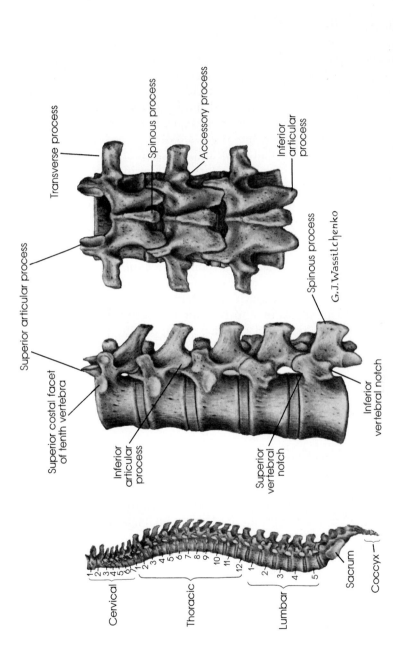

Fig. 17-1 Vertebral column and anatomic structure of vertebrae (From Rudy EB: *Advanced neurological and neurosurgical nursing,* St Louis, 1984, Mosby.).

occiput and assists in providing for normal flexion and extension of the neck. The axis, or C2, articulates at the odontoid process with C1 and provides for some of the normal rotation of the head (Fig. 17-2).

The spinal cord is a cylindric structure that passes through the bony spinal column. It begins at the level of the foramen magnum and ends at the lumbar vertebra 1 or 2. The cord is covered by the meningeal layers of dura, arachnoid, and pia mater and is protected by the meninges, vertebrae, and paravertebral muscles. Cerebrospinal fluid provides a cushioning effect for the spinal cord and provides a nutrient-rich environment for nerve function. Spinal nerves, of which there are 31 pairs, exit the spinal cord bilaterally and consist of a ventral root (anterior) and dorsal root (posterior). The spinal nerves provide pathways for involuntary reactions in response to stimulation. The dorsal root is responsible for the transmission of sensory impulses. The ventral root transmits motor impulses. Therefore each nerve is responsible for both motor and sensory function. For example, the first cervical nerve supplies the sensory region of the occiput and is also partially responsible for motor function of the sternocleidomastoid muscle. The fourth cervical nerve involves sensation in the neck and shoulder region and is also partially responsible for diaphragmatic contraction. The thoracic nerves innervate portions of the upper arm, epigastrium, abdomen, and buttocks. Lumbar nerves are responsible for sensation and function of the lower extremities and also innervate the groin region. Sacral nerves supply the perianal muscles that control bowel and bladder function. The term *sacral sparing* refers to preservation of S3, S4, and S5 function. This is important since preservation of distal function indicates an incomplete injury and is associated with a more favorable prognosis.

MECHANISM OF INJURY

Injury to the spinal cord and bony vertebrae can occur by a variety of mechanisms (Fig. 17-3). The predominant mechanisms of force are as follows:

- Hyperextension: forcing the head posteriorly beyond normal limits, causing tension to the anterior longitudinal ligaments and compression of the posterior elements.
- Compression (Axial Loading): the transmission of force in line with a straightened vertebral column.
- Flexion: forcing the head anteriorly beyond normal limits, causing compression of the bodies and discs anteriorly and disruption of the posterior ligaments and/or a posterior fracture.
- Distraction: separation of the surfaces of the joint, resulting in a malalignment of the vertebrae.
- Lateral Bending: bending of the head and neck to one or both sides beyond normal limits.

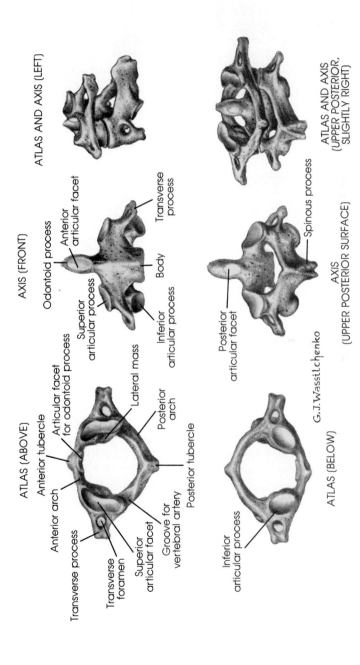

Fig. 17-2 Atlas and axis vertebrae (From Ruby EB: *Advanced neurological and neurosurgical nursing*, St Louis, 1984, Mosby.).

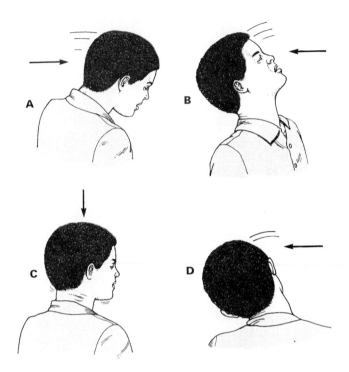

Fig. 17-3 Injuries of the vertebrae and spinal cord may be caused by a variety of mechanisms of injury, forcing the head and neck into unusual positions. **A,** Hyperflexion; **B,** hyperextension; **C,** axial loading; **D,** lateral bending.

SPINE INJURIES

Injuries can occur to the bony vertebrae from fracture, dislocation, and subluxation. Fractures are generally classified as simple, comminuted, teardrop, and compression. Fractures that involve C1 or C2 have the following special names:

- Simple Fracture: usually occurs without neurologic compromise and affects spinous or transverse processes, pedicles, or facets.
- Compression Fracture: occurs when a vertebral body is compressed, usually secondary to a hyperflexion injury.
- Burst Fracture/Comminuted Fracture: a shattering of the vertebral body. Since bone may be driven into the spinal cord, these fractures are more likely to result in neurologic compromise. Often comminuted fractures result from axial loading in which the patient sustains a blow to the top of the head.
- Jefferson Fracture: A burst fracture of C1; this fracture may not result in any neurologic deficit, but will require surgical intervention and stabilization.

- Hangman's Fracture: a fracture through the arch of C1; named after the fractures characteristically found after a judicial hanging.
- Odontoid Fracture: involves the odontoid process of C2, also known as the *dens.*
- Dislocation: dislocation of a vertebra occurs when one vertebra overrides another and is characterized by unilateral or bilateral facet dislocation. Atlanto-occipital dislocations are produced by an avulsion of the atlas from the occiput and usually result in immediate death. Fractures can occur in association with dislocations, and in these serious injuries SCI is usually present.
- Subluxation: occurs when there is partial or incomplete dislocation of one vertebra over another. Subluxed vertebra often require placement of the patient into cervical tongs and weights to realign the vertebrae.

ASSESSMENT

- Assess the ABCs.
- Palpate the entire spinal column, and check for pain, tenderness, deformity, and edema.
- Assess all four extremities for motor strength and weakness.
- Test for sensation of touch, pain, and proprioception. Note any areas of altered sensation.

DIAGNOSIS

- Clinical findings.
- Radiographic studies: Initial assessment begins with the lateral cervical spine film that must include all seven cervical vertebrae and the C7-T1 junction (Fig. 17-4). In addition, anteroposterior and odontoid views should be obtained. Anteroposterior views may best visualize injuries to the pedicles and facets; an odontoid, or open-mouth, view may best reveal fractures of the dens. If questions still exist regarding the stability of the cervical spine, CT scans or flexion-extension films may be performed. Flexion-extension views assist in identifying ligament damage. They are contraindicated in the patient in whom subluxation is identified in routine films, in patients with neurologic deficit, and in those not alert enough to cooperate during the test. Flexion-extension films should be used with caution during the acute stage of injury when spasm may mask ligament injury. Magnetic resonance imaging (MRI) may assist in identifying soft-tissue abnormalities resulting from hemorrhage, contusion, or compression of the cord. Clearance of the cervical spine includes radiographic and clinical evaluation. Generally only patients who are completely alert, oriented, and cooperative; do not have distracting injuries; and have a completely normal neurologic examination will not require x-ray examinations. Patients with significant falls or jumps, or those with a suggestive mechanism of injury, should have thoracic and/or lumbar spine radiographs.

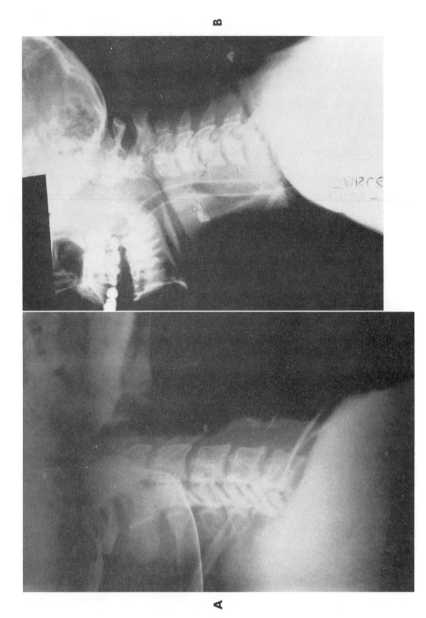

Fig. 17-4 **A,** Inadequate CTl film: visualizing only six cervical vertebrae is inadequate. One must be able to visualize all seven cervical vertebrae. **B,** All seven cervical vertebrae can be seen here.

- Maintain spinal immobilization until a spinal column injury is ruled out.
- Note the time of placement on backboard and pad pressure points to prevent skin breakdown.
- Assist with definitive stabilization if needed.

SPINAL CORD INJURIES

Injury to the spinal cord can occur secondary to concussion, contusion, transection, or decreased perfusion secondary to blood vessel damage or hemodynamic instability. Neurologic injury to the cord is described as complete or incomplete.

Complete injury

Defined as loss of conscious motor and sensory function below the level of the injury. This loss is because of interruption of the ascending and descending nerve tracts below the level of the lesion. Approximately 40% of all SCI are complete. Complete SCI are often seen in patients with thoracic fractures and dislocations resulting from the small size of the thoracic spinal canal in relation to the spinal cord. Patients with complete injuries that persist for 24 hours may later regain some sensory or motor function; however, the degree of recovery is usually negligible. Patients who sustain L1 or L2 complete injuries may have substantial recovery of the nerves that control the rectal and bladder sphincters and lower extremities.

Incomplete injury

Reflects some sparing of the sensory and/or motor fibers below the lesion. Incomplete lesions reflect a partial interruption of spinal cord function, manifested by a mixed loss of sensory or motor function. The two most common incomplete cord lesions are the central cord syndrome and Brown-Séquard syndrome.

INCOMPLETE SYNDROMES

Central cord syndrome

Central cord syndrome results from injury to the central segments of the spinal cord in the cervical region (Fig. 17-5, *A*). It is commonly seen in spinal injury in elderly patients who have cervical spinal canal stenosis and is usually secondary to hyperextension. These patients present with a motor deficit that is greater in the arms than in the legs and is most pronounced in the hands. Sensory deficits vary, although greater sensory loss is often noted in the upper extremities. Bowel and bladder dysfunction also vary. Complete or partial recovery is possible, although residual neurologic dysfunction is common.

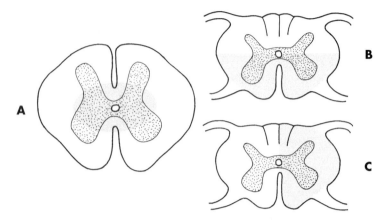

Fig. 17-5   A, Central cord syndrome. **B,** Anterior cord syndrome. **C,** Brown-Séquard syndrome.

Anterior cord syndrome

The anterior spinal cord syndrome most commonly occurs with cervical cord injuries secondary to flexion (Figure 17-5, *B*). Patients present with loss of motor, pain, and temperature sensation below the level of the injury while proprioception, sensory, and two-point discrimination remain intact.

Brown-Séquard syndrome

Brown-Séquard syndrome is most commonly seen after a penetrating injury to the spinal cord (Fig. 17-5, *C*). It is associated with a transverse hemisection of the spinal cord in which unilateral SCI occurs. The patient presents with loss of pain, sensation, and temperature opposite the side of injury (contralateral) and loss of motor function, proprioception, sensory, and two-point discrimination on the same side as the injury (ipsilateral).

KEY CONCEPTS

Management of the patient with a real or suspected SCI includes reduction of the existing neurologic deficit and prevention of any further loss of function. Spinal injury should be suspected in patients who have sustained significant trauma, have impaired level of consciousness after injury, complain of spinal pain, or present with motor or sensory impairment. The cervical spine is the most mobile portion of the spinal column and the most common site of SCI. If the cervical spine is unstable, it is at greater risk of causing SCI. Therefore complete spinal immobilization of the injured patient is a paramount consideration. The patient's entire spine should be immobilized during the prehospital phase and throughout the assessment and resuscitation phases. Turning these patients should be accomplished by logrolling while maintaining stabilization of the neck. Spinal cord injury patients are at enormously high risk of skin breakdown because of the lack of sensory warning mechanisms, the inability to move, and circulatory changes. Therefore immobilization time should be noted and efforts to reduce this time should be implemented. Stabilization devices may be placed in the Emergency Department by the neurosurgical team. Several devices may be used to place the spine in alignment and relieve compression. These devices generally consist of tongs or rings attached to weights. The amount of weight applied is determined by the location and type of injury. Rapid initiation or stabilization can relieve bony compression of the spinal cord and assist in maintaining spinal cord perfusion.

Respiratory compromise is a serious threat to the patient with a spinal cord injury. Cervical spine injuries have a high incidence of hypoxemia from hypoventilation. Hypoxemia can lead to further damage to the injured neurons and neuronal death. Patients who sustain an injury above the C4 level will have paralysis of the diaphragm and loss of phrenic nerve function. Patients with an injury below the C4 level may have respiratory compromise as a result of associated injuries, diaphragmatic or intercostal muscle paralysis, and/or aspiration. Patients with lesions in the upper cervical region may require early intubation and assisted ventilation. Increased cord edema, extension of injury, or fatigue may lead to respiratory compromise even in initially stable patients. The establishment of an airway in a patient with actual or potential SCI requires special consideration. Care must be taken not to manipulate the neck during establishment of the airway. Initially, a jaw thrust maneuver may be performed to open the airway. During intubation, an unstable cervical spine should be immobilized with manual immobilization. Complications from oral intubation are rare as long as manual, in-line stabilization is used. If available, fiberoptic bronchoscopy may be used.

Impairment of the sympathetic nervous system leads to loss of sympathetic innervation to the heart and loss of vasomotor tone, and may cause neurogenic shock. Vasodilatation leads to pooling of blood intravascularly and consequently hypotension. The loss of cardiac sympathetic tone leads to bradycardia. The combination of hypotension and bradycardia contributes to decreased spinal cord perfusion. This decrease in perfusion causes ischemia that can lead to further necrosis of the injured spinal cord segments. Therefore management of neurogenic shock includes treating initial hypotension with fluid replacement and early use of vasopressors to reverse the loss of vasomotor tone. The absence of vasoconstriction and loss of the ability to shiver, conserve heat, and sweat results in an inability to control internal body temperature. The SCI patient may exhibit poikilothermia, which is a condition in which the patient assumes the temperature of the environment.

The patient who has sustained an SCI requires extensive psychologic support. After SCI, many patients experience the same psychologic stages as those noted in a dying patient. Thus patients and families may exhibit denial during the early phases of care. Those who ask about prognosis may be told that the patient has a serious injury and that it is too early to predict the long-term outcome.

BOX 17-1

MUSCLE STRENGTH GRADING SYSTEM

5   Normal
4   Active movement through range of motion against resistance
3   Active movement through range of motion against gravity
2   Active movement through range of motion with gravity eliminated
1   Palpable or visible contraction
0   Total paralysis

ASSESSMENT

- Assess the airway for patency and for the presence of edema, blood, vomitus, or foreign material.
- Determine respiratory rate, depth of breathing, tidal volume, and use of accessory muscles.
- Check blood pressure, pulse, color, temperature, and skin moisture.
- Ascertain the mechanism of injury and the immediate history.
- Evaluate the entire spine for pain and tenderness.
- Evaluate motor strength and weakness utilizing the standard five-point grading system (Box 17-1).
- Assess sensory changes, including sensation to touch, pain, temperature, presence of paraesthesia, and proprioception. Begin at the area of no feeling, and progress to the area of sensation (Fig. 17-6).
- Evaluate rectal tone.
- Evaluate for the presence of other injuries.

NOTE: The strength of muscle groups of both upper and lower extremities should be systematically graded using a consistent scale to serve as a baseline for future neurologic assessment. When specifying the level of SCI, the accepted standard is to give the most caudal location with normal motor and sensory function.

DIAGNOSIS

- Clinical evaluation
- Radiographic studies, especially MRI
- Pulse oximetry
- Arterial blood gas

THERAPEUTIC INTERVENTIONS

- Provide and/or maintain neck and spine immobilization.
- Maintain a patent airway; if needed, open the airway using a jaw thrust maneuver and suction.
- Consider early intubation to reduce the effects of hypoxemia.

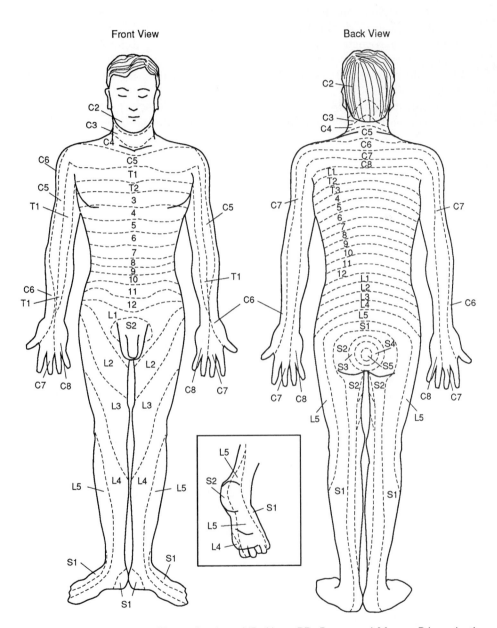

Fig. 17-6   Dermatomes (From Cardona VD, Hurn PD, Bastnagel Mason PJ, and others: *Trauma nursing from resuscitation through rehabilitation,* Philadelphia, 1994, Saunders.).

- Maintain a mean arterial pressure of 80 torr or greater.
- Place a urinary catheter, and monitor urinary output. (After SCI the bladder is areflexic-flaccid, and the patient will not be able to void.)
- Place a nasogastric or orogastric tube to prevent abdominal distention and emesis and to reduce respiratory compromises and the possibility of aspiration of gastric contents. (After SCI an acute paralytic ileus usually develops.)
- Administer methylprednisolone within 8 hours of SCI. Initial dose is a 30 mg/kg bolus over 15 minutes followed 45 minutes later by 5.4 mg/kg/hr for 23 hours.[4]
- Note time of placement on backboard and pad pressure points to prevent skin breakdown.
- Facilitate early neurosurgical consultation and more definitive stabilization.
- Provide psychologic support.
- Anticipate transfer to a Level I or II trauma center or spinal cord injury center.

NOTE: Recent evidence suggests that a 48-hour infusion of methylprednisolone in patients who receive their initial bolus more than 3 hours after injury may lead to improved outcome.[5]

Care of the SCI patient has improved dramatically over the past two decades. Future therapy will include improved pharmacologic interventions aimed at increased preservation of neurologic function and enhanced neural regeneration.

REFERENCES

1. Emergency Nurses Association: *Trauma nursing core course instructor manual,* ed 4, Park Ridge Il, 1995, Emergency Nurses Association.
2. DeVivo MJ, Ivie CS: Life expectancy of ventilatory-dependent persons with spinal cord injuries, *Chest* 108(1):226-232, 1995.
3. Berkowitz M: Assessing the socioeconomic impact of improved treatment of head and spinal cord injuries, *J Emerg Med* 11(Suppl 1):63-67, 1993.
4. Bracken MB, Shepard MJ, Collins WF, and others: A randomized, controlled trial of methylprednisolone or naloxone in the treatment of acute spinal-cord injury: results of the Second National Acute Spinal Cord Injury Study, *N Engl J Med* 322:1405-1411, 1990.
5. Bracken MB, Shepard MJ, Holford TR, and others: Administration of methylprednisolone for 24 or 48 hours or tirilazad mesylate for 48 hours in the treatment of acute spinal cord injury, *J Am Med Assoc* 277:1597-1604, 1997.

SUGGESTED READINGS

American College of Surgeons Committee on Trauma: *Advanced trauma life support manual,* Chicago, 1993, American College of Surgeon's Committee on Trauma.
Chiles BW, Cooper PR: Acute spinal injury, *N Engl J Med* 334:514-520, 1996.
Emergency Nurses Association: *Course in advanced trauma nursing: a conceptual approach,* Park Ridge Il, 1995, Emergency Nurses Association.

CHAPTER 18

Facial and EENT Trauma

Maureen Cullen

FACIAL INJURIES

Facial injuries may cause severe airway obstruction and may be a major cause of deformity. Soft tissue and bone structure damage to the face may result from motor vehicle crashes (Fig. 18-1), sports injuries, domestic violence, and other injuries that cause blunt and penetrating trauma to the face. Patients who suffer maxillofacial injuries as a result of blunt trauma should be maintained with cervical spine immobilization until clearance is assured.

ASSESSMENT

Because of the physical position of the face, clinical personnel should always conduct a thorough examination of the soft tissue and bony structures, including inside the mouth, nose, and ears. Anticipate the following:

- Airway compromise
- Cervical spine injury
- Hemorrhage
- Decreased level of consciousness because of intracranial bleeding and increased intracranial pressure
- Eye trauma
- Malocclusion of teeth
- Pain on palpation
- Facial asymmetry
- Cerebrospinal fluid (CSF) leak from the nose (rhinorrhea) or ear (otorrhea) or complaint of salty taste in throat

DIAGNOSIS

- Clinical observation
- X-ray

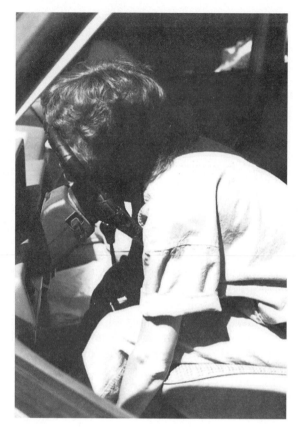

Fig. 18-1 Soft tissue and bone structure damage of the face may result from motor vehicle crash.

THERAPEUTIC INTERVENTIONS

- Ensure ABCs while maintaining cervical spine immobilization.
- Maintain an open airway, suctioning as needed.
- Administer supplemental oxygen.
- Initiate IV therapy if indicated.
- Control bleeding with pressure dressings as needed.

Facial lacerations

Blood loss can be significant from a facial laceration because of the dense vascularity of the soft tissue structures (Fig. 18-2). The patient may also be fearful of facial disfigurement as a result of this injury. Facial lacerations are usually caused by penetrating objects, such as glass, metal, knives, or from severe, blunt trauma to the face.

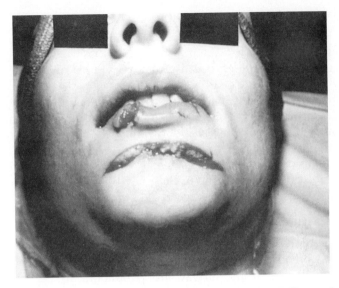

Fig. 18-2   Facial laceration. (Courtesy Dr. Daniel Cheney.)

ASSESSMENT

- Direct observation of the laceration
- Estimation of blood loss
- Exploration for foreign bodies

DIAGNOSIS

- Direct observation of the laceration

THERAPEUTIC INTERVENTIONS

- Apply local anesthesia (usually with epinephrine to control bleeding) or regional anesthesia.

NOTE: Do *not* use epinephrine for ear or nose lacerations because these are not highly vascularized and *necrosis* may occur.

- Cleanse the wound with normal saline. If antibacterial solutions are used to cleanse the wound, be sure to rinse the wound thoroughly afterward.
- Débride the wound, carefully remove foreign substances, and suture (usually done by a physician).
- Apply topical antibiotics.
- Assure tetanus prophylaxis.
- Assure discharge instructions are understood by patient.
- Consider discharge instructions regarding head trauma.

Special considerations for facial trauma patients

- The vermilion border of the lips should be carefully approximated when sutured.
- Never shave eyebrows, because they provide a landmark for repair and may not grow back.
- Approximate eyebrows as closely as possible before suturing.
- If a laceration is in the cheek area, the parotid duct and facial nerve should be checked carefully for disruption; if they are disrupted, they should be re-anastomosed before skin suturing.
- Explain to patient why sutures need to be reevaluated and removed on the prescribed day, because the patient may think it is better to leave them in longer, which may result in increased scarring.

Facial fractures

In major multiple trauma, facial fractures are given a low priority, except when a potential airway difficulty is present. Cervical spine precautions and surveillance of the airway are paramount in the early assessment of facial trauma. The mechanism of injury is usually blunt trauma to the face.

Zygomatic fractures (tripod)

The zygomatic arch may be fractured in three places: at the arch, at the posterior half of the infraorbital rim, and at the zygomatic suture (Fig. 18-3). This injury is caused by blunt trauma to the front and side of the face.

ASSESSMENT

- Palpation of infraorbital rim fracture
- Step defect
- Periorbital ecchymosis
- Facial edema
- Upward gaze
- Enophthalmos (sunken globe)
- TIDES
    Trismus
    Infraorbital hyperesthesia
    Diplopia
    Epistaxis (usually unilateral)
    Absence of symmetry
- Possible rhinorrhea
- Subconjunctival hemorrhage

DIAGNOSIS

- Palpable step defect of the inferior lateral orbital rim
- Clinical observation
- X-ray (Water's view is best) or computed tomography (CT) scan

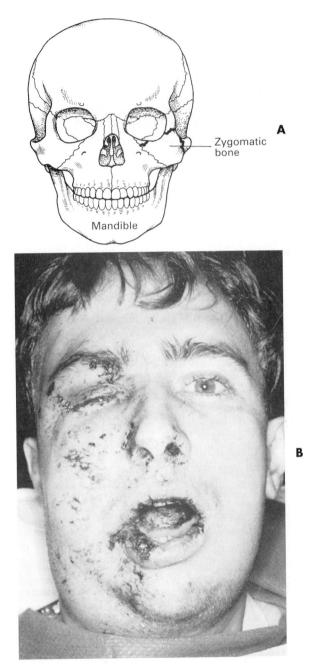

Fig. 18-3   A, The zygoma frequently fractures in three places; this is known as a tripod fracture. **B,** Patient with a zygomatic fracture. (Courtesy Dr. Daniel Cheney.)

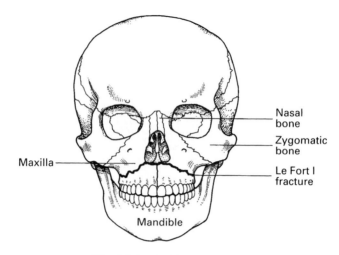

Fig. 18-4   Le Fort I fracture.

- Airway surveillance
- Elevate head of bed if cervical spine is cleared
- Anticipate vomiting
- Apply cold pack
- Consider preparing patient for surgery

Le Fort fractures

Patients with Le Fort fractures often have a history of severe blunt trauma to the face, usually caused by a motor vehicle crash. Le Fort fractures may be bilateral or unilateral and three types exist.

Le Fort I

A Le Fort I fracture is a fracture of the transverse alveolar process (Fig. 18-4). It is a horizontal fracture through the maxillary body that causes a detachment of the entire maxilla at the level of the nasal floor.

ASSESSMENT

- Epistaxis
- Malocclusion of teeth
- History of blunt trauma to the midface, just below the nose
- Maxilla mobile with palpation ("free floating maxilla")

DIAGNOSIS

- Clinical observation
- X-ray or CT scan

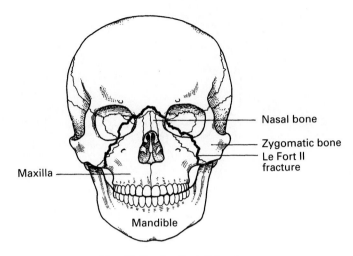

Fig. 18-5   Le Fort II fracture.

THERAPEUTIC INTERVENTIONS

- Check ABCs (especially airway management)
- Apply cold pack
- Internal fixation

Le Fort II

A Le Fort II fracture is a pyramid-shaped, midfacial fracture segment extending up through the superior nasal area (in the shape of an oxygen delivery face mask) (Fig. 18-5).

ASSESSMENT

- If manipulated, nose will move with dental arch; (midface appears caved in)
- Nasal fracture with epistaxis
- Periorbital ecchymosis
- Telecanthus (widening between eyes)
- Subconjunctival hemorrhage
- Rhinorrhea
- History of blunt trauma to the midface

DIAGNOSIS

- Clinical observation
- X-ray (Water's view) or CT scan

THERAPEUTIC INTERVENTIONS

- Check ABCs (especially airway management) with cervical spine precautions
- Apply cold pack

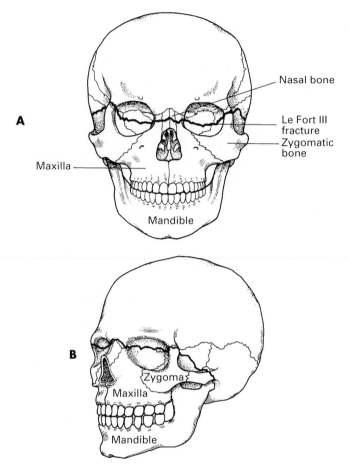

Fig. 18-6   Le Fort III fracture. **A,** Frontal view; **B,** lateral view.

- Prepare patient for surgery if open reduction and internal fixation exist
- Perform infection prophylaxis with IV antibiotics

Le Fort III

A Le Fort III fracture is a total craniofacial separation (Fig. 18-6).

ASSESSMENT

- Flattened and elongated appearance of face
- Usually significant bleeding occurs
- Massive facial edema and ecchymosis
- Patient often has loss of consciousness
- On manipulation, facial bones will move without frontal bone movement

- Possible rhinorrhea
- History of blunt trauma to the face

DIAGNOSIS

- Clinical observation
- X-ray (Water's view)
- CT scan
- Extraocular muscle entrapment

THERAPEUTIC INTERVENTIONS

- Check ABCs (especially airway management)
- Apply cold pack
- Prepare patient for open reduction and internal fixation
- Perform prophylaxis with IV antibiotics

NOTE: Midface maxillofacial fractures may also be associated with cribriform plate fractures. Therefore when a nasogastric tube is placed, it should be placed orally.

Mandible fracture

Mandible fractures are caused by severe blunt trauma commonly seen in contact sports and incidents of domestic violence (Fig. 18-7). These fractures are often accompanied by condyle fractures. A mandible fracture may be an open fracture if it involves the alveolar body. As a result of the shape of the mandible, more than 50% of the fractures are bilateral. Because the tongue is secured by muscles attached to the mandible, loss of control of the tongue and subsequent airway obstruction may occur. The nurse should be scrupulous in evaluating airway compromise in patients with this injury. In addition, the nurse should recall that the jaw is a very strong joint and that if the mandible has been struck with enough force to fracture it, soft tissue injury and edema is probably significant.

ASSESSMENT

- Airway compromise
- Observation of malocclusion of teeth
- Complaint of pain with jaw motion or tenderness on palpation
- Trismus
- Palpable fracture
- Soft tissue swelling with ecchymosis
- Loose or missing teeth and/or malalignment of teeth

DIAGNOSIS

- Clinical observation
- X-ray, Panorex x-ray, or CT scan

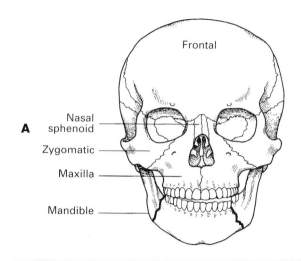

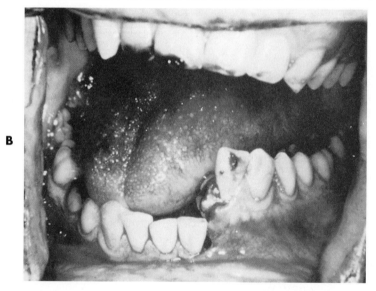

Fig. 18-7 **A,** Mandible fracture. **B,** May be identified by gross deformity or more subtle malocclusion of teeth. (Courtesy Dr. Daniel Cheney.)

THERAPEUTIC INTERVENTIONS

- ABCs (especially airway management) with cervical spine immobilization
- Cold pack
- Immobilize with a Barton dressing (bulk wrap surrounding the head)
- Possible open reduction and internal fixation

Dental trauma
Chipped or broken teeth

Chipped or broken teeth are most often caused by direct trauma to the teeth. The teeth most commonly injured are the four front upper teeth.

ASSESSMENT

- Observations of chips or fractures
- Bleeding from the pulp
- Bleeding from the gums
- Associated head or facial trauma
- Observation of foreign bodies (teeth fragments) in airway

THERAPEUTIC INTERVENTIONS

- ABCs (ensure airway clearance)
- Cover to reduce pain
- Dental consultation if bleeding from pulp

Avulsed teeth

Teeth usually are avulsed or subluxed by blunt trauma to the mouth and directly to the teeth.

ASSESSMENT

- Absence of teeth or loose teeth with fresh wounds underlying

DIAGNOSIS

- Clinical observation
- Panorex x-ray

THERAPEUTIC INTERVENTIONS

- Check ABCs (ensure airway clearance).
- Soak the tooth in milk, saline solution, or a commercially prepared tooth preservation solution.
- Obtain a dental consultation for consideration of possible tooth reimplantation.

NOTE: If a tooth is missing as a result of trauma, a chest or abdominal x-ray is indicated to rule out aspiration or swallowing of the tooth (Fig. 18-8).

EYE, EAR, AND NOSE TRAUMA

Although not generally considered to be major trauma, injuries to the eyes, ears, and nose are common types of associated traumatic injuries. In this chapter there is a brief review of some of the types of trauma that are frequently associated with major trauma.

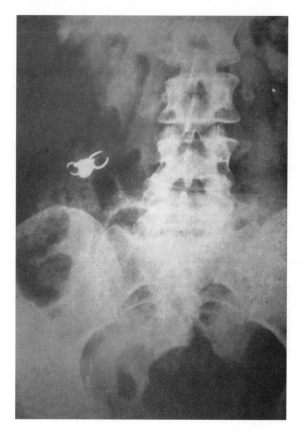

Fig. 18-8   Look for dentures. Patient may swallow or aspirate dental appliances or fractured teeth. (Courtesy Dr. Daniel Cheney.)

Eye trauma

If eye trauma is present, the patient should be assessed for other, more life-threatening injuries before focusing on the eye injury. The nurse may patch both eyes to minimize pain resulting from the trauma and to reduce the possibility of further injury by minimizing movement.

A majority of injuries to the eye are caused by industrial accidents that are blunt or penetrating. Others may be caused by contact with an inflating airbag (Box 18-1). The nurse should obtain a good patient history; including mechanism of injury, the presence of foreign bodies or chemicals, the care given before arrival at the Emergency Department, presence of contact lenses, and any other past medical history, especially that involving the eye, such as glaucoma or diabetes should be ascertained.

NOTE: Any patient involved in a motor vehicle crash with an airbag inflation should have visual acuity assessed.

BOX 18-1

AIRBAG-RELATED EYE INJURIES

Corneal abrasions and edema
Scleral rupture
Globe rupture
Hyphema
Angle recession
Lens subluxation
Retinal tear, detachment, or hemorrhage
Vitreous hemorrhage
Chemical keratitis
Eyelid contusion, abrasion, laceration
Periorbital fractures

ASSESSMENT

- Assess visual acuity.
- Assess the eye by first examining the area around the eye.
- Check the eyelid and the orbital rim before examining the eye itself.
- Check pupillary response and accommodation to light; document pupil size.
- Check for contact lenses and remove if present (Fig. 18-9).
- Keep the corneas moist.

DIAGNOSIS

- Clinical findings

THERAPEUTIC INTERVENTIONS

- Depends on the specific findings
- Ophthalmology consultation or referral for significant injuries

Orbital rim injury

Orbital rim injuries occur as a result of blunt or penetrating trauma to the orbital rim area.

ASSESSMENT

- Look for periorbital ecchymosis and edema.
- Palpate for tenderness and deformity (step off).
- Check visual acuity.
- Check for visual disturbances such as diplopia.
- Carefully assess for other associated injuries, especially to the globe of the eye.

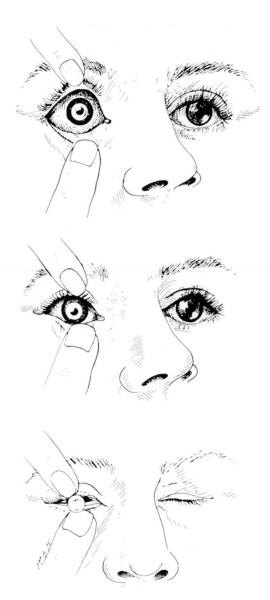

Fig. 18-9 Techniques for removing hard corneal contact lenses from a patient's eye. (From Barber JM, Stokes LG, Billings DM: *Adult and child care,* ed 2, St Louis, 1997, Mosby.)

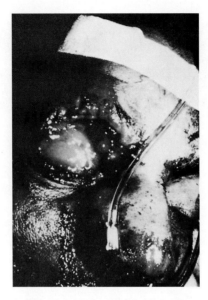

Fig. 18-10   Avulsed eyelid. (Courtesy Dr. Daniel Cheney.)

- Check for a fracture of the prominent supraorbital rim.
- Check for a CSF leak.
- Check for subconjunctival hemorrhage.

DIAGNOSIS

- Clinical observation
- X-ray or CT scan

THERAPEUTIC INTERVENTIONS

- Apply ice pack.
- Treat for specific fractures.
- Give aftercare instructions for head trauma.

Eyelid trauma

With eyelid trauma there is usually a history of penetrating trauma or other associated major trauma to the face or body (Fig. 18-10).

ASSESSMENT

- Assess for visual acuity if possible.
- Observe patient carefully.
- Check for possible eversion of the eyelid.
- Check for a laceration of the lacrimal duct.
- Check for other associated trauma.

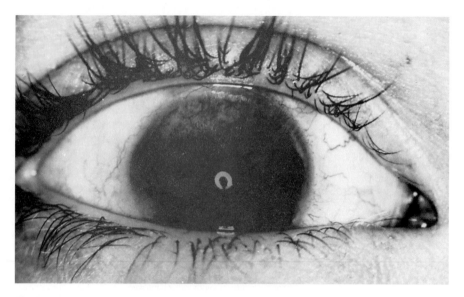

Fig. 18-11 Traumatic hyphema that obscures the iris. The blood in the anterior chamber has not clotted but, during rest, forms a fluid meniscus. (From Newell, Frank W: *Ophthalmology: principles and concepts,* St Louis, 1996, Mosby.)

DIAGNOSIS

- Clinical observation

THERAPEUTIC INTERVENTIONS

- Irrigate the wound with normal saline.
- Perform early approximation of edges before edema sets in (usually performed by a physician).
- Consider a plastic surgery consultation if there is a major deformity or any tissue missing.
- Assure tetanus prophylaxis.

Nonpenetrating blunt trauma to the globe

Blunt trauma to the globe causes aqueous humor to compress the iris and produce a hemorrhage or hyphema in the anterior chamber of the eye (Fig. 18-11).

ASSESSMENT

- Visual acuity
- Observation of hyphema in the anterior chamber of the eye

DIAGNOSIS

- Clinical findings

THERAPEUTIC INTERVENTIONS

- Limit patient to quiet activity or bedrest with head of bed elevated 45°.
- Sedation if needed.
- Patch affected eye with a Fox shield.
- Obtain ophthalmology consultation.
- Monitor for increased intraocular pressure.

Blowout fracture

A blowout fracture results from blunt trauma to the globe of the eye, causing increased intraocular pressure and a resultant fracture of the orbital floor.

ASSESSMENT

- Visual acuity
- Periorbital hematoma
- Subconjunctival hemorrhage
- Enophthalmos
- Periorbital edema
- Complaint of diplopia
- Limit in extraocular movements (usually upward gaze) caused by trapping of the inferior rectus muscle or the inferior oblique muscle

DIAGNOSIS

- Clinical findings
- X-ray or CT scan

THERAPEUTIC INTERVENTIONS

- Apply a cold pack.
- Consider antibiotic prophylaxis.
- Consider preparation for surgery.
- Patch affected eye.
- Assure tetanus prophylaxis.

Penetrating injuries to the globe of the eye

Perforation by a sharp object will cause direct trauma and possible tissue evisceration to the globe of the eye (Fig. 18-12).

ASSESSMENT

- Observation of the impaling object (should be secured in place)
- Observation of the perforation

DIAGNOSIS

- Clinical observation
- Observation of the opaque object on x-ray

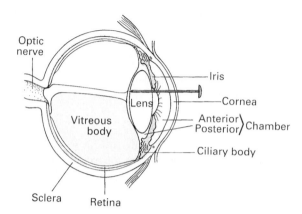

Fig. 18-12   Do not remove the impaled object from the globe, because this could result in the loss of humor from the anterior and posterior chambers.

THERAPEUTIC INTERVENTIONS

- Secure the impaled object.
- Patch the eyes bilaterally to minimize eye movement.
- Obtain an ophthalmology consultation.
- Administer IV antibiotics.
- Assure tetanus prophylaxis.

Ear trauma

The goal, when caring for a patient with trauma to the ear, is to repair current damage and prevent further damage. Circulation to the structures of the ear is poor, unlike the other structures of the head. Therefore much care should be taken to protect the injuries from possible necrosis.

General guidelines for therapeutic intervention are as follows:
- If using lidocaine, use it *without* epinephrine.
- Splint the ear posteriorly with soft padding and protect the inner areas from pressure and necrosis (Fig. 18-13).
- If blood is draining from the inner ear, assume that it is mixed with CSF and rule out a basilar skull fracture.

Simple laceration

A simple laceration is the most common type of ear injury. It is usually caused by a sharp penetrating object.

ASSESSMENT

- Observation of bleeding from ear structures

DIAGNOSIS

- Clinical observation

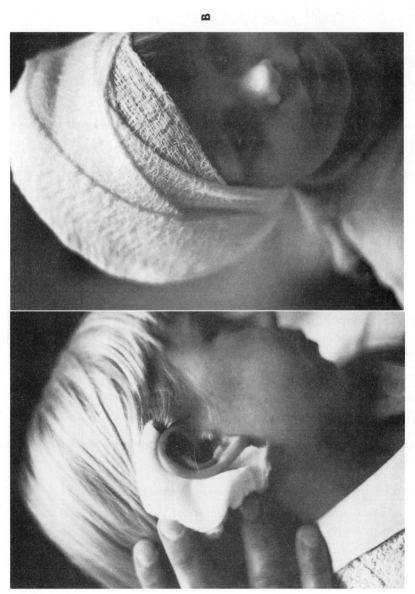

Fig. 18-13 **A,** Pad with fluffy dressing around the pinna. **B,** After padding the ear, dress it with a loose, bulky dressing.

THERAPEUTIC INTERVENTIONS

- Irrigate the wound with normal saline, cleanse, and débride.
- Edges of cartilage will be reanastomosed and skin will be sutured by the surgeon.
- Cover with a thin layer of topical antibiotic ointment.
- Assure tetanus prophylaxis.

Hematoma of the pinna

Hematoma of the pinna results from impact to the pinna of the ear from a blunt object.

ASSESSMENT

- Visible hematoma

DIAGNOSIS

- Clinical observation

THERAPEUTIC INTERVENTIONS

- Apply local anesthesia.
- Aspirate the hematoma.
- Drain may be placed to facilitate drainage.
- Small pressure dressing may be placed on the local area of the injury only.

Traumatic amputation of the ear

Traumatic amputation of the structures of the outer ear (also known as auriculectomy) usually occurs as a result of a knife fight or of the person being ejected from a car through a windshield (Fig. 18-14).

ASSESSMENT

- Observation of the amputation

DIAGNOSIS

- Clinical observation

THERAPEUTIC INTERVENTIONS

- Reanastomosis of cartilage and skin must be done with meticulous detail and is usually done in surgery.
- IV antibiotics may be prescribed.
- Patient may require skin grafts either immediately or at a later date.
- Assure tetanus prophylaxis.

Nose trauma

Injury to the nose may be associated with major trauma, or may be caused by interpersonal violence, sports injuries, and falls. It can be caused by both blunt and penetrating trauma.

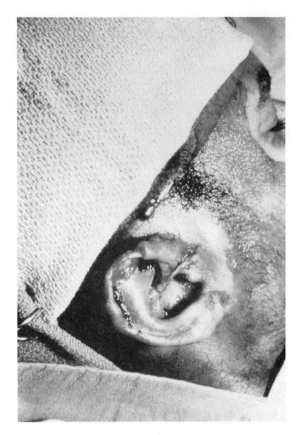

Fig. 18-14   Repair of partial traumatic amputation of the pinna. (Courtesy Dr. Daniel Cheney.)

Epistaxis

Traumatic epistaxis (nosebleed) may occur as the result of blunt or penetrating trauma to the nose. Trauma results in anterior epistaxis, usually caused by disruption of the anterior and inferior turbinates at the area of Kiesselbach.

ASSESSMENT

- Bleeding
- Observation of a deformity of the nose
- Other associated facial trauma
- Other associated trauma

DIAGNOSIS

- Clinical observation

THERAPEUTIC INTERVENTIONS

- Assure ABCs with particular attention to airway clearance.
- Reassure patient.
- Begin volume replacement if indicated.
- Check for anterior bleeding:
  - Slightly hyperextend neck (after cervical spine injury has been ruled out).
  - Suction clots.
  - Identify bleeding sites.
  - Apply a vasoconstrictor agent (usually cocaine 10% solution).
  - Cauterize with silver nitrate.
- May require nasal packing.
- Posterior bleeding usually requires a posterior pack.

Nasal fractures

A nasal fracture is usually caused by a blunt force to the front or side of the nose.

ASSESSMENT

- Observe for swelling.
- Observe for a deformity.
- Palpate for crepitus.
- Palpate for a fracture.
- Observe for a septal hematoma.

DIAGNOSIS

- Clinical observation
- X-ray

THERAPEUTIC INTERVENTIONS

- Apply a cold pack.
- Apply a splint.
- Control bleeding with pressure.
- Administer a local anesthetic (usually topical and subcutaneous).
- Fracture will be set by the physician.
- Septal hematoma may need to be drained in surgery.
- Pack (bilaterally if the septum is fractured).
- Assure tetanus prophylaxis.

Neck trauma

Neck trauma may be caused by either a blunt or penetrating mechanism. The neck is unique because it contains many vital structures in a small anatomic space.

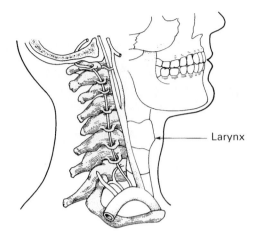

Fig. 18-15   A laryngeal fracture usually results from blunt trauma to the neck.

Laryngotracheal injuries

Fractured larynx and other laryngeotracheal injuries usually result from blunt trauma (Figs. 18-15 and 18-16). These injuries most commonly occur by a victim's neck striking the steering wheel or dashboard during a car crash. Other causes include sudden deceleration exerted by a rope or line and direct impact such as may be experienced in a karate chop.

ASSESSMENT
- Hoarseness
- Cough with hemoptysis
- Progressive respiratory stridor
- Respiratory distress
- Subcutaneous emphysema
- Pain and/or tenderness
- "Flattened" appearing larynx

DIAGNOSIS
- Clinical observation
- X-ray or CT scan
- Laryngoscopy

THERAPEUTIC INTERVENTIONS
- Closely check ABCS (especially airway management)
  - Intubation
  - Cricothyrotomy (always have a cricothyrotomy set at the bedside)
  - Tracheostomy

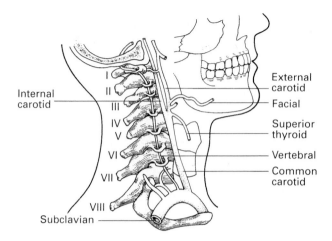

Fig. 18-16 Because of vascular anatomy and the closed space in the neck, penetrating trauma presents risk to the airway and circulation.

NOTE: The need to secure the airway must be balanced against the risk for further compromise in patients with altered anatomy. For stable or semistable patients, surgery may be the best plan. Endotracheal intubation should be avoided if possible, but if attempted, must be performed very gently. Cricothyrotomy is the next option; if the nature of the injury precludes this procedure, a formal tracheostomy is necessary.

• Administer high-flow humidified oxygen therapy.
• Administer broad-spectrum antibiotics
• Prepare patient for surgical repair.
• Have patient rest voice.
• Administer steroids if indicated.

Penetrating wounds

Penetrating objects, such as a bullet or the blade of a knife, can easily cause trauma to the structures of the neck. The presentation will be varied depending on the type of object that has penetrated and the angle and force of the penetrating object.

Low injuries (Zone I) may involve the major thoracic vessels, esophagus, thyroid, or trachea. High injuries (Zone III) may affect the internal carotid and/or vertebral arteries, pharynx, spinal cord, and/or salivary glands. The main portion of the neck (Zone II) is the most commonly injured, and any of the structures of the neck may be involved (Fig 18-16).

ASSESSMENT

• Obvious wound to neck
• Airway obstruction
• Signs and symptoms of hypovolemic shock

- Presence of expanding hematoma
- Potential associated spine or spinal cord injury
- Subcutaneous emphysema
- Presence of bruit

DIAGNOSIS

- Clinical observation
- Arteriography
- Possible exploratory surgery

THERAPEUTIC INTERVENTIONS

- Control ABCs with cervical spine immobilization if appropriate.
  - Airway management
  - Breathing management
  - Control of bleeding with direct pressure
- Establish IV lines of lactated Ringer's solution or normal saline.
- Consider preparations for surgery.

Blunt vascular injuries

Blunt vascular injuries may have significant sequelae, including exsanguination, stroke, air embolism, and airway obstruction. Diagnosis is a challenge. Some patients have little external evidence of trauma, and the onset of symptoms may be delayed until thrombosis or emboli develop and stenose or occlude an artery. Blunt vascular injuries most commonly occur as a result of the victim being involved in a car crash. The most common vessel injured is the internal carotid artery.

ASSESSMENT

- Soft-tissue trauma
- Hematoma
- Bruit
- Thrill
- Diminished pulse
- Decreased level of consciousness
- Neurologic deficits resembling transient ischemic attack or stroke

DIAGNOSIS

- Initial CT scan may be normal
- Arteriography
- Duplex ultrasound scan

THERAPEUTIC INTERVENTIONS

- Apply direct pressure to control bleeding.
- Anticoagulate if possible
- Prepare patient for surgical revascularization depending on the injury

Esophageal injuries

Esophageal injuries may be a result of either blunt or penetrating trauma. These injuries are rare and often difficult to diagnose, and the clinician must have a high index of suspicion. In blunt trauma, isolated esophageal injury is uncommon; rather, it usually occurs in combination with laryngotracheal and/or spine injuries.

ASSESSMENT

• Pain and/or tenderness
• Dysphagia
• Drooling
• Subcutaneous emphysema
• Air in the mediastinal or fascial spaces

DIAGNOSIS

• Soft-tissue neck x-rays
• Contrast esophagography
• Esophagoscopy

THERAPEUTIC INTERVENTIONS

• Prepare patient for surgical repair

SUGGESTED READINGS

Asensio JA, and others: Management of penetrating neck injuries: the controversy surrounding Zone II injuries, *Surg Clin North Am* 71(2):267, 1991.

Beirne JC, Butler PE, Brady FA: Cervical spine injuries in patients with facial fractures: a 1-year prospective study, *Int J Oral Maxillofac Surg* 24(1):26, 1995.

Campbell WH, Cantrill SV: Neck trauma. In Rosen P, editor: *Emergency medicine concepts and clinical practice,* vol 2, ed 3, St Louis, 1992, Mosby.

Duma SM, and others: Airbag-induced eye injuries: a report of 25 cases, *J Trauma* 41(1):114, 1996.

Emergency Nurses Association: *Trauma nursing core course,* ed 4, Park Ridge, IL, 1995, Emergency Nurses Association.

Gisness CM: Maxillofacial trauma. In *Sheehy's emergency nursing principles and practice,* ed 4, St Louis, 1997, Mosby.

Houdek DL, and others: Maxillofacial trauma: case managing patients with Le Fort I, II, or III fractures, *J Trauma Nurs* 4(2):33, 1997.

Linden JA, Renner GS: Trauma to the globe, *Emerg Med Clin North Am* 13(3):581-605, 1995.

Sargent LA, editor: Maxillofacial injuries, *Trauma Q* 9(1):1-140, 1992.

Weintraub BA: Airbag-mediated injury in the emergency department population, *Int J Trauma Nurs* 3(2):46-49, 1997.

CHAPTER 19

Chest Trauma

Linda Tatko Cooper

Chest injuries can create some of the most urgent situations that the trauma team faces. Because of the significance of the organs enclosed in the thorax and the large area of the body that is involved, life-threatening situations can result from seemingly small mechanisms. Approximately 25% of all trauma deaths in the United States each year are directly related to chest trauma. Injuries to the chest are the most frequently missed injuries in the first hour of care, and the development of a thorough chest examination technique is essential to the emergency nurse. Many chest trauma patients die after reaching the hospital.

Most injuries to the chest occur from blunt trauma, primarily caused by impact of the chest with a relatively immobile object, such as an automobile steering wheel. Presence of a seat belt with shoulder harness and deployment of an air bag affects the degree of energy transferred during a crash and needs to be taken into consideration.

Most penetrating wounds to the chest are caused by bullets or knives. Clinical personnel must consider the effect of the mechanism of injury and the patient's preexisting cardiac or pulmonary disease on the potential severity of chest injuries, so that diagnostic and therapeutic procedures can be administered before the patient's condition worsens.

GROSS ANATOMY OF THE CHEST

When assessing a patient and intervening for a possible injury to the chest, clinical personnel should be familiar with the gross anatomy of the chest. The thoracic cavity extends from the first rib to the diaphragm. The diaphragm may be anywhere from the fourth intercostal space on exhalation to the lower costal margin (about the tenth rib) on maximal inhalation (Fig. 19-1). Any injury that occurs between these areas should be considered as both chest and abdominal until each can be ruled out (Fig. 19-2).

249

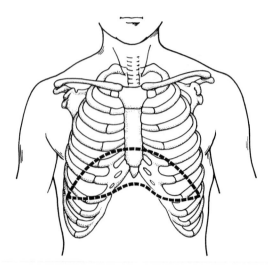

Fig. 19-1   Level of diaphragm on inspiration and expiration.

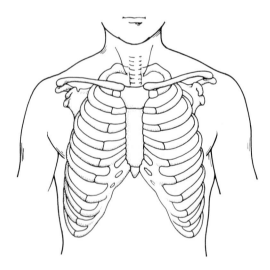

Fig. 19-2   Injuries in this area are considered chest and abdominal.

The thoracic cavity contains the heart, the great vessels (superior and inferior venae cavae and aorta), the lungs, and the lower airway (Fig. 19-3). It is surrounded by the ribs, the intercostal muscles, and the diaphragm. Movement of the thoracic cavity is assisted by the accessory muscles of respiration: the abdominal wall muscles, the pectoralis muscles, and the sternocleidomastoid muscles.

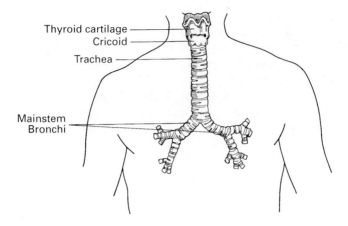

Fig. 19-3   The lower airway is included with the thoracic cavity.

If the mechanism of injury suggests a chest injury, the chest injury should be considered severe until proven otherwise. Hypoxia, a major cause of death associated with chest trauma, may have four causes:

Inadequate perfusion of unventilated lung
Inadequate ventilation of unperfused lung
Abnormal airway/lung relationship
Hypovolemia

ASSESSMENT

In the patient with chest injuries, careful assessment of the ABCs can affect the patient's survival.
- Check the patient's airway.
  - Check air movement at nose and mouth.
  - Be sure that airway is clear of obstruction(s)
- Check for breathing
  - Check breath sounds bilaterally.
  - Check tidal volume using hands.
  - Check for life-threatening injuries of the chest.[1]
    - Tension pneumothorax
    - Open pneumothorax
    - Massive hemothorax
    - Pericardial tamponade
    - Flail chest
  - Check for injuries that are potentially life-threatening:
    - Pulmonary contusion
    - Tracheobronchial disruption
    - Esophageal disruption
    - Traumatic diaphragmatic hernia

- Myocardial contusion
- Aortic disruption
- Check for use of intercostal and accessory muscles.
- Check for epigastric and supraclavicular indrawing.
- Check for circulation.
    Check vital signs (ascultate BP in both arms), skin color, turgor, temperature, and moisture, and other signs of hemodynamic status.
- Obtain a history of the event and mechanism of injury.
- Obtain an upright chest x-ray.
- Identify any entrance or exit wounds.
- Measure chest drainage.
- Measure urinary output.
- Monitor arterial oxygen saturation using pulse oximetry.
- Monitor arterial blood gases.
- Obtain 12-lead ECG.
- Monitor for dysrhythmias.

DIAGNOSIS

- Consider mechanism of injury
- Clinical observations
- Chest x-ray (preferably upright chest film)
- Evaluation of arterial oxygen saturation and/or arterial blood gases
- Observation of ECG

THERAPEUTIC INTERVENTIONS

Most patients with chest trauma require nonsurgical intervention to correct the hypoxic state, to improve circulation, or to remove a ventilatory obstruction.

- Assure an open airway.
    Use airway adjuncts, as indicated.
- Assure breathing.
    Administer oxygen at high flow.
- Initiate IV line(s) with large-bore cannulas and crystalloid solutions or blood.
- Prepare for chest tube placement.
- Prepare for autotransfusion.
- Prepare for emergency thoracotomy.
- Provide interventions for specific chest injuries as indicated. (See Therapeutic Intervention sections for specific chest injuries.)

CHEST WALL INJURIES

Rib fractures

Rib fractures are the most common chest injuries. They occur most frequently in the elderly and may cause subsequent problems secondary to inactivity and pain in this age group (Fig. 19-4).[1] Another population that deserves

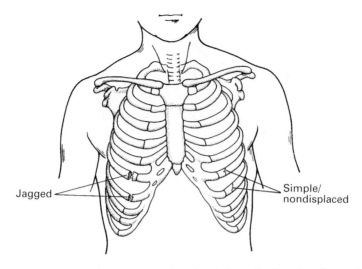

Fig. 19-4   A rib fracture may be simple/nondisplaced or jagged.

special consideration when rib fractures occur is children. Because children's ribs are so elastic, they do not frequently fracture. However, when a child does suffer a rib fracture, clinical personnel should be highly suspicious of underlying thoracic injuries. Rib fractures may be caused by blunt or penetrating trauma to the chest wall. If there is a first rib fracture or if there are multiple ribs fractured, personnel should suspect major underlying trauma to contents of the chest. Rib fractures may cause impaired ventilation, increased pulmonary secretions, atelectasis, and pneumonia.

ASSESSMENT

- Consider mechanism of injury.
- Patients will complain of pain upon inspiration or palpation.
- Patient will be splinting his or her chest.
- Chest wall ecchymosis.
- Ability to palpate fracture.

DIAGNOSIS

- Chest x-ray

THERAPEUTIC INTERVENTIONS

   Simple, nondisplaced fractures
- Administer analgesic agents
   Regional anesthesia may be considered for pain control.
   Avoid systemic analgesics and constrictive devices.
- Consider hospital admission for close observation if the patient is elderly or has a history of underlying lung disease or if the fracture is jagged.

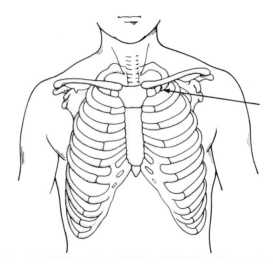

Fig. 19-5 A first rib fracture *(arrow)* is significant because of subclavian artery and vein location and the amount of force required to fracture the first rib.

First (Fig. 19-5), *second, or third rib fracture*

The patient must be hospitalized and an arteriogram should be considered. It takes significant force to break these ribs; therefore patients are at high risk for sudden death from CNS and tracheobronchial and vascular injuries.[2] The subclavian artery, vein, or aorta may be disrupted. It is difficult to visualize a first rib fracture on an anterior-posterior chest x-ray.

Fourth through twelfth rib fracture

The fourth through ninth ribs are most often injured in blunt trauma to the chest. In blunt trauma, a bowing effect occurs, resulting in a middle shaft fracture. With fractures of these ribs, clinical personnel must consider intrathoracic injuries and intraabdominal injuries. Fractures of ribs 10 to 12 are associated with a high incidence of liver and spleen injuries.

Flail chest

A flail chest results from two or more consecutive ribs being fractured in two or more places. Flail chest also results from a detached sternum, which causes an incongruity of the chest wall that responds directly to intrathoracic pressure (Fig. 19-6). When intercostal muscles contract and raise the rib cage, increased negative intrathoracic pressure causes the flail segment to draw inward. When the intercostal muscles relax, causing the rib cage to drop down, negative intrathoracic pressure decreases and the flail segment bulges outward. Because this motion is opposite that of the rest of the chest wall, it is known as *paradoxic motion.*

Flail chest is usually caused by a massive blunt force to the chest wall and results in rib fractures, as well as pulmonary contusion. Pain contributes to

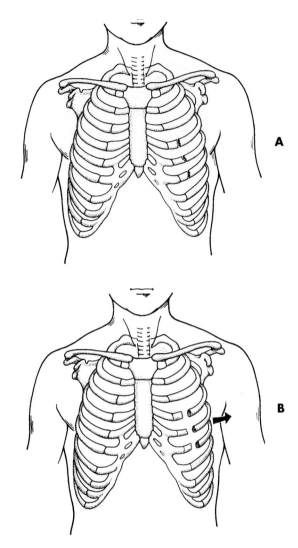

Fig. 19-6   A, Flail chest: More than two ribs fractured in consecutive places *B* and *C.* Paradoxic motion. **B,** On exhalation, the flail segment bulges outward.
Continued

hypoventilation.[3] Although work of breathing is greatly increased, the main cause of hypoxemia is the underlying lung contusion.[4]

ASSESSMENT

- Consider mechanism of injury
- Dyspnea/moves air poorly
- Chest wall pain

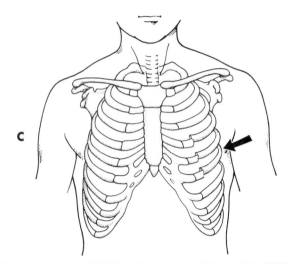

Fig. 19-6—cont'd   **C,** On inhalation, the flail segment sucks inward.

• Possible observation of movement of thorax as asymmetric and uncoordinated
• Palpation of subcutaneous emphysema

DIAGNOSIS

• Clinical observation
• Chest x-ray
• Arterial blood gases; these values demonstrate hypoxia and should be carried out to evaluate increasing size of contusion

THERAPEUTIC INTERVENTIONS

Good ventilation is imperative in the treatment of a person with a flail chest.
  • Perform selective endotracheal intubation
  • Administer supplemental, humidified oxygen
  • Control pain
  • Administer crystalloid IV solutions for volume replacement
    • In absence of hypotension, be careful not to fluid overload these patients. Injured lung tissue is sensitive to both underresuscitation of shock and fluid overload[1]
  • Consider stabilizing flail segment
  • Consider possible underlying injuries
  • Insertion of CVP to monitor fluid resuscitation

Sternum fracture

It takes a great force to fracture the sternum (Fig. 19-7). Of prime concern should be underlying structural damage. One of the injuries most commonly associated with a sternal fracture is a myocardial contusion. Common causes

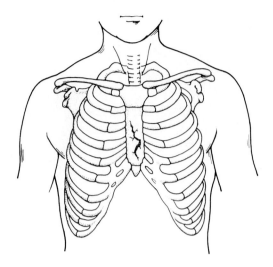

Fig. 19-7   Sternal fracture.

are the chest hitting a steering wheel or use of gas-powered chest compressor or aggressive manual chest compression.

ASSESSMENT

- Consider mechanism of injury
- Chest wall contusion, ecchymosis
- Complaint of chest pain
- Dysrhythmias (especially premature ventricular contractions, atrial fibrillation, right bundle branch block, ST segment elevations)
- Pain upon inspiration
- Palpation of fracture
- Assess for C-spine injury

DIAGNOSIS

- Palpation of fracture
- Chest x-ray

THERAPEUTIC INTERVENTIONS

- Observe patient
- Monitor PaO_2
- Administer analgesia
- Treat dysrhythmias, as prescribed
- Consider preparation for surgery for wiring if sternum is displaced

Clavicle fracture

A clavicle fracture is usually not a serious injury, but a jagged edge of the fracture may perforate the subclavian artery or vein, causing disruption, hema-

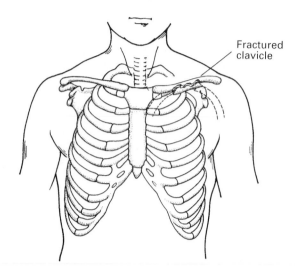

Fig. 19-8   A fractured clavicle may create concern because of the proximate anatomy of the subclavian artery and vein.

toma, or clot formation (Fig. 19-8). This injury is usually caused by blunt trauma directly to the clavicle or to the shoulder area laterally.

ASSESSMENT

• Consider mechanism of injury
• Pain on palpation
• Observation of deformity

DIAGNOSIS

• Clinical observation
• Chest x-ray

THERAPEUTIC INTERVENTIONS

• Apply a figure-eight splint.
• Consider an arteriogram.
• Administer analgesic agents, as prescribed.

LUNG INJURIES

Simple pneumothorax

A simple pneumothorax causes a ventilation/perfusion defect (Fig. 19-9). Blood is circulated to the nonventilated area and is not oxygenated. A loss of negative pressure in the intrapleural space causes a partial or total lung collapse. It may occur because of a tear in the lung tissue or from an opening in

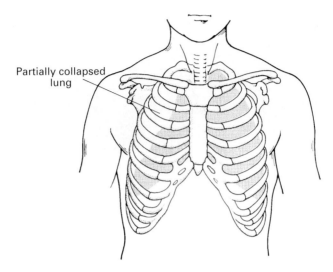

Fig. 19-9 Simple pneumothorax. One lung partially collapsed; other structures unaffected.

the chest wall. A simple pneumothorax usually results from blunt or penetrating trauma to the chest.

ASSESSMENT

- Consider mechanism of injury
- Complaint of sudden onset of chest pain
- Sudden onset shortness of breath, tachypnea
- Absence of or diminished breath sounds on affected side
- Hyperresonance on percussion on affected side

DIAGNOSIS

- Clinical observation
- Chest x-ray: upright, end-exhalation

THERAPEUTIC INTERVENTIONS

- Observe closely
- Administer high-flow oxygen
- Consider needle thoracostomy
- Prepare for chest tube placement
- Chest x-ray to confirm lung reexpansion

Tension pneumothorax

A tension pneumothorax is a life-threatening condition. There is usually good perfusion but poor ventilation, which will eventually cause poor perfusion (Fig. 19-10). A tension pneumothorax usually results from a penetrating injury

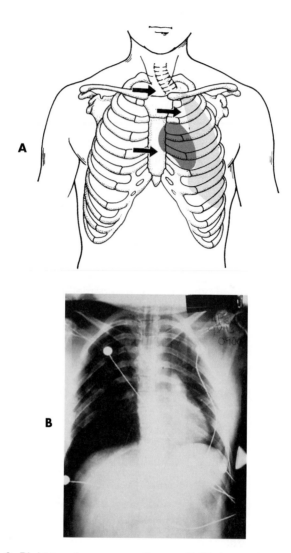

Fig. 19-10 **A,** Right tension pneumothorax. **B,** Right tension pneumothorax as seen on x-ray.

but may also be caused by blunt trauma. It may be caused by mechanical ventilation with positive end-expiratory pressure (PEEP), a nonsealing puncture, rupture of an emphysematous bulla, or a parenchymal lung injury.

A tension pneumothorax will form when pressure enters the thoracic cavity during inspiration but cannot exit during exhalation. As this process continues, pressure will not only collapse the affected lung but will also push the mediastinum toward the unaffected side (mediastinal shift). This movement, in turn, causes a decreased blood flow to the right side of the heart and consequently a decrease in cardiac output. It will also cause the unaffected lung to collapse. This condition may be aggravated by inflation of pneumatic antishock garment (PASG).[5]

ASSESSMENT

- Consider mechanism of injury
- Severe shortness of breath
- Deviated trachea (deviated toward unaffected side)
- Mediastinal shift, causing decreased venous return and impaired contralateral ventilation
- Distended jugular veins from impedance of blood return to right side of the heart
- Cyanosis
- Decreased blood pressure/hemodynamic deterioration
- Hyperresonance on percussion on affected side
- Unilateral absence of breath sounds

DIAGNOSIS

- Clinical observation
- Chest x-ray

THERAPEUTIC INTERVENTIONS

- Administer oxygen.
- Perform a needle thoracostomy using a large-bore (at least 16-gauge) needle.
- Prepare for chest tube placement.
    Be careful not to administer oxygen under positive pressure until after the chest tube is placed, because this may increase the tension.

NOTE: It is not necessary to await results of a chest x-ray before providing therapeutic intervention if signs and symptoms of the tension pneumothorax are present.

Hemothorax

A hemothorax may be caused by blunt or penetrating trauma to the chest (Fig. 19-11). If there is an injury to structures within the chest cavity (usually the lung or a vessel laceration) and bleeding occurs, this blood will collect in the intrapleural space, producing what is known as a hemothorax. The amount of collected blood will vary depending on the extent of the bleeding. A collection of greater than 1500 ml of blood is considered a massive hemothorax. An initial drainage of 1000 ml of blood followed by a consistent drainage of over 200 ml of blood for 4 hours or the initial loss of 1500 ml may be indicative of the need for emergency thoracotomy.[1]

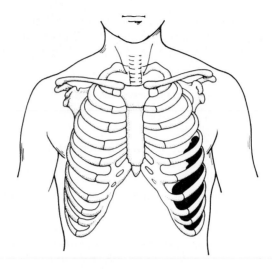

Fig. 19-11 Hemothorax.

ASSESSMENT

- Consider mechanism of injury
- Signs of hypovolemic shock
- Restlessness to unconsciousness
- Cool, clammy skin
- Cool distal extremities
- Increased pulse
- Increased, shallow respirations
- Decreased blood pressure
- Decreased breath sounds on affected side
- Dullness to percussion on affected side

NOTE: Jugular veins may be distended or flat and are not very useful in diagnosis.

DIAGNOSIS

- Clinical observation
- Chest x-ray
- May be seen in combination with tension pneumothorax

THERAPEUTIC INTERVENTIONS

- Administer oxygen.
- Establish IV lines administer crystalloids or blood products.
- Prepare for placement of a large-bore chest tube (36 Fr).
- Consider autotransfusion.
- Consider preparation for emergency thoracotomy.

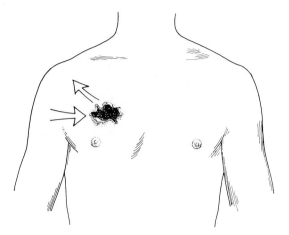

Fig. 19-12   Sucking chest wound/open chest wound. Air will preferentially enter and exit through the chest wall defect if the hole is greater than two thirds the diameter of the trachea. On expiration, air moves out of the defect. On inspiration, air preferentially enters the open wound.

Sucking chest wound/open pneumothorax

A sucking chest wound is caused by a penetrating force, especially that of a high-velocity missile (Fig. 19-12). If the diameter of the hole in the chest wall is greater than two thirds the diameter of the trachea, there will be preferential flow of air through the chest wall defect, the path of least resistance. Loss of negative pressure in the chest from the defect will cause immediate equilibration between intrathoracic pressure and atmospheric pressure, thus causing a pneumothorax to form. If the defect produces a one-way valve, as air enters the thoracic cavity but cannot escape, a tension pneumothorax will form.

ASSESSMENT
- Consider mechanism of injury
- Seeing defect/hearing sucking sound on inspiration
- Dyspnea
- Chest pain
- Signs of pneumothorax or tension pneumothorax

DIAGNOSIS
- Clinical findings

THERAPEUTIC INTERVENTIONS
- Administer oxygen.
- Seal the defect on three sides with a sterile, occlusive dressing.

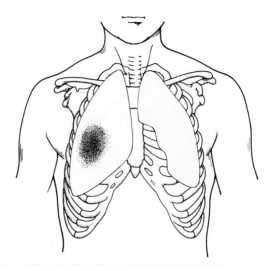

Fig. 19-13 Pulmonary contusion.

Leave one side open to act as a flutter valve to prevent the formation of a tension pneumothorax.

Observe for the development of tension pneumothorax and remove the seal if this occurs. If the patient is intubated, this procedure will not be necessary unless the wound is greater than the size of the trachea.

• Consider the placement of chest tubes, remote from area of injury
• Consider autotransfusion.
• Consider surgery for repair.

Pulmonary contusion

A pulmonary contusion is one of the most common types of chest injuries that occur in major trauma.[1] It is often seen in conjunction with a flail chest or severe rib fractures (Fig. 19-13). A pulmonary contusion is usually caused by severe blunt trauma to the chest. It may be slow to develop, so close, on-going observation of patients with mechanisms of injury that would suggest a pulmonary contusion is imperative.

A contusion forms when blood extravasates into the parenchyma, causing the patient to become hypoxic. There may also be resultant tracheal obstruction. The contusion may be localized or massive.

ASSESSMENT

• Consider mechanism of injury
• Ineffective cough
• Hemoptysis or blood suctioned from ET tube[2]
• Increasing hyperpnea
• Severe dyspnea

- Chest wall contusions or abrasions
- Additional severe injuries
- Hypoxemia on pulse oximetry or arterial blood gas

DIAGNOSIS

- High index of suspicion
- Clinical observation
- Chest x-ray

THERAPEUTIC INTERVENTIONS

- Maintain an adequate airway.
- Maintain adequate ventilation.
    - Administer humidified oxygen, as prescribed.
    - Selective endotracheal intubation may be necessary; consider the use of a ventilator.
- In the absence of hypotension, limit IV fluids during the resuscitative and early intensive care phase.
    - Use blood and colloids to maintain oncotic pressure and decrease pulmonary edema.
    - Consider administering diuretics.
    - Monitor pulse oximetry.
- Administer analgesics to keep the patient comfortable.
    - Give morphine sulfate in 1 to 2 mg increments intravenously, not intramuscularly.
    - Pay close attention to a decreased respiratory rate and increased hypoxia.[1]

Laceration of lung parenchyma

Laceration of lung tissue is usually caused by a jagged rib fracture or other penetrating injury (Fig. 19-14).

ASSESSMENT

- Often a small hemothorax or pneumothorax
- Hemoptysis
- Subcutaneous emphysema

THERAPEUTIC INTERVENTIONS

Usually none is required, because the process is usually self-limiting. If injury is severe, surgical repair is necessary.

OTHER STRUCTURAL INJURIES

Tracheobronchial injuries

Disruption of the tracheobronchial tree, most commonly near the bifurcation of the main stem bronchus 1 inch from the carina, may be the result of blunt or penetrating trauma. It may not be evidenced for up to 5 days after injury.

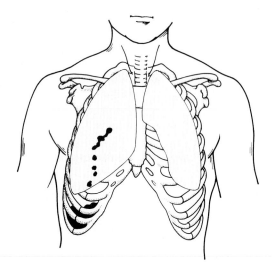

Fig. 19-14   Laceration of the lung parenchyma.

If the disruption is below the carina, a chest x-ray will show mediastinal air. Bronchoscopy is the most definitive diagnostic aid.

Bronchial injuries are subtle. Patients who arrive at the hospital with these types of injuries have a 30% mortality rate, often because of associated injuries.[1]

ASSESSMENT
- Consider mechanism of injury
- Observation for airway obstruction
- Noisy breathing
- Hemoptysis
- Cough
- Subcutaneous emphysema
- Progressive mediastinal emphysema
- Possible tension pneumothorax
- Air leak somewhere in chest

DIAGNOSIS
- Clinical findings
- Direct visualization on bronchoscopy
- Continuous air leak in chest tube drainage device

THERAPEUTIC INTERVENTIONS
- Maintain a patent airway.
- Administer high-flow oxygen.
- Prepare for chest tube(s).
- Prepare for surgery.

Diaphragmatic rupture

Diaphragmatic rupture may be a life-threatening injury.[6] A *diaphragmatic rupture* is a disruption of the diaphragm which is the main muscle of respiration, causing interference with the patient's ventilatory effort. It may occur with any chest or abdominal injury from the level of the fourth intercostal space to the tenth rib. Diaphragmatic rupture may be caused by a stiff, forceful blow to the left side of the stomach or by an increase in intraabdominal pressure, as occurs with lap seat belts. If the trauma is blunt, the rupture will usually result in large tears. If the trauma is penetrating, it will usually result in small perforations. It is usually associated with other massive injuries. This injury may be made worse by the use of PASG.[5]

ASSESSMENT

- Chest pain that may be referred to one shoulder
- Abdominal pain[3]
- Difficult breathing
- Decreased breath sounds
- Possible rhonchi (from the hemothorax)
- Bowel sounds auscultated in lower/middle chest[3]

DIAGNOSIS

- Supine x-ray (look for presence of bowel that has herniated into the chest cavity and elevated left hemidiaphragm) or the nasogastric tube in the thoracic cavity or loss of costophrenic angle on other side of injury[1]
- Contrast radiography (GI series)
- Bowel sounds in chest

THERAPEUTIC INTERVENTIONS

- Administer high-flow oxygen.
- Position patient to facilitate breathing.
- Place a nasogastric tube.
- Prepare the patient for surgery.

Esophageal rupture

Rupture of the esophagus is a very rare injury, but mortality is high if diagnosis is missed. A rupture of the esophagus usually results from penetrating trauma or a severe epigastric blow. It may be seen in conjunction with a pneumothorax or hemothorax without evidence of fractures, or it may be an iatrogenic injury that occurs during esophagoscopy.

ASSESSMENT

- Consider mechanism of injury
- Substernal pleuritic pain radiating to neck and shoulders[3]
- Mediastinal emphysema
- Mediastinal crunch sound
- Particulate matter in chest tube drainage

- Shock without associated pain
- Elevated temperature

DIAGNOSIS

- Clinical observation
- Contrast radiography (upper GI series)
- Endoscopy

THERAPEUTIC INTERVENTIONS

- Emergency surgery

CARDIAC AND GREAT VESSEL INJURIES

Myocardial contusion

Establishing the mechanism of injury is extremely important in suspecting the diagnosis of a myocardial contusion. One fourth of patients presenting with this injury will have no sign of physical injury.[3] It is usually caused by an impact of the myocardium on the chest wall, which causes a contusion to form. The contusion occurs as a result of a blunt trauma to the chest or a severe acceleration/deceleration force. Myocardial contusion can also occur following chest compression for cardiopulmonary resuscitation.

ASSESSMENT

- Consider mechanism of injury
- Complaints of severe chest pain, usually unaffected by vasodilatory drugs[6]
- Chest wall contusion/ecchymosis
- Dysrhythmias (usually within the first hour, but anywhere up to 24 hours), usually premature ventricular contractions, atrial fibrillation, right bundle branch block, or ST segment elevation in ECG; if there are premature ventricular contractions, there is possibility of ventricular injury

DIAGNOSIS

- High index of suspicion
- Mechanism of injury suggestive of severe blunt chest trauma (especially bent steering wheel)
- Possible signs of injury on 12-lead ECG (especially elevated ST segment in V_1, V_2, and V_3)
- Elevation of cardiac isoenzymes, similar to myocardial infarction

THERAPEUTIC INTERVENTIONS

- Assess and monitor this patient as if he or she were having a myocardial infarction.
- Administer oxygen.
- Administer an analgesia/narcotic for pain control.

- Administer the appropriate dysrhythmia therapy.
- Admit for observation and cardiac monitoring for at least 48 hours.

Pericardial tamponade

A pericardial tamponade is caused by bleeding myocardium, a ruptured coronary artery, or a lacerated pericardium. Blood from the wound is contained in the pericardial sac. This tamponade prevents the patient from hemorrhaging to death, but eventually it causes constriction of the heart, reducing cardiac output and causing hemodynamic deterioration. It is most frequently caused by a penetrating injury but may also be caused by a severe blunt trauma to the chest. Clinical personnel should think about the possibility of a pericardial tamponade whenever an unexplained pump failure is not responsive to volume replacement. This injury can be aggravated by inflation of PASG.[5]

ASSESSMENT

- Beck's triad
- Increased central venous pressure, evidenced by distended neck veins
  - Decreased arterial blood pressure
  - Muffled heart sounds
- Cyanosis
- Pulsus paradoxus
- Pulseless electrical activity (PEA)
- Patient unresponsive to resuscitation efforts

DIAGNOSIS

- High index of suspicion
- Clinical observation
- Chest x-ray; widened mediastinum
- Pericardiocentesis
- Echocardiography

THERAPEUTIC INTERVENTIONS

- Administer oxygen.
- Initiate an IV.
- Prepare for pericardiocentesis or minithoracotomy (Fig. 19-15).
- Monitor patient.

Aortic trauma

In aortic trauma the aorta tears, usually as a result of a blunt force to the chest at the point where the aorta is attached or fixed. It may also be caused by a penetrating force. It is most commonly associated with a motor vehicle collision (particularly lateral impact crashes) or a fall from a height where there is rapid deceleration.[7] The patient is critically injured and rarely survives long enough to reach the Emergency Department, and definitive care. There is an 85% mortality rate at the scene[8] and only a 50% chance of surviving after ar-

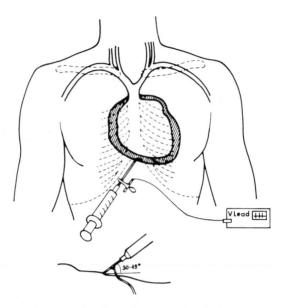

Fig. 19-15   Pericardiocentesis. (From Budassi SA, Barber J: *Mosby's manual of emergency care,* ed 3, St Louis, 1990, Mosby)

rival at the hospital.[2] The cause of death is exsanguination or massive pericardial tamponade.

The most common site for aortic rupture is at the ligamentum arteriosum (tethering point at junction between the aortic arch and the descending aorta). The integrity of the aorta may be maintained for a brief period by an intact adventitia or collateral circulation.

ASSESSMENT

- Consider mechanism of injury
- Trauma arrest
- Chest wall bruise
- Presence of a first or second rib fracture
- Left parascapular murmur
- Presence of upper extremity hypertension (if there is dissection)
- Decreased femoral pulses
- Sternal fracture
- Scapula or multiple rib fractures
- Paraplegia
- Tracheal deviation to the right
- Esophageal deviation (place nasogastric tube and observe deviation of tube)
- Lowered left main stem bronchus
- Elevated right main stem bronchus

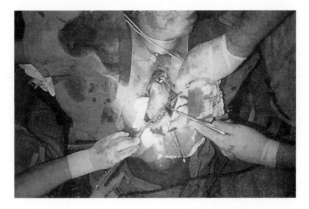

Fig. 19-16 Thoracotomy. (Courtesy Emanuel Hospital & Health Center, Portland, OR.)

DIAGNOSIS

Diagnosis of aortic trauma is made by a high index of suspicion because of the mechanism of injury.

- Visualized on x-ray

    Widened mediastinum, obliteration of aortic knob; and presence of pleural cap, hemothorax, or nasogastric deviation on x-ray[1]

- Visualized on thoracic aortogram
- Visualized on chest CT scan

THERAPEUTIC INTERVENTIONS

- CPR (even though it may not be effective)
- PASG, as indicated
- Administration of IV solutions and blood products
- Preparation for emergency thoracotomy (Fig. 19-16) and thoracic surgery consultation to

    Cross-clamp aorta

    Place patient on cardiopulmonary bypass

    Repair injury (resect and graft)

Subclavian artery injury

Subclavian artery injury may be a result of a blunt or penetrating force.

ASSESSMENT

- Consider mechanism of injury
- Observation of hematoma at base of neck
- Other signs of hemodynamic deterioration
- Difference in BP between right and left arm[6]

DIAGNOSIS

* Clinical observation
* Arteriography

THERAPEUTIC INTERVENTIONS

* Administer oxygen
* Administer IV fluids (place IV lines in lower extremities or on side opposite injury)
* Prepare patient for surgery

SUMMARY

Any patient with an obvious chest injury or a mechanism of injury suggestive of a chest injury should be treated as if he or she has a critical injury until such an injury can be ruled out. With a high index of suspicion and aggressive appropriate therapeutic intervention, these patients may be saved from death or permanent disability.

REFERENCES

1. American College of Surgeons Committee on Trauma: *Advanced trauma life support instructor manual,* Chicago, 1993, American College of Surgeons.
2. Laskowski-Jones L: Meeting the challenge of chest trauma, *Am J Nurs* 22-29, September 1995.
3. Jackimczyk K: Blunt chest trauma, *Emerg Med Clin North Am* 11:1, February 1993.
4. Wilson R, Walt A: *Management of trauma: pitfalls and practice,* ed 2, Philadelphia, 1996, Williams & Wilkins.
5. Ivatury R: *The textbook of penetrating trauma,* Philadelphia, 1996, Williams & Wilkins.
6. Emergency Nurses Association: *Emergency nursing core curriculum,* ed 4, Philadelphia, 1994, Saunders.
7. Katyal D, and others: Lateral impact motor vehicle collisions: significant cause of blunt traumatic rupture of the thoracic aorta, *J Trauma,* 42:5, May 1997.
8. Emergency Nurses Association: *Trauma nursing core course instructors manual,* ed 4, Chicago, 1995, Emergency Nurses Association.

CHAPTER 20

Abdominal, Genitourinary, and Pelvic Trauma

Andrea Novak

The abdominal cavity extends from the diaphragm to the pelvis and is highly susceptible to injury because of the lack of bony protection for underlying organs.[1] Free space in the abdomen can contain a large amount of shed blood before tamponade occurs, and exsanguination from abdominal injuries should be of utmost concern. Care of the patient with abdominal injuries on the surface appears simple yet may be complex.

Blunt trauma can cause severe injuries to abdominal contents as energy is diffused throughout the solid and hollow structures. Peritoneal injury and internal bleeding may not be recognizable immediately on arrival to the Emergency Department (ED). Frequent reassessment and a high index of suspicion based on mechanism of injury, history, and signs and symptoms should guide the healthcare provider in identification and management of the patient with abdominal trauma. Penetrating injury can be caused by any object that penetrates the abdominal wall. Underlying structures may or may not be affected, and diagnosis by clinical signs alone is unreliable. The patient demonstrating an altered mental status should always be evaluated for unknown injuries to the abdomen. An important factor in increasing survival from abdominal trauma is decreasing the time from the occurrence of the injury to definitive treatment. In the emergency setting it is more important to determine whether or not the patient requires surgery than to determine which organs or viscera have been injured. Advances in medical technology have expanded the diagnostic approach to the patient with abdominal injuries and resulted in more expeditious surgical treatment when required, and a decrease in the number of unnecessary exploratory operations. Such diagnostics as computed tomography (CT), magnetic resonance imaging (MRI), sonography (ultrasound [US]), and laparoscopic evaluation have aided in the diagnosis of abdominal injury. Ultrasound is being used more frequently in many Emergency Departments to diagnose abdominal injury. This relatively

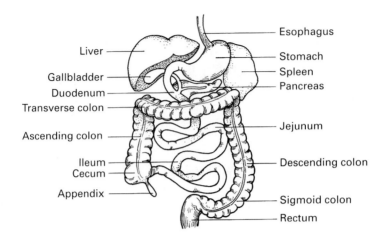

Fig. 20-1 Anatomy of the abdomen.

quick and simple procedure helps to decrease evaluation time in the ED and has an accuracy rate of 98.1%.[2]

ABDOMINAL ANATOMY

The liver and spleen are located in the intrathoracic abdomen (high up in the abdomen) (Fig. 20-1). The small bowel, large bowel, bladder, and pelvic organs are located in what is known as the true abdomen. The retroperitoneal abdomen contains the kidneys, ureters, duodenum, and pancreas. These locations are important when considering the appropriate diagnostic examinations to use.

BLUNT TRAUMA

The most common mechanisms of blunt trauma are motor vehicle crashes (MVC), injury from contact sports, violence/abuse, and falls. Blunt abdominal trauma should be suspected in any patient who has been involved in a traumatic event where the mechanism of injury was significant or where the patient has a decreased level of consciousness and may not be able to describe or demonstrate signs of pain.[3] Lack of pain sensation below a certain level may be indicative of spinal cord injury and may mask abdominal injury.[4]

ASSESSMENT

- Bruises on the abdominal wall (Fig. 20-2)
  - Circle ecchymotic area with marker to identify changes in size over time
- Auscultate for bowel sounds and bruits
  - Lack of bowel sounds may indicate ileus; presence of bruit in the presence of penetrating injury may indicate major vascular disruption

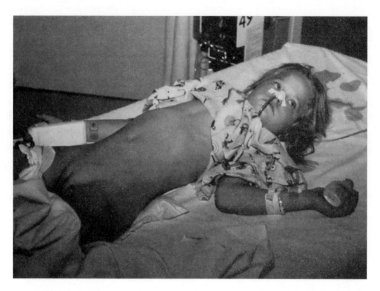

Fig. 20-2   Bruises on the abdominal wall are suggestive of intraabdominal injury. (Courtesy Karen Killian.)

- Pain, tenderness, or guarding
  - Referred pain, such as Kehr's sign (pain in the left shoulder) is a classic sign of splenic injury
- Abdominal wall rigidity or masses
- Crepitus
- Distended abdomen
- Signs of hypovolemia or hypovolemic shock/Vital signs
- Rectal exam
  - Check for sphincter tone and blood
  - Position of prostate (if appropriate)
- Other associated injuries: especially rib fractures, chest, and spinal cord injuries

DIAGNOSIS

Patients with blunt trauma to the abdomen are the most difficult to diagnose. The key to diagnosis is to obtain a good history, evaluate and reevaluate the patient's clinical signs, and conduct the appropriate diagnostic studies.
- ED Ultrasound to identify the presence of free fluid in the abdomen.
- X-rays: Flat plate of abdomen, Pelvis, Chest, to observe for free air in the peritoneum, displacement of abdominal organs, fractures, and level of the diaphragm.
- CT scan (with and/or without contrast) to observe for hematomas, free blood, and displacement of abdominal organs.

- Cystogram (suspected bladder injury) to identify displacement of the bladder or leakage of urine.
- Guaiac test on any specimen from the rectum, bladder, or stomach to detect occult bleeding.
- Retrograde urethrogram to look for interruption of the urethra.
- Laboratory evaluation should include Complete Blood Count (CBC), liver enzymes, serum amylase, clotting factors, renal function studies, pregnancy test (if appropriate), urinalysis, and toxicology as indicated.
- Diagnostic peritoneal lavage (DPL) to rule out blood and fecal contamination of the peritoneal fluid and possible intraabdominal injury.
- Intravenous pyelogram (IVP) look at kidney perfusion, placement, and/or extravasation of blood or urine from the urinary tract.
- Laparoscopic exam
- Exploratory surgery

THERAPEUTIC INTERVENTIONS

- **Assure ABCs**—Administer 100% oxygen; initiate IV therapy (two large-bore) with lactated Ringer's or normal saline solution; and stabilize the cervical, thoracic, and lumbar spine.
- **Insert nasogastric/orogastric tube**—To decompress the stomach and avoid aspiration.
- **Insert Foley catheter**—If no contraindications, that is blood at urinary meatus, high-rising prostate on rectal exam.
- **Prepare for surgical intervention**—Prophylactic antibiotic IV therapy preoperatively.
- **Consider extra peritoneal injuries**

Specific types of injuries from blunt trauma

Spleen

The spleen is a dense organ, located on the left side of the abdomen, just behind the eighth through twelfth ribs in the left upper quadrant. The spleen is the most commonly traumatized solid organ, with the liver and kidney next in line. Injury to the spleen may cause hypovolemia, shock, and death if unrecognized. The patient may complain of pain radiating to the left shoulder (Kehr's sign) when the spleen is ruptured. The definitive diagnosis of splenic rupture is made by a CT scan of the abdomen/spleen or by exploratory laparoscopy or laparotomy. The presence of blood in the DPL fluid should raise the index of suspicion for injury.

Liver

The liver, a solid organ, is also frequently injured in blunt abdominal trauma because it is large, dense, only partially protected by the anterior ribs, and is anteriorly located. Suspect liver injury when there is trauma to the eighth through twelfth ribs on the right side of the body or trauma to the upper central part of the abdomen. A patient with liver injury may also demonstrate

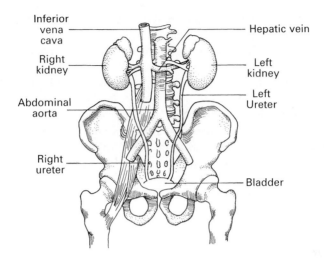

Fig. 20-3   Location of the hepatic vein, inferior vena cava, and abdominal aorta.

signs of respiratory difficulty because of the liver's close proximity to the lung, on the opposite side of the diaphragm. A bloody return of peritoneal lavage fluid may be indicative of liver injury as well. Small lacerations of the liver may heal without surgical intervention; however, large or stellate lacerations should be considered for surgical repair.

Pancreas

The pancreas is a solid organ that is rarely injured in blunt trauma because of its protective placement in the posterior upper abdomen. A common mechanism of injury is from a blow to the midepigastrum from a steering wheel or handlebar of a bicycle.[5] If the pancreas is injured, the injury is usually discovered because of a high index of suspicion, worsening abdominal pain or signs of peritonitis, or because serum amylase or serum lipase is high or rises over a 24-hour period. The use of DPL or Emergency Department ultrasound in diagnosing pancreatic injury may not be reliable. Peritoneal lavage fluid should be sent to the laboratory for amylase analysis, as well as for blood, feces, bile, and white blood cell counts.

Hepatic vein, inferior vena cava, and abdominal aorta

Disruption of these major vessels can be lethal if not corrected with emergency surgery (Fig. 20-3). The patient will demonstrate signs and symptoms of hypovolemic shock. Diagnosis is usually made on angiography or at surgery.

Stomach

The stomach is a hollow organ. Injury to the stomach is rare in blunt abdominal trauma because the stomach is flexible and can readily be displaced without damage. However, if the stomach is full at the time of the incident, there is a higher likelihood of stomach or diaphragmatic injury. Insertion of a nasogastric or orogastric tube allows for testing of gastric contents for blood. Free air in the abdomen on x-ray should lead one to suspect either a stomach or an intestinal injury. Definitive diagnosis is made on exploratory laparotomy.

Large and small intestines

The large and small intestines are hollow organs that are frequently injured in both blunt and penetrating trauma. These injuries may lead to sepsis caused by the release of intestinal contents into the abdominal cavity. Patients may initially present with signs of peritoneal irritation. Definitive diagnosis is made on exploratory laparotomy.

Diaphragm

When the diaphragm is ruptured and left uncorrected, death may ensue rapidly. If the injury is small and goes undetected, leakage of abdominal contents into the chest cavity may take place over a period of several days to weeks. Since signs and symptoms of this injury are so nonspecific, it is important to rule out other injuries and keep in mind the possibility of diaphragmatic rupture throughout the initial assessment and resuscitation. Diagnosis is usually made by observation on x-ray of an air bubble in the stomach or intestine above the diaphragm.

GENITOURINARY TRAUMA

The genitourinary (GU) system is subject to injury from external forces just like the rest of the abdomen. The integrity of the urinary system and male reproductive organs is easily disrupted from either blunt or penetrating trauma.[6]

ASSESSMENT

- Always begin with the ABCs.
- During the secondary assessment inspect the perineum—lacerations may be indicative of open pelvic fracture.[5]
- Rectal exam—check prostate gland, check for blood and sphincter tone (decreased sphincter tone may indicate spinal cord injury). Perform rectal exam *before* insertion of Foley catheter in a patient with suspected GU/pelvic injury.
- Check urinary meatus for blood.
- Scrotum—look for edema, ecchymoses, hematomas, testicular disruption.
- Vaginal exam.
- Ability to void spontaneously.
- Flank area for tenderness, presence of hematomas, masses.
- Impaled objects—do not remove, stabilize and prepare for surgical removal.

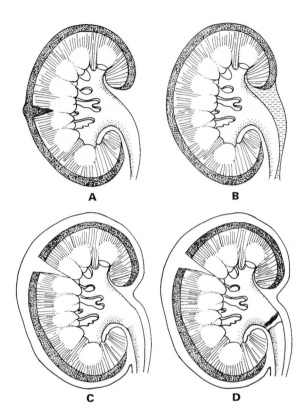

Fig. 20-4 **A,** Lacerated kidney, bleeding contained in capsule. **B,** Fracture with extravasation of urine. **C,** Laceration through the capsule with blood extravasation. **D,** Fracture/laceration with extravasation of blood and urine.

Kidney

The kidneys are located in the retroperitoneal space at the level of T12 to L3 (Fig. 20-4). The right kidney is slightly lower than the left because of the position of the liver. They are not fixed to the abdominal wall. They are held in place by fascia and renal vessels. The kidneys are the most frequently injured structure in the GU system.[6] Two types of injuries generally occur to the kidneys.

- A *contusion* is usually self-limiting. It is diagnosed by history and by urinalysis that detects the presence of blood. Therapeutic intervention includes bed rest, fluids, monitoring hematocrit, vital signs, and frequent urine checks.
- A *fracture/laceration* of the kidney is more severe and may require surgery (a partial or total nephrectomy) for repair. There may be a hemorrhage or urine extravasation or both. The extent of injury depends on which part of the kidney is damaged. Diagnosis is made by contrast CT,

urinalysis, and/or IVP. Depending on the extent of the injury, therapeutic intervention varies, ranging from bed rest and fluids to surgery for repair, or nephrectomy.

Ureter

Ureters are hollow and are rarely injured in blunt abdominal trauma. Suspect uretal injury with gunshot wounds where the entrance or exit wound is in the lower abdomen or flank area. Gunshot wounds account for 95% of penetrating urethral injuries.[6] Diagnosis of urethral injuries is made by IVP. Therapeutic intervention is surgical reanastomosis.

Bladder

The bladder is a hollow organ and may rupture as a result of penetration from a pelvic fracture or as the result of blunt trauma when the bladder contains a large amount of urine. This injury is diagnosed on cystogram, and if the bladder is ruptured, surgical repair is most likely indicated.

Urethra

Disruption of the urethra is more common in males than in females. This type of injury is rare with blunt trauma, but is seen frequently in association with extensive pelvic fractures. It is diagnosed by the clinical finding of a high-floating prostate gland in men, or on a retrograde urethrogram. The retrograde urethrogram should be done before insertion of a Foley catheter in patients with a high index of suspicion of urethral injury.

GENITAL TRAUMA

Testicular and scrotal injury

Blunt trauma to the testicles may cause a hematocele to form, which appears blue on the tender scrotum. Doppler studies can help identify the extent of testicular trauma.[5] Management is with elevation, cold packs, analgesics, and rest, or with testicular rupture surgical exploration and removal of blood clots.

Penile trauma

Trauma to the penis may result from self-inflicted wounds (stabbings, amputations, vacuum cleaner injuries) or blunt trauma. Contusions are treated with elevation of the scrotum, cold packs, and rest. With penile rupture, the patient may report hearing a cracking sound followed by intense penile pain with swelling and discoloration. Urethral injuries may also be present. This condition requires immediate surgical evacuation of the blood clot and repair of torn vessels.[5] Strangulation of the penis from an object (condom, ring, etc.) can result in ischemia, necrosis, and gangrene. The object needs to be removed immediately. Conservative treatment may include débridement of necrotic tissue.

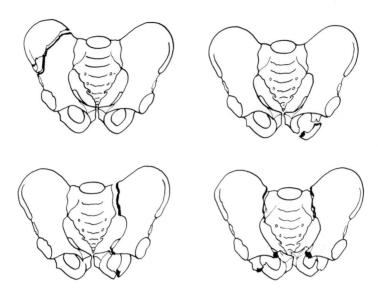

Fig. 20-5   Types of pelvic fractures.

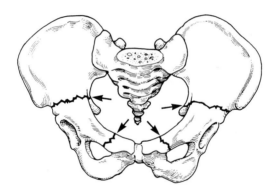

Fig. 20-6   Fractured pelvis. Because of its ring formation, the pelvis usually fractures in two places. The common areas of fracture are indicated.

Pelvic fracture

Pelvic fractures are usually the result of a crush injury or rapid acceleration/deceleration injury that might occur in MVCs or motorcycle crashes, penetrating trauma, falls from a significant height, or from a sudden contraction of muscle against resistance (Fig. 20-5).

   If a pelvic fracture is present (Fig. 20-6), one should anticipate the potential for a massive amount of internal bleeding and prepare for blood volume replacement. Rule of thumb is that one to two units of blood are lost for every pelvic fracture.[3] Timely stabilization of the fractured pelvis helps control bleeding. Concurrently, clinical personnel should search for other associated injuries while observing the patient carefully for hemodynamic compromise. Assume that there is major soft tissue abdominal injury as well until proven otherwise, as a result of the tremendous amount of energy that is required to fracture the pelvis. Diagnosis is made on x-ray. Therapeutic intervention ranges from bed rest to internal or external reduction and fixation.

ASSESSMENT

- ABCs
- Evaluate for hypovolemic shock
- Pain or inability in leg movement
- Tenderness over pubis or when iliac wings are compressed
- Paraspinous muscle spasm
- Sacroiliac joint tenderness
- Paresis or hemiparesis
- Pelvic ecchymosis
- Hematuria and/or inability to void spontaneously
- Rectal exam—check for blood
- Vaginal exam—check for penetrating wounds or bony fragments

THERAPEUTIC INTERVENTIONS

- Administer 100% oxygen
- Treat hypovolemia
- Consider early stabilization with pelvic external fixation
- Stabilize spine and legs
- Monitor vital signs frequently (every 5 minutes)
- Consider angiography and embolization of pelvic vascular structure
- Monitor output—insert Foley catheter if no contraindications or suprapubic cystotomy
- Check for other fractures and injuries (especially of the spine, abdomen, and knees)
- Prophylactic IV antibiotics when considered an open fracture
- Assist with diagnostics: x-ray, CT, laboratory work; type and crossmatch for blood and blood products
- Orthopedic consult

Complications may be internal bleeding (up to 8 units possible), bladder trauma, genital trauma, lumbosacral trauma, ruptured internal organs, shock, and death.

PENETRATING TRAUMA

The extent of injury from penetrating trauma depends on the entry and exit sites of the penetrating object, its size and velocity, and the distance and angle of projection. Injury may range from minimal to severe and may not be confined to the direct path of the object between the entry and exit sites. Therefore penetrating injuries to the abdomen should also be considered penetrating trauma to the chest until proven otherwise. Clinical personnel should consider the mechanism of injury and observe very carefully for hemodynamic compromise. If the mechanism of injury is suggestive of severely underlying trauma or if the wound was caused by a high-velocity missile, exploratory surgery is indicated so that a definitive diagnosis and appropriate therapeutic interventions can be applied.

ASSESSMENT

Assessment varies depending on the nature and extent of the injury. The patient should be observed very closely for signs and symptoms of hypovolemic shock. Intraabdominal bleeding usually manifests early with signs of peritoneal irritation.

THERAPEUTIC INTERVENTIONS

- ABCs
- Administer supplemental oxygen
- Initiate two large-bore IVS with Ringer's lactate or normal saline
- Stabilize spinal column
- PASG if indicated
- Saline dressings on eviscerated tissue
- Stabilize impaled objects for later surgical removal
- Prepare for surgery to repair injuries

Abdominal trauma is a frequent occurrence. Careful attention to assessment details is key to diagnosis and appropriate interventions.

REFERENCES

1. Emergency Nurses Association: *Trauma nursing core course,* Chicago, 1995, Emergency Nurses Association.
2. Clevenger F, Tepas III J: Preoperative management of patients with major trauma injuries, *AORNJ* 65(3):592, 1997.
3. American College of Surgeons Committee on Trauma: *Advanced trauma life support,* Chicago, 1993, American College of Surgeons.
4. Wachtel TL: Current concepts in the management of the trauma patient, *Crit Care Nurs Quart* 17(2):34-50, 1994.
5. Tintinalli J, editor: *Emergency medicine: a comprehensive study guide,* New York, 1996, McGraw-Hill.
6. Karlowicz K, editor: *Urologic nursing: principles and practice,* Philadelphia, 1995, Saunders.

SUGGESTED READINGS

Cardona V, and others, editors: *Trauma nursing,* ed 2, Philadelphia, 1994, Saunders.
Sheehy SB: *Manual of emergency care,* ed 5, St Louis, 1997, Mosby.
Sommers M: Missed injuries: a case of trauma hide and seek, *AACN Clinical Issues* 6(2):187-195, 1995.

CHAPTER 21

Extremity and Vascular Trauma

Kathleen J. Burns

EXTREMITY TRAUMA

Injuries to arms and legs are more frequent and generally considered less life-threatening than injuries to the torso. When the patient has suffered multiple injuries, it is important to recall the principles of the trauma assessment and first identify and focus on life-threatening injuries and not be distracted by the deformities that frequently accompany extremity injuries. However, a great number of the disabilities and days of missed work that are suffered every year are the direct result of limb trauma. Prompt and appropriate management may not only be life- and limb-saving but may also prevent subsequent disabilities and reduce the costs of those disabilities to individuals and society.

DEFINITIONS*

- *Skeleton*   Forms framework of body; provides support and protection.
- *Bone*   Two types: (1) cancellous (spongy) bone, found in skull, vertebrae, pelvis, and long-bone ends and (2) cortical (dense) bone, found in long bones. Bone has its own blood and nerve supply and is usually capable of healing itself. Bones serve to protect vital organs and serve as levers for movement.
- *Ligament*   Fibrous connective tissue that connects bone to bone.
- *Tendon*   Fibrous connective tissue that connects muscle to bone.
- *Cartilage*   Dense connective tissue between ribs; in the nasal septum, ear, larynx, trachea, and bronchi; between vertebrae; and on the articulating surfaces of bones. Cartilage has no neurovascular supply.
- *Joints*   Connection of two bones for mobility and stability; may provide flexion and extension, medial and lateral rotation, abduction and adduction. Consists of articulating bone surfaces that are covered with carti-

---

*Definitions from Budassi SA: *Mosby's manual of emergency care*, ed 4, St Louis, 1998, Mosby.

lage, a two-layered sac containing synovial membranes (to lubricate), and a capsule that thickens and becomes a ligament. Muscle that overlies joints attaches the bone surfaces to one another and provides movement.

EMERGENCY MANAGEMENT

After identifying injuries that are more life-threatening, it is important to assess and stabilize all limb injuries. Obtain a brief history, and discover the mechanism of injury. Consider patterns of injury to assist with diagnosis. For instance, a fractured right humerus and a fractured left femur in a patient who was struck by debris in an explosion would suggest that the plane of injury may also include the chest, abdomen, and pelvis, the structures that lie between the two obviously injured parts. Early treatment includes:

- ABCs
- Quick assessment for other major trauma (head, cervical spine, chest, and abdomen)
- Protection of head and cervical spine
- Immobilization of traumatized limb to include joints above and below trauma site
- Evaluation of vascular status of limb distal to injury before and after immobilization:
    Pulses distal to trauma
    Color
    Temperature
    Capillary refill
- Evaluation of neurologic status of limb before and after immobilization
    Voluntary movement
    Sensation
- Reduction of the fracture *only* if vascular status is compromised
- Elevation and support of limb, if possible
- Application of cold pack to area
- Transportation to hospital

Immobilization is accomplished before movement or transport to prevent further damage and to reduce the amount of pain and avoid further discomfort.

Clinical personnel should note any swelling, discoloration, contusions, abrasion, or obvious deformities. If the injury includes an open fracture:

- Irrigate wound site with normal saline
- Apply sterile, normal saline dressing; cover with dry sterile dressing
- Apply slight compression dressing to control hemorrhage
- Splint limb
- Do not attempt to reduce fracture in field
- Assess need for tetanus shot; administer booster, if needed

If a puncture wound is present but no bone is protruding, clinical personnel should assume that the wound was made by a jagged bone end or missile and treat it as an open fracture. To control bleeding:

- Apply pressure over bleeding site or on edges of wound
- Elevate extremity, if possible

A tourniquet should be used only as a life-saving measure. The limb may have to be amputated if all circulation ceases for an extended period of time.

When the patient arrives in the Emergency Department, he or she should be undressed to avoid missing any injuries. The patient should be turned to examine front and back, stabilizing the injured limb throughout the maneuver.

SOFT-TISSUE INJURIES

Strains

A strain is a weakening or stretching of a muscle at the tendon attachment. It may be the result of any trauma that stresses the attachment or injures the muscle in that area.

Mild strain

ASSESSMENT

- Local pain
- Point tenderness
- Spasm

THERAPEUTIC INTERVENTIONS

- Compression bandage
- Elevation for 12 hours
- Cold pack for 12 hours
- Weight bearing as tolerated, but with as much rest and elevation as possible

Moderate strain

ASSESSMENT

- Point tenderness
- Local pain
- Swelling
- Discoloration
- Inability to use for short time

THERAPEUTIC INTERVENTIONS

- Compression bandage
- Elevation for 24 hours
- Cold pack for 24 hours
- Consider need for analgesic

- Light weight bearing as tolerated
- Assistive device for ambulation

Severe strain

ASSESSMENT

- Point tenderness
- Local pain
- Swelling
- Ecchymosis
- Snapping noise at time of injury

THERAPEUTIC INTERVENTIONS

- Compression bandage
- Elevation for 24 to 48 hours
- Cold pack for 48 hours
- Consider need for analgesia
- No weight bearing for 48 hours
- Assistive device for ambulation

Sprains

A mild sprain is a ligament that has been stretched. A moderate sprain is a ligament that has been partially torn. A severe sprain is a ligament that has been completely torn. The mechanism of injury may be the same as for a strain, but usually one with exaggerated force. Joint motion exceeds its normal limits. Most common sprains are in the shoulders, knees, wrists, and ankles.

Mild sprain

ASSESSMENT

- Slight pain
- Slight swelling

THERAPEUTIC INTERVENTIONS

- Compression bandage
- Elevation for 12 hours
- Cold pack for 12 hours
- Light weight bearing as tolerated

Moderate sprain

ASSESSMENT

- Pain
- Point tenderness
- Swelling
- Inability to use for short time
- Ecchymosis

THERAPEUTIC INTERVENTIONS

- Compression bandage
- Rigid splint
- Elevation for 24 hours
- Cold pack for 24 hours
- Minimal weight bearing for 3 days
- Consider need for analgesia
- Assistive device for ambulation

Severe sprain

ASSESSMENT

- Pain
- Point tenderness
- Swelling
- Ecchymosis
- Inability to use

THERAPEUTIC INTERVENTIONS

- Compression bandage
- Rigid splint or cast
- Elevation for 48 hours
- Cold pack for 48 hours
- No weight bearing for 3 days
- Consider need for analgesia
- Assistive device for ambulation

Achilles' tendon rupture

An Achilles' tendon rupture occurs most often in athletes over 30 years old. The injury usually occurs in stop-and-start sports (such as tennis or racquetball) in which one steps off abruptly on the forefoot with the knee forces in extension. The patient will usually describe a "snap" or "pop" noise and little or no pain at the time of injury. Many athletes who suffer this injury do not seek immediate care because of the lack of pain.

ASSESSMENT

- Inability to extend foot (will not be able to stand on toes of affected side)
- Deformity
- Palpable gap in tendon
- Positive Thompson's sign*

---

*Positive Thompson's sign: With the leg extended and the foot over the end of a table, squeeze the calf muscle; no heel pull or upward movement will be seen.

- Compression
- Elevation
- Cold pack
- Consider need for analgesia
- Surgical repair
- Toe-to-knee plaster splints and nonweight bearing
- Assistive device for ambulation

PERIPHERAL NERVE INJURIES

Peripheral nerve injuries can be caused by trauma (mechanical, chemical, or thermal), toxins, malignancy, metabolic disorders, or collagen disease (Table 21-1). In the emergency situation, they are usually associated with lacerations, fractures, dislocations, and penetrating wounds.

Accurate assessment requires an understanding of the distribution of nerves, the origin of motor branches, and the muscles they supply.

The clinician should recognize that motor loss tests are accurate only if he or she can palpate or visualize the tendon or muscle belly under consideration. Diagnostic tests such as electromyography, nerve conduction tests, and electrical stimulation are of little or no value in the emergency evaluation of peripheral nerve injury.

Repair of peripheral nerves should not be undertaken as an Emergency Department surgical intervention.

Table 21-1   Modes for Assessing Common Peripheral Nerve Injuries

Nerve	Frequently associated injuries	Assessment technique*
Radial	Fracture of humerus, especially middle and distal thirds	Inability to extend thumb in "hitchhiker's sign"
Ulnar	Fracture of medial humeral epicondyle	Loss of pain perception in tip of little finger
Median	Elbow dislocation or wrist or forearm injury	Loss of pain perception in tip of index finger
Peroneal	Tibia or fibula fracture, dislocation of knee	Inability to extend great toe or foot; may also be associated with sciatic nerve injury
Sciatic and tibial	Sciatic nerve injuries should be considered in patients with hip fractures or dislocations; tibial nerve injuries are associated with knee injuries	Loss of pain perception in sole of foot

*Test is invalid if extension tendons are severed or if severe muscle damage is present.

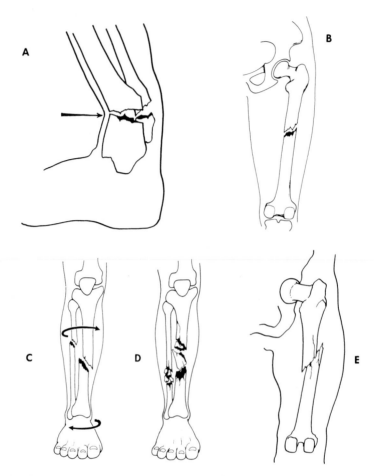

Fig. 21-1 Types of fractures. **A,** Transverse; **B,** oblique; **C,** spiral; **D,** comminuted; **E,** impacted.

Continued

FRACTURES

Fractures are divided into two general categories:
- *Closed* (simple): the skin is not disrupted
- *Open* (compound): the skin is disrupted by
  Bone puncturing from inside out
  Object puncturing from outside in, with resultant fracture

There are many different types of fractures (Fig. 21-1):
- *Transverse*   Results from angulation force or direct trauma
- *Oblique*   Results from twisting force
- *Spiral*   Results from twisting force with firmly planted foot
- *Comminuted*   Results from severe direct trauma; has more than two fragments

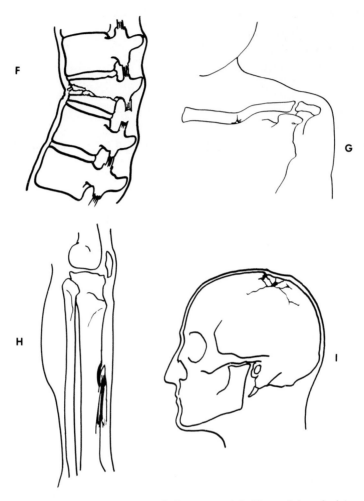

Fig. 21-1—cont'd **F,** compressed; **G,** greenstick; **H,** avulsion; **I,** depression.

- *Impacted*   Results from severe trauma causing fracture ends to jam together
- *Compressed*   Results from severe force to top of head or os calcis or from acceleration-deceleration injury
- *Greenstick*   Results from compression force; usually occurs in children under 10 years of age and middle school or high school athletes
- *Avulsion*   Results from muscle mass contracting forcefully, causing bone fragment to tear off at insertion
- *Depression*   Results from blunt trauma to flat bone; usually involves much soft-tissue damage

ASSESSMENT

When treating a patient with a suspected limb fracture, one should always assess for the *five Ps:*

Pain and point tenderness
Pulse (distal to fracture site)
Pallor
Paresthesia (distal to fracture site)
Paralysis (distal to fracture site)

The following factors should also be included in assessment:

Deformity
Swelling
Crepitus
Discoloration
Open wounds
Other injuries

Clinical personnel should always suspect a fracture in limb trauma until proven otherwise. The patient's inability to move the limb or the presence of pain on movement should make the examiner suspicious of fracture. X-ray examination is the most definitive way of detecting a fracture. The film should include the joints above and below the suspected fracture and should be taken in both anterioposterior and lateral views.

THERAPEUTIC INTERVENTIONS

- ABCs
- Assess patient (as described above)
- Determine mechanism of injury
- Immobilize limb (above and below fracture site)
- Reassess neurovascular status
- Apply traction if circulatory compromise is present
- Elevate injured limb, if possible (to decrease swelling and hemorrhage)
- Apply cold pack (to cause vasoconstriction and reduce swelling, spasm, and pain)

Complications of fractures include:

Blood loss causing hypovolemia and shock
Injury to vital organs
Neurologic and/or vascular damage
Infection (in open fractures)
Fat embolism
Deep vein thrombosis
Rhabdomyolysis
Compartment syndrome

Fat embolism

Fat embolism may occur 24 to 48 hours after trauma and usually comes from a pelvic, tibial, or femoral fracture, but it may come from any other fracture site. Fat embolism has a high mortality rate and is a life-threatening situation.

- Elevated temperature
- Rapid pulse
- Decreasing level of consciousness
- Inefficient respirations, leading to respiratory failure
- Cough
- Dyspnea
- Cyanosis
- Pulmonary edema
- Petechiae

- Oxygen at high flow
- Close observation and monitoring
- Supportive therapy

Rhabdomyolysis

Rhabdomyolysis may be seen with fractures and crush injuries when there is major muscle destruction along with ischemia and edema, causing the release of potassium and myoglobin. Patients who are also hypotensive and hypovolemic may develop tubular necrosis and renal failure.

Compartment syndrome

Compartment syndrome should be suspected in patients with severe fractures or crush injuries. This syndrome develops secondary to an increase in the pressure of the joint, resulting in a decrease blood supply to the muscles and nerves, leading to ischemia and necrosis if the pressures are not reduced. Compartment syndrome usually occurs within 6 to 8 hours of injury. It may occur in any soft-tissue compartment but is most commonly seen in the forearm and lower extremities.

- Throbbing pain out of proportion to injury that is not relieved by analgesia
- Increased pain with passive stretching
- Firmness over compartment

- Ongoing assessment of compartment for pain, firmness
- Compartment pressures checked by orthopedics
- Fasciotomies for elevated pressures

VASCULAR TRAUMA

A person who sustains trauma to the vascular system is at risk of losing an extremity or his or her life. Vascular trauma is often the consequence of blunt or penetrating injury. It may be seen in conjunction with fractures, deceleration injuries, crush injuries, and many other mechanisms. Injuries may involve veins, arteries, or both. Usually, when penetrating trauma, such as a gunshot wound, stab wound, or blast injury, occurs, the resulting vascular trauma is a laceration or transection. Blunt trauma, such as occurs with deceleration injuries, crush injuries, and joint disruptions may cause dissections, hematomas, or disruptions.

Signs and symptoms of vascular injury may include:
• Internal hemorrhage
• External hemorrhage
• Audible bruit

Arterial injuries may cause
• Pain
• Pallor
• Pulselessness
• Paresthesias
• Paralysis (neurologic deficit)
• Cold distal extremity
• Pale distal extremity

When a trauma patient presents at the Emergency Department, clinical personnel should think about the mechanism of injury, the location of the injury, and the proximity of the injury to arterial structures while they are completing a primary and secondary survey.

During the secondary survey, clinical personnel should check the affected part for:
• Pulses (to be described as normal, diminished, absent, or Doppler) (Box 21-1)
• Capillary refill
• External blood loss
• Skin color, temperature, and moisture
• Type of wound
• Neurovascular status

BOX 21-1

PROMINENT PULSES

• Carotid
• Brachial
• Radial
• Ulnar
• Femoral
• Popliteal
• Dorsalis pedis
• Posterior tibial

- Hematoma (and pulsations of hematoma)
- Bruits
- Differences in extremities

Definitive diagnosis of arterial injury can be made by:
- Pulselessness
- Angiography
- Computed tomography (CT scan)

TYPES OF VASCULAR INJURIES

Vascular laceration

A vascular laceration will usually bleed until a thrombus forms or the vessel is repaired. An artery that is lacerated may continue to have pulses unless it is transected.

Vascular transection

A vascular transection is a complete disruption of the vessel. When a vessel is transected, particularly an artery, bleeding may be minimal because transection causes the vessel to contract and go into spasm. A transection usually occurs from penetrating trauma or from a shearing or stretch injury.

Vascular contusion

When a contusion has occurred in the lining of the vasculature, a thrombus usually forms. This thrombus may cause an obstruction or may break loose and become an embolus. A vascular contusion occurs as the result of a stretching injury or a tear in the adventitia from an acceleration/deceleration injury.

Vascular crush

A vascular crush injury usually involves the surrounding soft tissues (skin and muscles), nerve, and bone. The entire injured area becomes edematous and causes compression that leads to severely compromised circulation. If a crush injury is large with no associated hemorrhage, lab studies might show an increase in hematocrit and hemoglobin. (As plasma leaks into the surrounding tissues, the percentage of hematocrit and hemoglobin left in whole blood will increase proportionally.) Also, serum potassium increases as injured cells release potassium. Myoglobin is also released from injured muscles. Victims of vascular crush injury present with the possibility of compartment syndrome.

Vascular pseudoaneurysm

Occasionally an artery will be lacerated, and the laceration will become temporarily closed by a blood clot. The inside lining communicates with the arterial lumen. The clot will begin to deteriorate, and the hematoma near the clot will increase in size. This hematoma does not occlude the artery. Because it does not encompass all the layers of the arterial wall, it is known as a *pseudoaneurysm.*

Pseudoaneurysms may increase in size and eventually rupture. They can usually be identified on angiography and should subsequently be surgically repaired.

THERAPEUTIC INTERVENTIONS ▰▰▰▰▰▰▰▰▰▰▰▰▰▰▰▰▰▰▰▰▰▰▰▰

- ABCs
  - Direct pressure
  - Use of pressure cuff
  - IV fluid replacement
  - Angiogram to assess location and extent of injury or to provide means for inducing intentional embolization
- Splint fractures
- Surgery for vascular repair; patient may require surgery before angiography if situation is urgent

COMPLICATIONS OF VASCULAR INJURIES (BEFORE AND AFTER REPAIR)

- Spasms
- Edema
- Compartment syndrome
- Stenosis
- Thrombosis
- Emboli
- Hemorrhage
- Pain
- Decreased mobility
- Infection
- Disseminated intravascular coagulation (DIC)
- Arteriovenous fistula
- Gangrene
- Contractures
- Failure of repair site

SPECIFIC FRACTURES AND ASSOCIATED VASCULAR INJURIES

Clavicular fracture

A clavicular fracture is common in all age groups (Fig. 21-2). It is usually the result of a fall on the arm or shoulder or direct trauma to the shoulder laterally (contact injury in which athletes run into one another). Clavicular fracture is a common athletic injury.

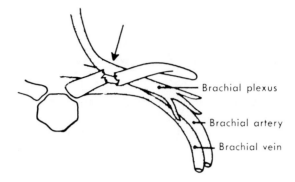

Brachial plexus

Brachial artery

Brachial vein

Fig. 21-2 Clavicular fracture.

ASSESSMENT

- Pain in clavicular area
- Point tenderness
- Inability to raise arm or make sawing motion
- Swelling
- Deformity
- Crepitus
- Head tilted toward side of injury, chin to opposite side

THERAPEUTIC INTERVENTIONS

- Assessment of neurovascular status
- Close observation for hematoma at base of neck that may suggest injury to subclavian vessels; any patient who is hypotensive with no other injury should be considered for arteriography to rule out subclavian vessel injury
- Arm support
- Sling and swath
- Cold pack
- Padding axillary area well to avoid damage to brachial plexus and artery
- Consider need for analgesia
- Orthopedic consult

Subclavian artery disruption

Because of the anatomic location of the subclavian artery and vein between the clavicle and the first rib, one or both vessels may be disrupted when there is a fracture of the first rib or a severely fractured clavicle. In addition, clinical personnel may see a scapular fracture.

ASSESSMENT

- Signs of shock
- Unilateral diminished pulse

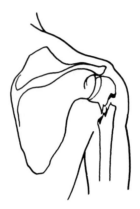

Fig. 21-3 Shoulder fracture.

- Unilateral cold, clammy, pale upper extremity
- Subclavicular hematoma
- Possible widened mediastinum on chest x-ray
- Possible airway obstruction (from expanding hematoma)

DIAGNOSIS

- Arteriogram
- CT scan

THERAPEUTIC INTERVENTIONS

- ABCs
- Surgical repair

Shoulder fracture (glenoid, humeral head, or humeral neck)

Shoulder fractures can occur from a fall on an outstretched arm or from direct trauma to the shoulder (Fig. 21-3). They occur in trauma to the shoulder in the elderly because of weaker bone structure; the same mechanisms of injury in a younger person would probably cause shoulder dislocation. A humeral neck fracture frequently causes axillary nerve damage.

ASSESSMENT

- Pain in shoulder area
- Point tenderness
- Refusal to move arm
- Gross swelling
- Ecchymosis

THERAPEUTIC INTERVENTIONS

- Assessment of neurovascular status
- Sling and swath

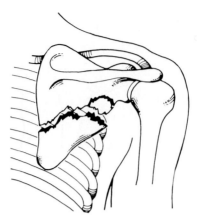

Fig. 21-4   Scapular fracture.

- Cold pack
- Consider need for analgesia
- Orthopedic consult

Scapular fracture

A scapular fracture may be caused by direct or indirect trauma (Fig. 21-4). Underlying injury of ribs and viscera may accompany this fracture.

ASSESSMENT

- Point tenderness
- Bone displacement
- Pain on shoulder movement
- Swelling

THERAPEUTIC INTERVENTIONS

- Assessment of neurovascular status
- Sling and swath
- Cold pack
- Consider need for analgesia
- Orthopedic consult

Upper arm (humeral shaft) fracture

An upper arm fracture is common in the elderly and children (Fig. 21-5). It may be caused by a fall on the arm, direct trauma, or dislocation.

ASSESSMENT

- Pain
- Point tenderness

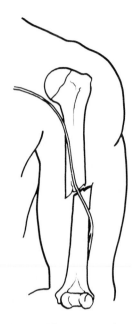

Fig. 21-5 Upper arm fracture.

- Swelling
- Inability or hesitance to move arm
- Severe deformity or angulation
- Crepitus

THERAPEUTIC INTERVENTIONS

- Assessment of neurovascular status
- Sling and swath
- Traction if there is vascular compromise
- Assessment for other injuries, especially to chest
- Cold pack
- Consider need for analgesia
- Orthopedic consult
- Recognize potential need for surgical intervention

Radial nerve damage may also occur if fracture occurs in the middle or distal portion of the shaft. Hemorrhage may be a complication, particularly if other fractures are present.

Elbow fracture

Elbow fracture is common in children and young athletes because of a fall on an extended arm or a fall on a flexed elbow (Fig. 21-6).

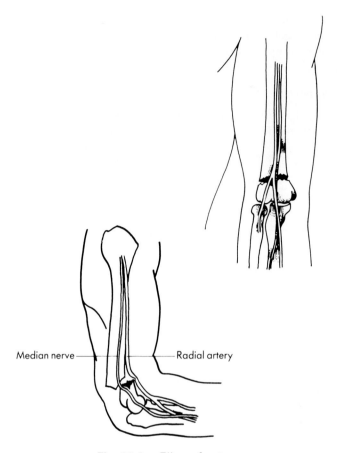

Median nerve — — Radial artery

Fig. 21-6 Elbow fracture.

ASSESSMENT

- Pain
- Point tenderness
- Swelling
- Refusal to move elbow
- Deformity
- Decreased circulation to hand

THERAPEUTIC INTERVENTIONS

- Assessment of neurovascular status
- Splinting "as it lies," usually with pillow, blanket, or sling and swath
- Cold pack
- Flexing of arm to greater degree if there is neurovascular compromise
- Consider need for analgesia

- Orthopedic consult
- Recognize potential need for surgical intervention

Additional complications associated with this injury are brachial artery laceration, median or radial nerve damage, and Volkmann's contracture.*

Brachial artery

The brachial artery may be injured during severe upper extremity trauma. It is the most frequently seen vascular injury in the upper extremities.

ASSESSMENT

- Pain in upper extremity
- Fracture, dislocation, or penetrating injury in upper extremity
- Loss of pulses unilaterally in upper extremity
- Pale, cold upper extremity
- Paresthesias or paralysis in upper extremity

DIAGNOSIS

- Arteriography

THERAPEUTIC INTERVENTIONS

- ABCs
- Surgical intervention

Forearm (radius or ulna) fracture

A forearm fracture may be caused by a fall on an extended arm or by a direct blow (Fig. 21-7). It is common in children and adults. Volkmann's contracture may be an additional complication.

ASSESSMENT

- Pain
- Point tenderness
- Swelling
- Deformity or angulation
- Shortening

THERAPEUTIC INTERVENTIONS

- Assessment of neurovascular status
- Splint
- Sling
- Cold pack
- Consider need for analgesia

---

*In Volkmann's contracture, degeneration and contraction of muscles occur because of ischemia caused by decreased arterial blood flow.

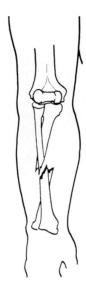

Fig. 21-7 Forearm fracture.

• Orthopedic consult
• Recognize potential need for surgical intervention

Wrist (distal radius, distal ulna, and carpal bone) fracture

Wrist fracture is common in the elderly, usually because of a fall on an extended arm and open hand (Fig. 21-8). Clinical personnel should be aware of the mechanism of injury. The patient may have had a fall from a height that originally resulted in a heel (os calcis) fracture, a lumbodorsal compression fracture, and a fall forward onto the open hand as a reaction to back pain, resulting in fracture of the distal radius and ulna (known as a *Colles' fracture* or *silver fork deformity*).

ASSESSMENT

• Pain
• Swelling
• Deformity

THERAPEUTIC INTERVENTIONS

• Assessment of neurovascular status
• Splint "as it lies"
• Sling
• Cold pack
• Consider need for analgesia
• Compression

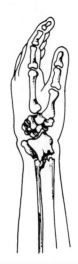

Fig. 21-8 Wrist fracture.

- Orthopedic consult
- Recognize potential need for surgical intervention

Rare aseptic necrosis may be a complication of this injury.

Hand (carpals and metacarpals) or finger (phalanges) fracture

Hand or finger fracture is common in athletes (in contact sports) (Fig. 21-9). It could be the result of fighting (a fracture of the first metacarpal [boxer's fracture]), throwing a baseball (a tearing loose of the distal attachment of the extensor tendon, which also breaks off a small piece of bone), or an industrial crush injury.

ASSESSMENT

- Pain
- Severe swelling
- Deformity
- Inability to use hand
- Often open fracture

THERAPEUTIC INTERVENTIONS

- Assessment of neurovascular status
- Control of bleeding
- Dry, bulky dressing on open wounds
- Splint in functional position
- Cold pack
- Pressure
- Orthopedic consult
- Recognize potential need for surgery

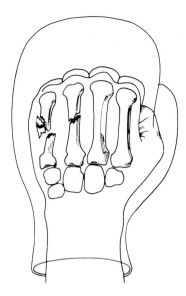

Fig. 21-9   Hand or finger fracture.

If a hematoma appears beneath the fingernail, the patient will complain of severe throbbing pain. Therapeutic intervention is nail trephination.

Hip fracture

Hip fractures are common in the elderly, usually from a fall or minor trauma (Fig. 21-10). In younger people, hip fractures are usually from major trauma.

ASSESSMENT

- Pain in hip or groin area
- Severe pain with movement
- Inability to bear weight
- External rotation of hip and leg
- Minimal shortening of limb
- If injury is extracapsular and associated with trochanteric fracture:
    Pain in lateral area of hip
    Increased shortening
    Greater external rotation

THERAPEUTIC INTERVENTIONS

- Immobilization
- Splint (backboard or one leg to the other)
- Check of pulses distal to injury
- Frequent (every 5 minutes) monitoring of vital signs
- Consider need for analgesia

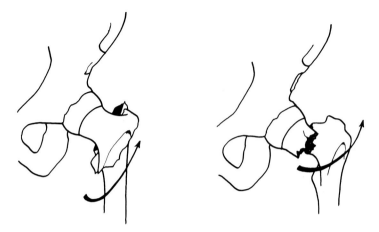

Fig. 21-10 Hip fracture.

- Orthopedic consult
- Recognize potential need for surgical intervention

Femoral fracture

The mechanism of injury of femoral fractures is usually major trauma (Fig. 21-11). These patients are at risk for hemorrhage and shock.

ASSESSMENT

- Severe pain
- Inability to bear weight on leg
- Swelling
- Deformity
- Angulation
- Shortening of limb and severe muscle spasm
- Crepitus

THERAPEUTIC INTERVENTIONS

- ABCs
- Hare traction or long-leg splint (Thomas or other); do not use long-leg air splint or other leg as splint
- Two large-bore IV lines
- Serial assessment of distal pulses
- Serial assessment of distal neurologic status
- Examination for other injuries
- Frequent (every 5 minutes) monitoring of vital signs
- Cold pack
- Consider need for analgesia
- Orthopedic consult

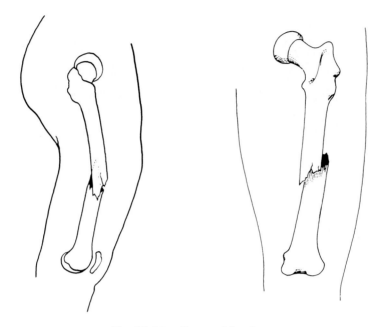

Fig. 21-11   Femoral fracture.

- Recognize potential need for surgical intervention
- Ongoing assessment for compartment syndrome

Femoral artery

The femoral artery is most frequently injured because of a displaced midshaft femur fracture or of penetrating trauma. It is the most common vascular injury in the lower extremities.

ASSESSMENT

- Pain in extremity
- Pale extremity
- Diminished pulses in extremity distal to injury
- Paresthesias in extremity
- Paralysis of extremity
- Hematoma near/over the injury site
- Possible external hemorrhage
- Signs of shock
- Compartment pressures

DIAGNOSIS

- Doppler studies
- Arteriogram

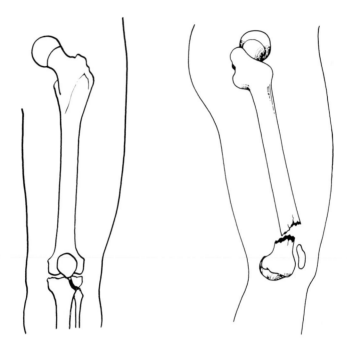

Fig. 21-12 Knee fracture. **A,** At the proximal tibia. **B,** At the distal femur.

THERAPEUTIC INTERVENTIONS

- ABCs
- Consider need for analgesia
- Splint extremity (if midshaft femur, use Hare traction splint)
- Surgical manipulation

Knee fracture (supracondylar fracture of femur, intraarticular fracture of femur or tibia)

Knee fracture is usually the result of an automobile, motorcycle, or automobile-pedestrian collision, with direct trauma to the knee area (Fig. 21-12). Because the anatomy of the nerve and vascular supply is complicated through the joint, knee fracture can be a limb-threatening injury, and the patient should be transported very carefully with the limb splinted in the position in which it was found. The patient will usually have this fracture reduced in surgery under general anesthesia. Knee fracture should not be confused with fracture of the patella, which is relatively benign.

ASSESSMENT

- Knee pain
- Inability to bend or straighten knee
- Swelling

- Tenderness
- Loss of neurologic and vascular supply to extremity distal to injury

THERAPEUTIC INTERVENTIONS

- Long-leg splint or one leg splinted to other
- Serial assessment of distal pulses
- Serial assessment of distal neurologic status
- Consider need for analgesia
- Orthopedic consult
- Preparation for reduction under general anesthesia
- Recognize potential need for surgical intervention
- Anticipate potential need for lower extremity angiography

Popliteal artery

A popliteal artery disruption usually occurs because of a knee dislocation. It can also occur when a severe proximal tibial fracture occurs. This is a very serious injury, which may result in amputation of the distal lower extremity, even following surgical repair.

ASSESSMENT

- Absent popliteal pulses (and other more distal pulses)
- Severe pain in lower extremities
- Pale, cold lower extremity
- Paresthesias or paralysis of lower extremity

DIAGNOSIS

- Doppler studies
- Arteriography

THERAPEUTIC INTERVENTIONS

- Consider need for analgesia
- Splint extremity in alignment
- Surgical repair

Patellar fracture

Patellar fracture is usually caused by direct trauma (fall or impact with dashboard) or indirect trauma (severe muscle pull) (Fig. 21-13).

ASSESSMENT

- Pain in knee
- Frequently open fracture

THERAPEUTIC INTERVENTIONS

- Apply long-leg splint
- Cover open wound

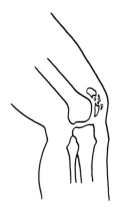

Fig. 21-13   Patellar fracture.

- Apply cold pack
- Consider need for analgesia
- Orthopedic consult
- Recognize potential need for surgical intervention, especially if wound is open

Tibial and/or fibular fracture

Tibial or fibular fracture results from direct trauma, indirect trauma, or a twisting injury (Fig. 21-14).

ASSESSMENT

- Pain
- Point tenderness
- Swelling
- Deformity
- Crepitus

THERAPEUTIC INTERVENTIONS

- Splint as found, if no pulse deficit (long-leg splint)
- Check distal pulses; gentle traction if pulse deficit
- Place sterile dressing over open fracture; gentle pressure if actively bleeding
- Consider need for analgesia
- Orthopedic consult
- Recognize potential need for surgical intervention, especially if there is open fracture
- Ongoing assessment for compartment syndrome

Ankle fracture

Ankle fracture results from direct trauma, indirect trauma, or torsion (Fig. 21-15).

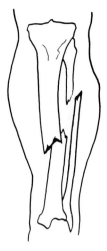

Fig. 21-14   Tibial and fibular fracture.

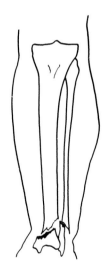

Fig. 21-15   Ankle fracture.

ASSESSMENT

- Pain
- Inability to bear weight
- Point tenderness
- Swelling
- Deformity

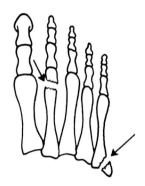

Fig. 21-16   Foot fracture.

THERAPEUTIC INTERVENTIONS

• Splint (soft)
• Serial assessment of distal pulses; gentle traction if pulse deficit
• Serial assessment of distal neurologic status
• Elevation
• Cold pack
• Consider need for analgesia
• Orthopedic consult
• Recognize potential need for surgical intervention

Foot fracture (metatarsal fracture)

A foot fracture may result from an automobile collision, athletic injuries, crush injuries, or direct trauma (Fig. 21-16).

ASSESSMENT

• Pain
• Hesitancy to bear weight
• Point tenderness
• Deformity
• Swelling

THERAPEUTIC INTERVENTIONS

• Compression dressing
• Soft splint

Heel (os calcis) fracture

Heel fracture occurs frequently in young adults (Fig. 21-17). It is usually caused by a fall from a height, and the patient lands directly on the feet. It is frequently accompanied by compression fractures of the thoracic or lumbosacral spine.

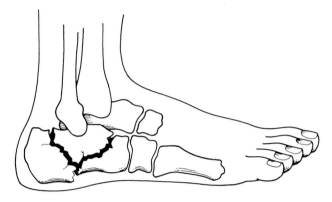

Fig. 21-17   Heel fracture.

ASSESSMENT

- Pain
- Swelling
- Point tenderness
- Dislocation

THERAPEUTIC INTERVENTIONS

- Compression dressing
- Elevation
- Cold pack
- Consider need for analgesia
- Orthopedic consult
- Recognize potential need for surgical intervention

Fracture of toes (phalanges)

Toe fracture results most often from kicking a hard object, "stubbing" the toe, or dropping a heavy object (Fig. 21-18).

ASSESSMENT

- Pain
- Swelling
- Ecchymosis

THERAPEUTIC INTERVENTIONS

- Compression dressing
- Rigid splint
- Elevation
- Cold pack

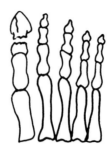

Fig. 21-18   Phalanges fracture.

DISLOCATION

Dislocation occurs when a joint exceeds its range of motion and the joint surfaces are no longer intact. This type of injury is generally accompanied by a large amount of soft-tissue injury in the joint capsule and surrounding ligaments; much swelling; and possible vein, artery, and nerve damage. When obtaining a history, clinical personnel should determine the force that caused the injury to project a diagnosis.

ASSESSMENT

• Severe pain
• Joint deformity
• Inability to move joint
• Swelling
• Point tenderness

THERAPEUTIC INTERVENTIONS

• Palpate joint area carefully
• Splint joint "as it lies"
• Do *not* reduce dislocation in field
• Early reduction with adequate anesthesia is required in Emergency Department, but only after x-ray examination to rule out accompanying fracture
• Compare injured side to other side for symmetry, droop, edema, deformity
• Orthopedic consult

Acromioclavicular separation

Acromioclavicular separation is a common athletic injury produced by a fall or a force on the point of the shoulder (Fig. 21-19).

ASSESSMENT

• Great pain in joint area
• Inability to raise arm or bring arm across chest
• Deformity
• Point or area tenderness

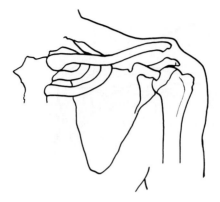

Fig. 21-19   Acromioclavicular separation.

- Swelling
- Hematoma

THERAPEUTIC INTERVENTIONS

- Neurovascular assessment
- Sling and swath
- Cold pack
- Consider need for analgesia
- Orthopedic consult
- Need for early reduction
- Recognize potential need for surgical intervention

Shoulder dislocation

Shoulder dislocation is a common athletic injury (Fig. 21-20). An anterior dislocation is usually an athletic injury from a fall on an extended arm that is abducted and externally rotated, resulting in the head of the humerus locating anterior to the shoulder joint. A posterior dislocation is a rare form of dislocation, usually found in patients with seizure, in which the extended arm is abducted and internally rotated, or from a direct blow.

ASSESSMENT

- Severe pain in shoulder area
- Inability to move arm
- Deformity (difficult to see in posterior dislocation)
- Recurrent in 55% to 60% of cases

THERAPEUTIC INTERVENTIONS

- Support in position found or position of greatest comfort
- Apply cold pack
- Reduce recurrent dislocation *if* it is easy to do

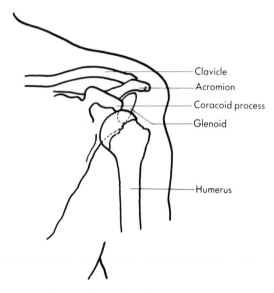

Fig. 21-20   Shoulder dislocation.

- Check distal pulses
- Check distal neurovascular status
- Consider need for analgesia
- Orthopedic consult
- Need for early reduction

Much soft-tissue damage and occasional axillary nerve damage may accompany a shoulder dislocation. Axillary artery damage and brachial plexus damage are rare complications.

Elbow dislocation

An elbow dislocation is a common athletic injury (Fig. 21-21). It occurs most frequently in children, teenagers, and young adults. The injury may result from a fall on an extended arm or from the jerking or lifting of a child by a single arm, which causes displacement of the ulna *(nursemaid's elbow)*.

ASSESSMENT ▬▬▬▬▬▬▬▬▬▬▬▬▬▬▬▬▬▬▬▬▬▬▬▬▬▬

- Pain
- Swelling
- Deformity or lateral displacement
- May feel locked
- Severe pain produced by movement

THERAPEUTIC INTERVENTIONS ▬▬▬▬▬▬▬▬▬▬▬▬▬▬▬▬▬▬▬▬

- Cold pack
- Immobilization in position of greatest comfort
- Serial assessment of distal pulses

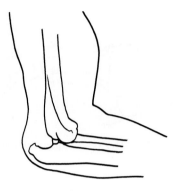

Fig. 21-21   Elbow dislocation.

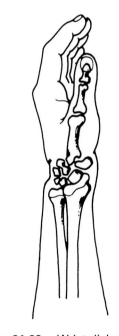

Fig. 21-22   Wrist dislocation.

- Serial assessment of distal neurologic status
- Consider need for analgesia
- Orthopedic consult
- Need for early reduction

Wrist dislocation

Wrist dislocation is usually the result of a fall on an outstretched arm and hand. It is seen commonly in athletes (Fig. 21-22).

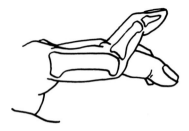

Fig. 21-23   Finger dislocation.

ASSESSMENT

- Pain
- Swelling
- Point tenderness
- Deformity

THERAPEUTIC INTERVENTIONS

- Splint
- Sling
- Cold pack
- Consider need for analgesia
- Orthopedic consult
- Need for early reduction

Hand or finger dislocation

Hand or finger dislocation is common in athletes (Fig. 21-23). It is usually the result of a fall on an outstretched hand or finger, of direct trauma, or of a jamming force on the fingertip.

ASSESSMENT

- Pain
- Inability to move joint
- Deformity
- Swelling

THERAPEUTIC INTERVENTIONS

- Splint in position of comfort
- Apply cold pack

Hip dislocation

Hip dislocation is usually the result of a major trauma (with extended leg and foot on brake pedal before impact or with knee hitting dashboard), falls, or crush injuries (Fig. 21-24).

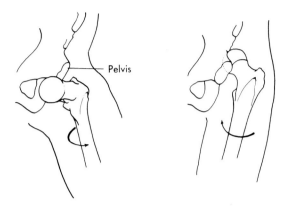

Fig. 21-24 Hip dislocation.

ASSESSMENT

- Pain in hip area
- Pain in knee
- Hip flexed, adducted, and internally rotated *(posterior dislocation)*
- Hip slightly flexed, abducted, and externally rotated *(anterior dislocation; rare injury)*
- Joint feeling locked
- Inability to move leg

THERAPEUTIC INTERVENTIONS

- Observe for signs of blood loss and shock
- Splint in position found or in position of comfort
- Assess distal pulses serially
- Assess distal neurologic status serially
- Check for other injuries
- Apply cold pack
- Consider need for analgesia
- Orthopedic consult
- In hospital, urgent reduction or necrosis of femoral head may occur
- Recognize potential need for surgical intervention

Sciatic nerve damage and femoral artery and nerve damage may be complications of hip dislocation.

Knee dislocation

See Fig. 21-25.

ASSESSMENT

- Severe pain
- Much swelling

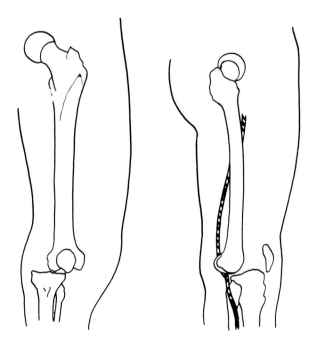

Fig. 21-25 Knee dislocation.

- Deformity
- Inability to move joint

THERAPEUTIC INTERVENTIONS

- Splint in position of comfort
- Assess distal pulses serially
- Assess distal neurologic status serially
- Apply cold pack
- Consider need for analgesia
- Orthopedic/vascular consult
- In hospital, urgent reduction may be needed to avoid arterial damage
- Recognize potential need for surgical intervention
- Anticipate potential need for lower extremity angiography

Peroneal nerve damage, posterior tibial nerve damage, and popliteal artery damage may be complications of knee dislocation.

NOTE: Consider the possibility of popliteal artery disruption when the patient has a very recent history of knee dislocation (even if the knee has been reduced).

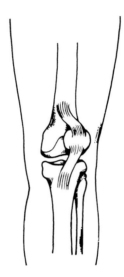

Fig. 21-26   Patellar dislocation.

Patellar dislocation

Patellar dislocation is a common athletic injury resulting from direct trauma or rotation injury on the planted foot (Fig. 21-26). Bleeding into the knee joint (hemarthrosis) may be a complication.

ASSESSMENT

- Pain
- Knee usually in flexed position with inability to function
- Tenderness
- Swelling

THERAPEUTIC INTERVENTIONS

- Splint in position found
- Apply cold pack
- Consider need for analgesia
- Orthopedic consult
- Consider need for early reduction

Ankle dislocation

Ankle dislocation is usually an athletic injury that is associated with a fracture (Fig. 21-27).

ASSESSMENT

- Pain
- Swelling

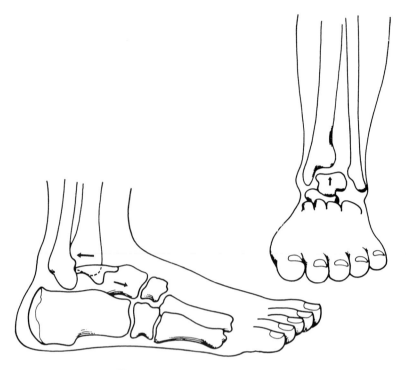

Fig. 21-27 Ankle dislocation.

- Deformity
- Inability to move joint

THERAPEUTIC INTERVENTIONS ▬▬▬▬▬▬▬▬▬▬▬▬▬▬▬

- Splint in position of comfort
- Check distal pulses
- Check distal neurologic status
- Apply cold pack
- Consider need for analgesia
- Orthopedic consult
- Consider need for early reduction

Foot dislocation

Foot dislocation is a rare injury, usually resulting from an automobile or motorcycle collision. It is most often associated with an open wound.

ASSESSMENT ▬▬▬▬▬▬▬▬▬▬▬▬▬▬▬▬▬▬▬

- Pain
- Tenderness
- Swelling

- Deformity
- Inability to use foot

THERAPEUTIC INTERVENTIONS ▰▰▰▰▰▰▰▰▰▰▰▰▰▰

- Sterile dressing on open wound
- Soft splint
- Serial assessment of distal pulses
- Serial assessment of distal neurologic status
- Cold pack
- Consider need for analgesia
- Orthopedic consult
- Consider need for early reduction
- Recognize potential need for surgical intervention if there is open wound

PEDIATRIC LIMB TRAUMA

Special attention should be paid to pediatric limb trauma when fractures occur at the epiphysis, or growth center. A fracture at the epiphysis may cause an early closure of the plate, which results in a short extremity as the child grows, or it may stimulate long-bone growth resulting in unequal limb length. If the fracture is a partial fracture, an angular deformity may result. A child with such a fracture should be followed by an orthopedic surgeon for several months, because it is difficult to predict the outcome at time of injury.

TRAUMATIC AMPUTATIONS

Traumatic amputations are common to farm workers, factory workers, and motorcyclists. They occur under many different circumstances. Common types of traumatic amputations are:

Digits (fingers and toes)	Hand
Transmetatarsal	Forearm
Tarsometatarsal	Arm
Below knee	Ears
Through knee	Nose
Above knee	Penis

THERAPEUTIC INTERVENTIONS ▰▰▰▰▰▰▰▰▰▰▰▰▰▰

- Assure ABCs
- Control bleeding
- Support limb in functional position if amputation is partial
- Initiate fluid replacement with two large-bore IV lines
- Type and crossmatch for possible blood replacement
- Administer high-flow oxygen
- Transport patient to hospital
- Prepare patient for surgery

Preservation of amputated part

- Use hypothermia; do not freeze amputated part
- Soak or dress part in sterile normal saline or Ringer's lactate solution
- Place part in dry container; then place container—but *not* part—on ice
- Maintain correct anatomic position of severed limb, if limb is partially attached

Care of stump

- Treat for shock
- Apply direct pressure to reduce blood loss
- Apply ice and elevate
- Consider débridement, if wound is contaminated

Limiting factors in reimplantation

- Availability of reimplantation team
- Severity of damage to amputated part *(including damage during preservation technique)*
- Amount of time since incident occurred
- Physical status of patient

Upper extremity reimplantations have been more successful than lower extremity reimplantations.

SPLINTING

Splinting prevents further damage to soft tissues, arteries, and veins; decreases pain; and minimizes muscle spasm.

Clinical personnel should always splint above and below the injury site. For example, if the ankle is injured, also splint the foot and knee. If the knee is injured, also splint the lower leg and the trunk on the injured side.

Splints are divided into four basic types:

Soft splint: soft, not rigid, such as a pillow

Hard splint: firm surface; rigid, such as a board

Air splint: inflatable; provides rigidity without being hard*

Traction splint: provides support, decreased angulation, traction

There are many varieties of splint materials and uses:

- Thomas†
- Reel†
- Hare†
- Sagar†

---

*With a closed-end air splint, it is impossible to assess the distal pulses and neurovascular status after the splint is in place.

†Use for femoral shaft fractures or fractures of the upper third of the tibia; these splints should not be used on fractures of the hip, lower tibia, fibula, or ankle.

- Backboard
  Short board (or Kendrick extrication device)
  Long board
- Aluminum long-leg
- PASG

General principles of splint application

- Immobilize injured part, including joint above and below injury and proximal and distal to injury
- Correct severe angulation only if it is impossible to splint or if vascular compromise is present
- Use at least two people for splinting: one to maintain manual alignment and one to apply splinting apparatus
- Secure injured part to splint (do *not* use elastic bandage)
- Monitor extremity for swelling
- Monitor neurovascular exam

Application of air splint (open on both ends)

- Slip splint backward over rescuer's arm
- Grasp distal portion of injured limb with arm that has air splint in place
- Slide splint onto injured limb
- Inflate splint

SUMMARY

When a patient presents with limb trauma, the caregiver needs to do a thorough assessment. Clinical personnel must assess for potential fractures and think about the underlying vascular supply. Keeping the fracture and underlying structures in mind will help the caregiver anticipate the diagnostic signs and symptoms particular to that limb. When these signs and symptoms are detected early, the caregiver can provide appropriate, timely interventions and optimize the patient's care.

SUGGESTED READINGS

Bucholz RW: *Orthopaedic decision making,* ed 2, St Louis, 1996, Mosby.
Cardona VD, and others, editors: *Trauma nursing: from resuscitation through rehabilitation,* Philadelphia, 1994, Saunders.
Crosby LA, Lewallen DG: *Emergency care and transportation of the sick and injured,* ed 6, Rosemont, Ill, 1995, American Academy of Orthopaedic Surgeons.
Farrell RG: Conservative management of fingertip amputations, *JACEP* 6:6, 1977.
Feliciano DV: Peripheral vascular injury. In Moore EE, editor: *Early care of the injured patient,* ed 4, Philadelphia, 1989, BC Decker.
Gomez GA, and others: Suspected vascular trauma of the extremities: the role of arteriography in proximity injuries, *J Trauma* 26(11):1005-1008, 1986.

Klafs CE, Arnheim DD: *Modern principles of athletic training,* ed 3, Philadelphia, 1991, JB Lippincott.

Neff J, Kidd P: *Trauma nursing,* St Louis, 1992, Mosby.

Rich NM: Peripheral vascular injury. In Mattox K, Moore EE, Feliciano DV, editors: *Trauma,* Norwalk, Conn, 1988, Appleton-Lange.

Richardson JD, Vitale GC, Flint LM Jr: Penetrating arterial trauma: analysis of missed vascular injuries, *Arch Surg* 122(6):678-683, 1987.

Rockwood CA, Wilkins KE, King RE: *Fractures in children,* ed 3, Philadelphia, 1991, JB Lippincott.

Ruiz E, Cicero JJ: *Emergency management of skeletal injuries,* St Louis, 1995, Mosby.

Sheehy SB: *Emergency nursing,* ed 3, St Louis, 1992, Mosby.

Sheehy SB: *Emergency nursing: principles and practice,* ed 3, St Louis, 1992, Mosby.

CHAPTER 22

Burn Injuries

Mary-Liz Bilodeau

Evaluation of the patient with a major burn injury is initially the same as for any other trauma victim. The patient should be evaluated for life-threatening conditions and problems with ABCs: airway, breathing, and circulation. A careful assessment using the ABC primary survey should also aid in the identification of other life-threatening injuries. A secondary head-to-toe assessment is necessary to diagnose other injuries such as fractures, abdominal injuries, and closed head injuries. The burn wound itself should receive low priority during the initial survey except that all clothing should be removed and, if the wound is the result of a chemical burn, it should be thoroughly irrigated with water to stop the burning process. Clinical personnel should exercise caution so that they do not get the chemical on themselves and thus sustain an injury.

ETIOLOGY AND INCIDENCE

Burn injuries occur because of exposure to flame, flash, hot liquids, hot objects, chemicals, electrical current, or radiation (Fig. 22-1). There is no national reporting system for burn injuries, but best estimates suggest that approximately 60,000 hospitalizations and 10,000 deaths annually are from burns. Most of the available data come from the National Fire Data Center, under the auspices of the National Fire Prevention and Control Administration. Most of their data are related to fires and the injuries they cause and do not include data on burn injuries related to scalds, chemicals, and electric current. Although fires, especially residential fires, cause most burn-related deaths, scald injuries are the single most common type of burn injury, accounting for 40% to 50% of patients seen in most burn centers. The most common cause of death in the first 48 hours after burn injury is from respiratory complications related to smoke inhalation. After 48 hours, sepsis becomes the most common cause of death.

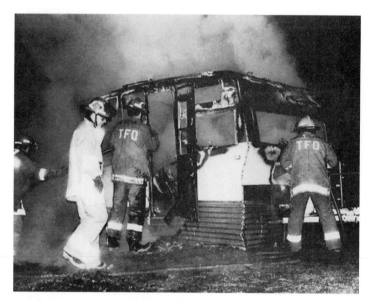

Fig. 22-1 Burn injuries occur as a result of exposure to flame and smoke. (Courtesy Tacoma Fire Department.)

ASSESSMENT OF DEPTH AND EXTENT OF BURN

Depth of burn

The depth of the burn injury is referred to as first, second, or third degree or partial-thickness or full-thickness injury (Table 22-1). Initial identification of the depth of injury is often difficult. Unless the burn area is very superficial, as with a first-degree burn, or very deep, as with a third-degree burn, there is little need to identify the depth of injury during the initial survey and the initial therapeutic interventions. The depth of the injury may actually increase over time as edema forms and circulation to the area of the injured tissue is compromised. The extent of the burn area is usually complete at about 48 hours, and at 48 to 72 hours a more accurate determination of depth of the burn can be made.

Extent of burn

The extent of injury for thermal and chemical injuries is assessed by using guides such as the rule of nines (Fig. 22-2) or the Lund and Browder charts (Figs. 22-3 and 22-4). For the rule of nines, it is important to remember that the formula must be modified for children. As noted in Fig. 22-2, *B*, the head and neck of an infant, represent 19% of the body surface area (BSA), and the legs represent a correspondingly smaller percentage of BSA (that is, 13% for each lower extremity). To correct for age, subtract 1% from the head for each year of age through 10 years and add 0.5% to each lower extremity. To obtain a more accurate estimate of the extent of burn, calculate both the area burned

Table 22-1 Classification of Burn Injury

Depth of burn	Sensitivity	Appearance	Healing time and results	Treatment
Partial thickness				
First degree				
Epidermal	Hyperalgesia	Erythema	3-5 days; no scarring	Moisturizers
Superficial dermal	Hyperalgesia to pink	Blisters, red, moist	6-10 days; minimal scarring	Topical antibacterial agents or biologic dressings required
Second degree				
Moderate dermal	Normal algesia	Blisters, pink, moist	10-18 days; some scarring	Topical antibacterial agents or biologic dressings required
Deep dermal	Hypoalgesia or analgesia	Blisters, opaque, with less moisture	>21 days; maximal scarring if not excised and grafted	Topical antibacterial agents and early excision and grafting
Full thickness				
Third degree				
Loss of all dermal elements with extension into fat, muscle, and bone	Analgesia	White, opaque, brown, or black, occasionally deep red; very dry, leathery; may or may not have blisters or thrombosed veins	Never heals if area is larger than 3 cm^2; The longer the wound is open, the more hypertrophic the scar	Topical antibacterial agents and early excision and grafting

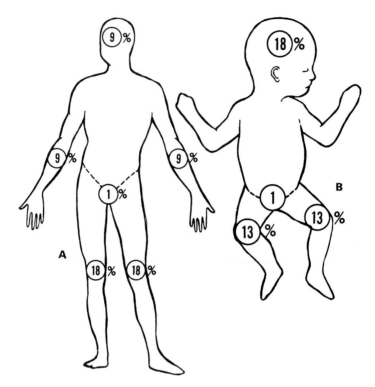

Fig. 22-2 Rule of nines. **A,** Adults. **B,** Children.

and the area not burned. The two estimates should then be compared. If the total is more or less than 100%, the areas should be reestimated. When estimating burn size, assess the posterior aspects of the body, as well as the anterior aspects. When an electrical injury has occurred, it is much more difficult to assess the extent of injury because surface damage may be minimal, whereas deeper injuries that cannot be visualized may be extensive. Thus, when describing an electrical injury, it is more important to describe the injury anatomically and by the amount of voltage (if known), rather than try to calculate a percentage of burn.

Severity of burn

The severity of a burn injury is based on an assessment of the extent and depth of injury, as well as the age of the patient, the presence of concomitant injuries, smoke inhalation, and preexisting diseases. The American Burn Association's categories for burn injuries are listed in Table 22-2.

Care of patients with burns of different severity is determined by the availability of specialized care facilities. Initial assessment and stabilization of the patient who has been burned must be available in any community

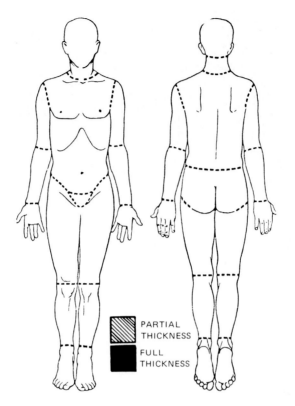

Percent Surface Area Burned

AREA	1 YEAR	1-4 YEARS	5-9 YEARS	10-14 YEARS	Y 15 YEARS	ADULT	2°	3°
Head	19	17	13	11	9	7		
Neck	2	2	2	2	2	2		
Ant. Trunk	13	13	13	13	13	13		
Post Trunk	13	13	13	13	13	13		
R. Buttock	2½	2½	2½	2½	2½	2½		
L. Buttock	2½	2½	2½	2½	2½	2½		
Genitalia	1	1	1	1	1	1		
R. U. Arm	4	4	4	4	4	4		
L. U. Arm	4	4	4	4	4	4		
R. L. Arm	3	3	3	3	3	3		
L. L. Arm	3	3	3	3	3	3		
R. Hand	2½	2½	2½	2½	2½	2½		
L. Hand	2½	2½	2½	2½	2½	2½		
R. Thigh	5½	6½	8	8½	9	9½		
L. Thigh	5½	6½	8	8½	9	9½		
R. Leg	5	5	5½	6	6½	7		
L. Leg	5	5	5½	6	6½	7		
R. Foot	3½	3½	3½	3½	3½	3½		
L. Foot	3½	3½	3½	3½	3½	3½		
TOTAL								

Fig. 22-3 Lund and Browder formula. (From Artz CP, Moncrief JA: *The treatment of burns,* ed 2, Philadelphia, 1969, Saunders)

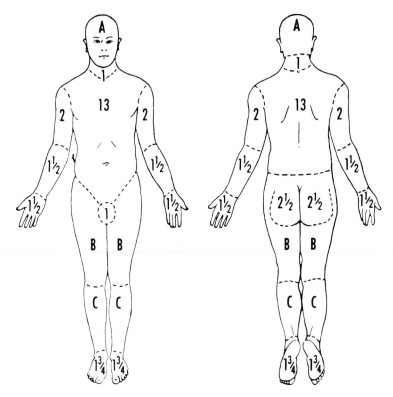

Relative Percentage of Areas Affected by Growth

	Age in Years					
	0	1	5	10	15	Adult
A—½ of head	9½	8½	6½	5½	4½	3½
B—½ of one thigh	2¾	3¼	4	4¼	4½	4¾
C—½ of one leg	2½	2½	2¾	3	3¼	3½

Fig. 22-4   Lund and Browder formula.

hospital with 24-hour emergency capabilities. Patients with minor burns may be treated as outpatients or admitted to the community hospital. Patients with moderate burns may be treated either in a community hospital with appropriate staff and facilities to deliver burn care or in a hospital with a specialized burn care facility. Patients with major burns should be cared for in a hospital where specialized burn care is available. Transfer agreements with hospitals with special burn care units should be developed in advance to facilitate timely and uneventful transfer of the burn patient.

Table 22-2   Categories of Burn Injuries

	Major burn* (%BSA)	Moderate burn† (%BSA)	Minor burn† (%BSA)
Adults			
Second degree	>25%	15%–25%	<15%
Third degree	>10%	3%–10%	<3%
Children			
Second degree	>20%	10%–20%	<10%
Third degree	>10%	3%–10%	<3%

Data from the American Burn Association, 8th annual meeting: Specific optimum criteria for hospital resources for care of patients with burn injuries, San Antonio, TX, April 1976.

*In both adults and children, burns involving hands, face, feet, or perineum, or burn injuries complicated by smoke inhalation, major associated trauma, or preexisting illnesses.
†Not involving face, hands, feet, or perineum.

PHYSIOLOGIC RESPONSE TO BURN INJURY

Initial circulatory changes

When major electrical burn injuries and thermal or chemical injuries greater than 15% to 20% of BSA occur, fluid shifts may cause hypovolemic states. Circulatory fluid deficits will be directly proportional to the extent of the burn injury: the more extensive the injury, the greater the amount of fluid that will shift from the intracellular to the extracellular space. The more fluid that shifts, the more severe the physiologic derangements that occur. A graphic description of this physiologic response is presented in Fig. 22-5.

When injury to the skin occurs, the normal host defense response is activated. This involves the release of histamines and other vasoactive substances that cause an increase in capillary permeability and localization of white blood cells and plasma proteins in the area to fight infection. If the wound is greater than about 15% of BSA, the capillary leak may involve other areas of the body besides the injured area. As a result, the patient develops generalized edema that causes a loss of intravascular volume. Because of translocation of the fluid portion of blood (*plasma*) from the intravascular to the interstitial space, the patient will develop a resultant increase in hematocrit, and the blood will become more viscous. The body's compensatory response to this functional fluid loss is to increase peripheral resistance so that blood will be shunted from the peripheral to the central circulation. This causes the cool, pale, clammy extremities that are evidenced in burn patients. This response maintains central circulation for a short period of time, but eventually the patient will develop a decrease in cardiac output and exhibit signs of hypovolemia.

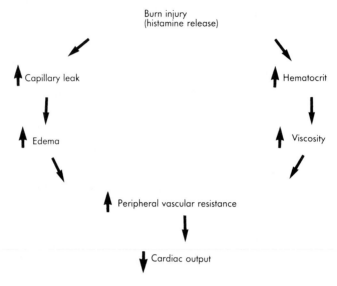

Fig. 22-5   Physiologic response to burn injury.

Response of lung to smoke inhalation

Inhalation injury or smoke inhalation is a syndrome composed of three distinct problems: carbon monoxide intoxication, upper airway obstruction, and a chemical injury to the lower airways and lung parenchyma.

Carbon monoxide intoxication is the most common cause of death in victims of fires. Most people who die in a fire are overcome by carbon monoxide before they sustain a burn injury. In the body, carbon monoxide has 200 times the affinity for hemoglobin than does oxygen, thus causing inadequate tissue oxygen delivery. Carbon monoxide also combines with myoglobin in muscle cells, resulting in muscle weakness. These two factors, tissue hypoxia resulting in mental confusion and muscle weakness, are said to be the major reasons most fire fatalities occur. In addition, carbon monoxide combines with the cytochrome oxidase system of the brain and may result in prolonged coma in some fire victims.

Upper airway obstruction is the result of intrinsic or extrinsic edema that may lead to airway occlusion at or above the vocal cords (Fig. 22-6). This injury is primarily a thermal injury, resulting in tissue damage in the posterior pharynx. It is rare to have actual thermal injury below the vocal cords, because the posterior pharynx is a very efficient heat exchange system. True thermal injury below the vocal cords is usually the result of injury from superheated steam, in which water vapor carries heat into the lungs, or of injuries that occur in either an oxygen-enriched atmosphere or one in which the victim was inhaling gases that exploded during inhalation anesthesia. A true thermal injury to the lungs is almost always fatal. A thermal injury to

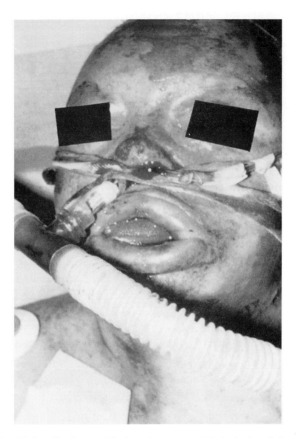

Fig. 22-6   Patient with face burns and inhalation injury.

the upper airway is usually associated with facial burns. With this type of injury, edema progresses rapidly, causing total occlusion of the airway in a very short time (minutes to hours). Early management for airway edema is intubation.

Chemical injury to the lower airways occurs when smoke has been inhaled. Chemical injury from acids and aldehydes in the smoke may damage the lung parenchyma. These chemicals are attached to carbon particles in the smoke, and, because they are heavier than air, the chemicals are readily inhaled and find their way down the bronchi into the alveoli. This chemical injury results in hemorrhagic tracheobronchitis, increased edema formation, decreased surfactant levels, and decreased pulmonary macrophage function. This in turn leads to the rapid development of acute respiratory distress syndrome (ARDS) in 24 to 48 hours. Severe inhalation injury may increase the patient's fluid needs in the first 24 hours by as much as 50% of calculated values.

GENERAL MANAGEMENT CONSIDERATIONS

The patient should initially be assessed using the ABC assessment tool for trauma. Then assessment for specific burn injuries should be performed.

Airway

ASSESSMENT

- History of smoke inhalation/high index of suspicion
- Visual inspection of oropharynx and vocal cords for redness, blisters, carbonaceous particles
- Increasing restlessness
- Complaints of difficulty breathing or swallowing
- Increasing difficulty handling secretions
- Increasing hoarseness
- Rapid, shallow respiration

NOTES: Blood gas values, although appropriate for assessing oxygenation problems related to chemical injury to lower airway, will reveal little about impending airway obstruction.

THERAPEUTIC INTERVENTIONS

- Early intubation (before complete occlusion)

A tracheostomy can and should be avoided initially because edema in the neck area makes this procedure especially difficult.

Breathing
Circumferential chest wall burns

ASSESSMENT

Initially, the major, specific, burn-related problem that may impair breathing is a circumferential, full-thickness burn of the thorax. This may limit chest wall excursion and prevent adequate gas exchange.

- Visual inspection of chest
- Tight, leathery eschar circumferentially around chest
- Inadequate expansion of chest
- Rapid, shallow respirations
- Restlessness/confusion
- Decreased oxygenation
- Decreased tidal volume

THERAPEUTIC INTERVENTIONS

Escharotomies of the chest are surgical incisions made along the lateral borders of the chest halfway between the midaxillary line and the midnipple line. If the abdomen is also involved, an incision can be made over the diaphragm to connect the two lateral incisions.

Escharotomies are made deep enough only to release the eschar and expose the underlying subcutaneous tissue. This procedure should allow for immediate improvement in the excursion of the chest wall. These incisions will cause bleeding. Clinical personnel should have an electrocautery unit or 10 to 20 small hemostats available to control the bleeding.

General anesthesia is not necessary because the incisions are made only in the area of the full-thickness burn. Narcotic analgesia given intravenously is sufficient to relieve any pain.

Carbon monoxide (CO) intoxication

ASSESSMENT

- Decreased respirations or apnea at scene
- Cherry-red, normal skin
- Confusion or coma
- Increased CO in measurement of carboxhyemoglobin (HgbCO) level
- Carbonaceous sputum

THERAPEUTIC INTERVENTIONS

- Administer oxygen at 100% or at as high a percentage as possible
- If not breathing, intubate and ventilate
- If unconsciousness continues after 1 to 1½ hours with adequate resuscitation and no evidence of head injury, hyperbaric oxygen therapy should be considered
- Chest x-ray

Chemical injury or ARDS

ASSESSMENT

ARDS is usually not a problem for at least 8 hours after injury.
- Decreased oxygenation
- Increased secretions
- Rapid respirations
- Increased patchy infiltrates on x-ray
- Confusion

THERAPEUTIC INTERVENTIONS

- Intubation and ventilation
- Positive end-expiratory pressure (PEEP)
- Bronchodilators, as indicated
- *No steroids* (steroids given to patients with burns plus smoke inhalation increase morbidity and mortality at least threefold)

Clinical personnel should assess for other trauma-related causes for problems in breathing, especially pneumothorax or hemothorax, tension pneumothorax, and flail chest. These problems should be expected when burn victims have been in car accidents or explosions or have jumped or fallen. History of chronic pulmonary problems that may complicate therapy should also be noted.

Circulation

ASSESSMENT

These assessment parameters should be followed closely. If present, they indicate a low-flow state.

- Tachycardia
- Hypotension
- Tachypnea
- Central venous pressure (CVP) below 3 cm H_2O
- Oliguria
- Hematocrit above 50 mg/dl
- Diminished capillary refill
- Restlessness or confusion
- Nausea
- Vomiting
- Ileus

THERAPEUTIC INTERVENTIONS

- Start 1 or 2 large-bore IV lines (1 if less than 40% BSA; 2 if greater than 40% BSA or if patient is to be transferred)
- Avoid leg veins when possible in adults because of increased risk of thrombophlebitis
- Administer fluid replacement by one of many accepted formulas; more popular are Baxter formula and modified Brooke formula

Baxter formula

First 24 hours: 4 ml lactated Ringer's/kg body wt/% BSA
- ½ first 8 hours
- ¼ second 8 hours
- ¼ third 8 hours

Time is calculated from time of injury, not time IV therapy was initiated.
Second 24 hours:
- D5W in sufficient quantities to keep serum Na^{++} below 140 mEq/liter
- Potassium to maintain normal serum K^+ level
- Plasma or plasma expander to maintain adequate volume with normal pulse, blood pressure, and urine output

Modified Brooke formula

First 24 hours: 2 ml lactated Ringer's/kg body wt/% BSA
- ½ first 8 hours
- ¼ second 8 hours
- ¼ third 8 hours

Time is calculated from time of injury, not time that IV therapy was initiated.
Second 24 hours: Same as Baxter formula

NOTE: These and other formulas are intended only as a guideline for fluid replacement and may need to be adjusted up or down as personnel monitor the signs of adequate resuscitation. These signs are:
- Pulse in upper limits of normal range for age
- Urine output
    - 30 to 50 ml/hr for adults
    - 20 to 30 ml/hr for children
    - 1–1½ ml/kg body wt for infants
- Urine sugar < 2+
- Mentally alert
- Absence of ileus or nausea

For electrical injuries, there is no formula for fluid resuscitation. Lactated Ringer's solution is administered rapidly, 1 to 2 liters per hour in the average adult, until the patient shows signs of adequate resuscitation.
- Urine output is usually maintained at 2 to 3 times normal to facilitate excretion of myoglobin
- Once urine output is established, mannitol may be given to increase urine flow and aid excretion of myoglobin
- Acidosis (pH 6.8–7.0) is an early complication and may require repeated administration of sodium bicarbonate ($NaHCO_3$) to prevent dysrhythmias until fluid therapy can correct acidosis
- Draw blood for CBC, electrolytes, and type and crossmatch
- Place Foley catheter
- Send urine for urinalysis and myoglobin level
- Monitor hourly urine output
- Monitor urine sugar and acetone every 2 to 4 hours
- Monitor cardiac rhythm.
- Obtain 12-lead ECG

Prevention of infection
Aseptic technique
- Gloves, mask, cap, and gown should be worn by all personnel.
- All invasive procedures should be treated as sterile procedures.
- Wounds should be kept covered with clean sheets while other care is provided.

Antibiotics
- Topical antibiotics should be applied as soon as possible after wound is débrided.
- Systemic antibiotics are rarely indicated even in severe burns until the patient has a culture-proven infection. Exceptions to this may be young children, elderly patients, diabetic persons, or patients with immune deficiency diseases.

Tetanus prophylaxis

- For all burns, give tetanus immunization if previous immunization has been given more than 5 years ago.
- In patients who have never been immunized or in whom there is no clear history of immunization, give tetanus hyperimmune globulin (Hypertet), in addition.

Management of pain

ASSESSMENT ▰▰▰▰▰▰▰▰▰▰▰▰▰▰▰▰▰▰▰▰▰▰▰▰▰

- Patient complains of pain specific to burn injury or other injuries
- Patient is restless, tachycardic with rapid respirations (rule out other potential causes)
- Ask patient to rate pain on an established scale

THERAPEUTIC INTERVENTIONS ▰▰▰▰▰▰▰▰▰▰▰▰▰▰▰▰▰▰▰▰

- Administer morphine.
    Small doses (3 to 5 mg in adults)
    Frequently (every 20 to 40 minutes)
- Always administer IV analgesia in burns greater than 15% of BSA
- Explain procedures
- Administer anxiolytic drug such as diazepam (Valium) if patient is severely agitated for no apparent reason

---

NOTE: Burn wounds are exquisitely painful, especially partial-thickness injuries. Careful titration of morphine, either as needed or as a morphine drip, can be used effectively to control pain initially.

Obtain history

- How did injury occur (flame, scald, or other)?
- Was smoke involved? Was it in closed space?
- Who was involved? What happened to others?
- What was patient doing before accident? (may lead to early diagnosis of stroke or myocardial infarction)
- What previous medical problems or allergies did patient have?

Burn wound care

Burn wound care can wait until the patient's condition is stabilized.

Circumferential full-thickness injuries

ASSESSMENT ▰▰▰▰▰▰▰▰▰▰▰▰▰▰▰▰▰▰▰▰▰▰▰▰▰

- Assess all full-thickness, circumferential burns for circulatory problems
- Check distal pulses with Doppler
- Assess capillary refill
- Note paresthesia

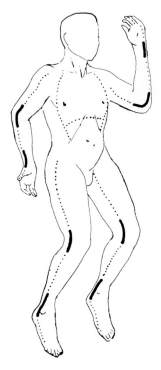

Fig. 22-7 Placement of escharotomies.

THERAPEUTIC INTERVENTIONS ▬▬▬▬▬▬▬▬▬▬▬▬▬▬▬▬▬▬

- If patient develops signs of circulatory compromise, escharotomy will be performed (Fig. 22-7 shows placement of surgical incisions).
- Be prepared for significant bleeding with either electrocautery unit or 10 to 20 small hemostats to control bleeding (Fig. 22-8).
- Once procedure is completed, apply topical antibacterial to open wound, dress with light pressure dressing, and keep arms and legs slightly elevated.

Thermal burns: flames, flashes, scalds, and hot objects (Fig. 22-9)

- Cleanse wounds with sterile or clean water, 0.25 strength Betadine, and clean cloths or coarse mesh gauze dressings.
- Keep blisters intact; unroof only when they have spontaneously broken.
- Shave all hairy areas of burns and adjacent areas.
- Cover wound immediately with prescribed topical antibacterial agent and apply dressing.
- Elevate extremities slightly to reduce swelling.

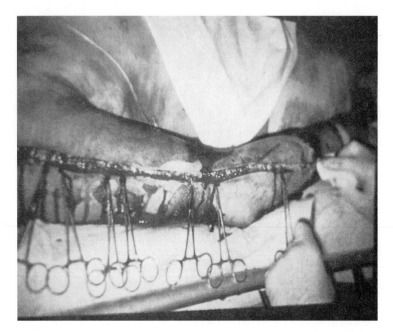

Fig. 22-8 Control of bleeding from escharotomy.

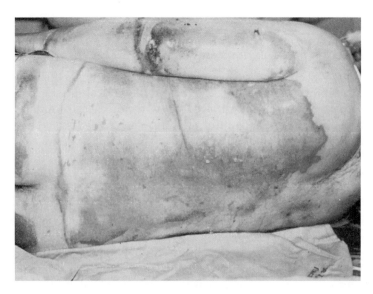

Fig. 22-9 Flame burns to back.

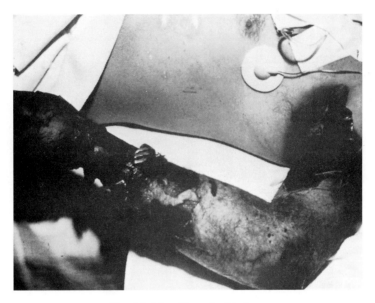

Fig. 22-10   Electrical injury.

Chemical burns

• Thoroughly rinse chemical wounds immediately with tap water or saline to remove the chemical. Remember to remove clothing and jewelry and rinse the nonburned areas, because some areas of chemical exposure may not begin to hurt, blister, or even become red immediately.
• Then treat wound as if it were a thermal burn.
• Chemical burns of the eyes are ophthalmologic emergencies.

As with other chemical wounds, thoroughly rinse the eye with copious amounts of water or saline. If the patient is wearing contact lenses, wash the eye before trying to remove lenses. Then if the lens does not come out during irrigation, carefully remove the lens with a lens removal suction cup. If the lens is adherent, leave it in place for the ophthalmologist to remove and continue irrigation of the eye. When the lens is removed, the eye should be thoroughly irrigated again.

Electrical injuries

• These wounds are different from thermal or chemical wounds because there may be little superficial tissue loss with massive muscle injury underlying normal-looking skin (Fig. 22-10).
• These wounds should be gently cleansed with water or saline and 0.25 strength Betadine.
• There is rarely any need to débride the wound immediately.
• These wounds should be handled minimally. Cadaver-like limbs should not

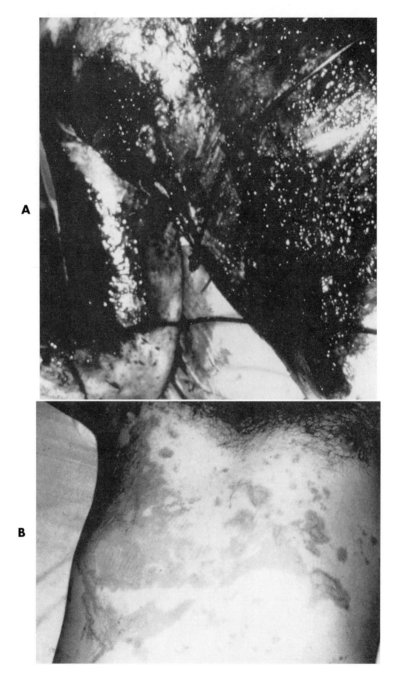

Fig. 22-11   **A,** Tar burns to chest before removal of tar. **B,** Tar burns after removal of tar.

be moved about or manipulated, because large patent vessels may be torn and massive hemorrhage may occur.
- Topical agents, such as silver sulfadiazine (Silvadene) and/or silver nitrate, should be used to cover the wound.
- Light dressings may be applied to cover these often grotesque wounds, taking care not to impair observation of extremities for development of compartment syndrome.
- Because of possible muscle damage, injured extremities should be observed for compartment syndrome. Symptoms may include:
    Pain
    Pallor
    Paresthesia
    Decreased motor function
    Decreased pulse
- Fasciotomies are performed to relieve compartment syndrome.
    These procedures are usually carried out under general anesthesia so that all compartments can be completely explored. Fasciotomy can be a very painful procedure, because the incisions are often made through normal skin.
- Fasciotomies are left open, covered with a topical antibacterial agent, and dressed with a light dressing postoperatively.

Tar or asphalt burns

Tar wounds may be deep or superficial, depending on the temperature of the tar, which may range from 150° to 600° F or higher (Fig. 22-11).
- Cool tar with cool liquids.
- Do not try to peel off tar.
- Remove tar by loosening with:
    Mineral oil
    Petroleum jelly (Vaseline)
    Solvent, such as Medi-Sol
    Removal of tar can be accomplished in areas of noncircumferential burns by applying oil or ointment and a light dressing and removing the dressing after 4 to 12 hours and reapplying the oil or ointment and a dressing.
- For circumferential areas, the oil or ointment can be applied with light dressings and changed every 20 to 30 minutes until the tar is removed.
- Then the wound can be treated as a thermal or chemical wound.

INTERFACILITY TRANSFER

Once the injury has been identified as a significant burn, the team should consider transfer to a regional burn center. Patients should be considered for transfer based on their age, the percentage of TBSA of burn, and any associated factor that would decrease their chances for optimal outcome (Box 22-1). Prehospital providers and community Emergency Department personnel

---

BOX 22-1

TRANSFER CRITERIA FOR BURN PATIENTS TO A BURN CENTER

Second-degree burns 10%-20%
    TBSA
    Children <10 years old
    Adults >50 years old
Second- and third-degree burns
    20% TBSA
    All age groups
Third degree burns >10%
    All age groups
Second- and third-degree burns
    and chemical burns to the fol-
    lowing areas:
    Face

Hands
Feet
Genitalia
Perineum
Major joints
Electrical burns, including light-
    ning strikes
Burns with associated factors:
    Major trauma
    Inhalation injury
    Comorbid/preexisting medical
      problems

---

should establish a network with their regional burn center to ensure a consistent approach to clinical management from injury to definitive care.

SUGGESTED READINGS

Carrougher GT: Burn care and therapy, St Louis, 1998, Mosby.

Gordon M, Goodwin C: Initial assessment, management, and stabilization, *Nurs Clin North Am* 32(2):237-249, 1997.

Hemdon D: *Total Burn Care,* Philadelphia, 1996, Saunders.

Jordan B, Harrington D: Management of the burn wound, *Nurs Clin North Am* 32(2):251-273, 1997.

PART IV

Special Populations

CHAPTER 23

Pediatric Trauma

Anne Phelan Bowen

> *"If diseases were killing our children in the proportions that accidents are, people would be outraged and demand that this killer be stopped."*
>
> C. EVERETT KOOP

More than half of all childhood deaths (ages 1 to 14) are due to injury. Mechanisms of injury causing pediatric deaths include unintentional injuries, such as motor vehicle incidents, falls, drowning, and burns, as well as intentional injuries like homicide, suicide, and child abuse. Millions of children require Emergency Department (ED) treatment annually as a result of trauma, many of whom suffer permanent disability.

The principles of trauma assessment and management are the same for the child victim as the adult. However, there are some issues unique to children, with which the care provider should be familiar. The vast majority of pediatric trauma is due to blunt trauma (85%) as opposed to penetrating injury (15%). The injured child is best cared for in an ED prepared to meet their unique needs.

PRIMARY SURVEY

This rapid initial assessment is used to identify and treat life-threatening injuries.

Airway with full spine immobilization

DEVELOPMENTAL/ANATOMIC CONSIDERATIONS:

- Oral cavity is small in comparison to tongue size.
- Young infants less than 3 months of age are obligate nasal breathers.
- Narrowest portion of child's airway is the cricoid cartilage.

ASSESSMENT

- Assure patency of airway
- Look for oral foreign bodies
- Maintain full spine immobilization

THERAPEUTIC INTERVENTIONS

- Use the jaw thrust maneuver to open the airway in an unconscious child.
- Suction any obstructing matter, such as blood, emesis, or secretions from the airway.
- Oral airways, when required, are inserted using a forward motion with the tongue depressed outward. Rotation of the airway is contraindicated since it may cause trauma to the soft tissues of the palate and hypopharynx.
- Nasal airways are better tolerated by the conscious child. These are to be used in the absence of maxillofacial injuries or suspected basilar skull fractures.
- Intubation is recommended when respiratory distress or poor ventilation persist, or when the child has a Glasgow Coma Score (GCS) of 8 or less. Use an uncuffed tube for children less than 8 years old to avoid vocal cord trauma, subglottic edema, and pressure necrosis.

Breathing

Children have high metabolic rates, resulting in a higher rate of oxygen consumption than adults. When breathing becomes inadequate, hypoxemia occurs more rapidly.

ASSESSMENT

- Observe respiratory rate, depth, symmetry, and quality.
- Observe for signs of respiratory distress or air hunger; grunting, nasal flaring, retractions, head bobbing, or shoulder lifting.
- Auscultate breath sounds for equality and adventitious sounds.
- Palpate the position of the trachea gently, noting the presence of any crepitus.
- Check the integrity of the chest wall.

THERAPEUTIC INTERVENTIONS

- During the initial assessment administer 100% oxygen to all children.
- Monitor oxygen saturation, via pulse oximetry, noting that readings are unreliable in children with poor peripheral perfusion.
- Provide assisted ventilation with bag-valve-mask or positive pressure ventilation.
- Decompress suspected tension pneumothorax with needle thoracostomy and prepare for chest tube insertion.
- Prepare for intubation for optimal long-term aggressive airway management.

Circulation

Children have a circulating blood volume of approximately 80cc/kg and a strong, young heart muscle. In the presence of a decrease in circulating blood volume, a child's primary mechanism to increase their cardiac output is to increase their heart rate. Hypotension is a late sign of shock in children, usually occurring after a circulating blood loss of about 25%.

ASSESSMENT

- Palpate the quality and effectiveness of a peripheral and central pulse.
- Observe for areas of external hemorrhage.
- Observe skin color and temperature.
- Check capillary refill time.

THERAPEUTIC INTERVENTIONS

- *If pulseless,* initiate CPR and follow pediatric advanced life support protocols.
- If pulse is present, but ineffective, obtain vascular access using 2 large bore IV catheters (or obtain intraosseus access) and administer a 20 cc/kg bolus of warmed RL or NS. If response is unsatisfactory, repeat the bolus and administer 10cc/kg of packed red blood cells (RBCs) (type specific or O negative).
- Apply direct pressure to areas of uncontrolled external hemorrhage.

Disability—neurologic evaluation

The child's large head size in relation to body size, accompanied by more lax neck muscles, makes him or her more susceptible to head injuries. Head injuries are the leading cause of traumatic death and disability in children.

ASSESSMENT

- Assess pupillary size, shape, and response.
- Determine level of consciousness using the GCS or AVPU scale.
    A-alert and oriented
    V-responsive to verbal stimuli
    P-responsive to painful stimuli
    U-unresponsive

THERAPEUTIC INTERVENTIONS

- In selected cases, consider pharmacologic intervention to improve mental status, such as Narcan or D25.
- Once the child is hemodynamically stable, restrict IV fluids to ⅔ maintenance.

SECONDARY SURVEY

On completion of the primary survey and resuscitation, the secondary survey is performed to identify the extent of all injuries present. Frequent reassessment is also made of the child's respiratory, circulatory, and neurologic status. Since the remaining injuries are not immediately life threatening, interventions identified in the secondary survey are performed at the end of the assessment.

- *Expose* the child by removing all clothing so that a complete assessment can be performed.
- *Fahrenheit,* children lose body heat more quickly than adults, so they should be kept warm by blankets, radiant warmers, and warmed IV fluids.
- *Get a full set of vital signs,* including a blood pressure and rectal temperature.
- *History* should be obtained from the care giver and emergency medical service (EMS) personnel. The history should include; mechanism of injury, treatment before arrival in the ED, past medical history, allergies, medications, immunization status, and last food/fluid intake.
- *Head to toe assessment* is performed in detail including both anterior and posterior body surfaces.
- *Interventions* after the secondary survey may include:
  - Sending trauma labs
  - Preparing for trauma imaging
  - Dressing lacerations or débriding burn wounds
  - Splinting suspected fracture sites
  - Placing Foley catheter and/or naso/orogastric tube

SELECTED INJURIES

Head trauma

Head injuries are very common in children largely as a result of their large head size in relation to body mass. Most childhood head trauma is blunt in nature, and head injuries account for most of the permanent disabilities seen.

- A significant volume of blood can be lost via scalp laceration.
- An infant can have a significant intracranial bleed resulting in hypotension and shock, rarely experiencing brain stem herniation as seen in older children. Observe the infant up to age 12 to 18 months for bulging anterior fontanelle.
- Occasionally depressed skull fractures may be palpable. Boggy crepitant swelling associated with subgaleal hematomas are often felt over linear skull fractures.
- Seizures can occur as a result of head injuries. Children with significant intracranial bleeds or diffuse cerebral edema are often given prophylactic anticonvulsant medications.
- Cerebral perfusion pressure is produced by subtracting the intracranial pressure (normal is less than 15 mmHg) from the mean arterial pressure. If the mean arterial pressure is low and the intracranial pressure is high, cerebral perfusion pressure will be low and the brain will not receive an adequate supply of oxygen and nutrients.

- Children often suffer cerebral hyperemia following significant head injuries. The etiology of this increased cerebral blood flow is not known. One method of decreasing the amount of blood flowing to the brain is to hyperventilate the child to a Pco_2 of 30 to 35 mmHg.
- In children with penetrating neck injuries, careful attention must be paid to ongoing assessment of their airway. The bleeding and swelling resulting from this trauma often cause airway compromise.

Blunt abdominal trauma

The intraabdominal organs in children are less protected because of an immature cartilaginous rib cage and less firm musculature than adults.
- The most common sites of injury in the abdomen are the liver, spleen, and intestines.
- Blunt abdominal trauma in children is difficult to assess. Use of computed tomography (CT) scan is advisable. Ultrasound (US) imaging is also emerging as a valuable assessment tool.
- Early placement of an orogastric or nasogastric tube will decompress the stomach, reduce diaphragmatic irritation, and improve respiratory effort. The stomach can often become distended when children swallow air while crying.
- In the absence of blood at the urinary meatus, insertion of a Foley catheter will enable the nurse to carefully monitor urinary output.
- Measurement of the abdominal girth at the level of the umbilicus will enable the team to detect more subtle abdominal distention.

Extremity trauma

Sprains, strains, and limb fractures are frequent occurrences in childhood injuries.
- Comparison views of the uninjured side may be required.
- Fractures occurring near the epiphyseal (growth) plates require specialized attention.
- Always obtain x-rays of the joint above and below a subtle or suspected fracture site in children not yet able to communicate the pinpoint level of their pain to the care provider.
- Document the peripheral neurovascular assessment before and after any manipulation or splinting of the injured extremity.

OTHER GENERAL INFORMATION

Common trauma laboratory tests in children under 6 years of age

Type and crossmatch
CBC + differential
Serum electrolytes
Prothrombin time
Partial thromboplastin time

BUN

Glucose

The laboratory should be able to run all the specimens listed above with 7 to 10 ml of blood.

Standard trauma x-rays

Cervical spine

Chest

Pelvis

CT as indicated

Child abuse

Clinical personnel should suspect child abuse when a child is injured and:

- The story does not fit the injury.
- Much time has elapsed since the injury.
- There is repeated trauma.
- Parents respond inappropriately.

Clinical personnel should look for:

- Perioral injury
- Subdural hematoma in a child under 1 year old
- Spiral fractures of long bones in a child not yet walking
- Burn abuse patterns; glove, stocking burns, or dunk burns of buttocks
- Malnutrition
- Intraabdominal bleeding without history of trauma
- Perineal/genital injury
- Bizarre injuries (i.e., strangulation or gag marks, inflicted tattoos, circumferential tie marks)

Children suspected of being abused should be admitted and the suspected abuse should be reported. The reader is referred to texts and hospital protocols specific to child maltreatment.

SUGGESTED READINGS

Baker S: Advances and adventures in trauma prevention, *J Trauma* 42(3):369, 1997.

Buntain W: *Management of pediatric trauma*, Philadelphia, 1995, Saunders.

Cardona V, and others: *Trauma nursing: from resuscitation through rehabilitation*, ed 2, Philadelphia, 1994, Saunders.

Girotti M: Reengineering trauma care: the challenge of the nineties, *J Trauma* 40(6):855, 1996.

Givens T: Pediatric cervical spine injury: a three-year experience, *J Trauma* 41(2):310, 1996.

Hulka F, and others: Influence of a statewide trauma system on pediatric hospitalization and outcome, *J Trauma* 42(3):514, 1997.

Moront M, and others: The injured child an approach to care, *Pediatr Clin North Am* 41(6):1201, 1994.

Pieper P: Pediatric trauma, an overview, *Nurs Clin North Am* 29(4):563, 1994.

Rhoads J: Trauma care, trauma prevention, and the role of the American Trauma Society, *J Trauma* 41(3):375, 1996.

Scaletta T, Schaider J: *Emergent management of trauma*, New York, 1996, McGraw-Hill.

CHAPTER 24

Trauma in Pregnancy

Lorelei B. Camp

Trauma is a leading cause of death in women, with motor vehicle crashes being the leading cause of death in women ages 15 to 44, during the "childbearing years."[1] It has been estimated that 7% of pregnant women will sustain a traumatic injury during pregnancy.[2] The most common cause of trauma in pregnant women is motor vehicle crashes, followed by falls, penetrating injuries/domestic violence, and burns/smoke inhalation.

When a female of childbearing age presents to the emergency care setting as a victim of trauma, she must be assumed to be pregnant until proven otherwise, since early signs of pregnancy may not be readily visible or assessable. The physiologic changes that occur in pregnancy must be considered when the patient has been traumatized. When a pregnant woman has been injured, two lives are affected—the mother and the fetus.

It is important to remember that the initial assessment and interventions will remain the same: airway, breathing, and circulation. Clinical personnel should perform a primary and secondary survey, just as on any other trauma patient. It would be wise to have the obstetric team evaluate the patient and assist with care.

Blood pressure

A pregnant woman is normally hypervolemic resulting from a total blood volume increase of nearly 50% by the third trimester. If she presents hypotensive, it may be because of her body position. If she is supine, the vena cava may be compressed by the uterus/fetus, causing cardiac output to drop as much as 30% to 40%.[3] This is known as *supine hypotension* or *vena cava syndrome*. Clinical personnel should turn the patient onto her left side by tilting the backboard 15 to 30 degrees with pillows or blankets.[4,5] If tipping is inappropriate the uterus can be displaced manually.

A pregnant woman can tolerate an acute blood loss of 10% to 20% or a gradual blood loss of 35% without changes in vital signs.[4] Maternal hypovolemia can trigger a reduction in uterine blood flow up to 20% without changes in blood pressure.[4] The fetus is dependent on maternal blood flow for survival (about 700 ml per minute).[6] Thus blood pressure may be an unreliable indicator of fetal and maternal well being.[4]

Pulse

By the middle of the second trimester, heart rate will increase by 15 to 20 beats per minute. An average heart rate in a pregnant woman is 90 to 100 beats per minute.[3] A rate of 70 may actually be bradycardic for a pregnant woman.

Respirations

The respiratory rate in a pregnant woman must be monitored carefully, since pregnant women are prone to hypoxia.[7] This is due to a 40% increase in tidal volume, a 100 to 200 ml increase in vital capacity, an elevated diaphragm, and a reduction in residual capacity by about 20%.[8] A PCO_2 of 30 is normal in the third trimester as is a PO_2 of 101 to 104 mmHg.[4] At this point, the patient will be very sensitive to changes in PCO_2. Note that pH is usually the same as in the nonpregnant patient.

Temperature

Temperature usually remains the same as that of the nonpregnant patient.

Capillary refill

Capillary refill will usually remain normal, even in the face of shock, because of the increase in overall blood volume.

Skin signs (color, temperature, moisture)

Intense vasodilation occurs in pregnancy. Even when in shock, the patient may continue to have good skin color and feel warm and dry.

Cardiovascular

By the third trimester there will be a left axis shift of 15 degrees resulting from the leftward tilt of the heart caused by the elevation of the diaphragm by the enlarged fetus. Clinical personnel may also see Q waves or elevated ST segments or T wave inversion in leads II, III, and aVF. There will also be an S_3 sound on cardiac auscultation in the third trimester and a normal increase in ectopy.[3] By the time the pregnant woman reaches the term of her pregnancy, she is experiencing nearly maximum cardiac output and there is little ability to compensate in the event of a hemodynamic insult.

Blood components/laboratory values

The hypervolemia of pregnancy causes plasma volume to increase by 40% to 50%; red blood cell volume increases by less. This causes a dilution of red blood cells, which causes hematocrit to drop to approximately 31% to 35% (physiologic anemia).[8]

By the second trimester the white blood cell count has increased to 5000 to 15,000/cu mm.[4] Serum fibrinogen and clotting factors (factors VII, VIII, and IX) increase, causing prothrombin time and partial thromboplastin time to decrease. However, if there is total placental separation, clotting factors (especially fibrinogen) will decrease drastically.

GENERAL THERAPEUTIC INTERVENTIONS FOR THE TRAUMATIZED PREGNANT WOMAN

- Perform standard trauma care (ABCs).
- Administer high-flow oxygen.
- Position the patient with her right side elevated.
- If fluids are required, give blood products early.
   Avoid large volumes of crystalloid solutions.
   Type and crossmatch blood.
- Check the patient's Rh status and determine the need for RhoGam.
- Assure current tetanus prophylaxis.
- If pneumatic antishock garment (PASG) is being used, inflate leg chambers only.
- Diagnostic peritoneal lavage has been deemed safe to perform in the pregnant patient.[8-11]
- Shield the abdomen during radiologic procedures whenever possible.
- Insert a gastric tube as gastric emptying is prolonged.
- Provide continuous fetal/uterine monitoring.

SPECIFIC INJURIES AND INDICATIONS IN PREGNANCY

In addition to standard therapeutic interventions for trauma to any patient, caregivers should be particularly cognizant of the following in the injured pregnant patient:

Head

There is a 10% to 15% possibility of abruptio placentae associated with severe head injury.[6] This is thought to result from a greatly enlarged pituitary gland (twice normal size during pregnancy) and increased pressure on the gland. Clinical personnel should closely observe the patient and prepare for the possibility of an emergency cesarean section.

Chest

Pulmonary volume may be decreased as a result of anatomic changes in the second and third trimesters. The diaphragm is elevated and vital capacity is decreased. Chest trauma that causes even small changes in lung volumes and expansion may be lethal.

Gastrointestinal

- Caregivers should assume that the patient has a full stomach and, therefore at risk for aspiration. Bowel sounds may be absent.
- Lower abdominal injuries usually do not cause intestinal trauma, as intestines are relocated high anatomically.
- There may be aberration in referred pain resulting from relocation of the abdominal contents.
- There is a 5% to 10% incidence of disseminated intravascular coagulation (DIC) that occurs with significant blunt abdominal trauma.[6]
- If there has been massive abdominal trauma and a pelvic floor "blow out," there will be *massive* vaginal bleeding and profound hypovolemic shock. In this case, consider the use of a PASG, including the abdominal chamber, while preparing the patient for emergency surgery.

Genitourinary

- The bladder is pushed out of the pelvic ring and is less protected in late pregnancy.
- BUN and creatinine will decrease to 50% of normal adult values and urine glucose will increase.[6]
- Any blood found in the urine—gross or microscopic—is not normal and further investigation should occur to determine its cause.

Vaginal/fetal

- Ultrasound procedures may be extremely advantageous in this situation because they can help determine fetal well being, gestational age, and placental and uterine injuries.[5]
- Pelvic examination should be performed by a person who understands obstetric findings in trauma.
- Contractions may occur prematurely. Uterine activity must be monitored carefully.
- Any fluid coming from the vaginal vault should be tested to determine whether it is amniotic fluid. The pH of amniotic fluid is 7 to 7.5. If it has been determined that the fluid is amniotic fluid, a stat cesarean section should be considered.
- Check for frank blood or hemorrhage. This may be indicative of abruptio placentae or fetal injury. Signs and symptoms of abruptio placentae include premature labor, abdominal pain, fetal distress, uterine tenderness, or maternal shock. Obvious vaginal bleeding may or may not be present. Stat cesarean section should be considered.
- Fetal trauma is also not common, except in massive abdominal trauma, because of the cushioning effect of amniotic fluid.
- There may be damage to the fetal skull from an acceleration/deceleration motion (when the mother is wearing only a lap seatbelt).

Burns/smoke inhalation

- The patient with a burn injury will have increased fluid needs.
- The rule of nines may not apply to the pregnant patient when measuring body surface area because of the great increase in body surface area during pregnancy. One may use the area of the palm of the patient's hand to estimate the amount of body surface area burned (palmar surface of the patient's hand is approximately 1% of total body surface area).
- There is an increased risk of preterm labor in the patient who has sustained a large thermal burn.
- If smoke inhalation has occurred, it is essential to administer high-flow oxygen and obtain an O_2 saturation measurement and arterial blood gases.

Fetal assessment

- Estimate gestational age by using a measurement of the height of the fundus, fetal heart tones, and, if available, the date of the patient's last menstrual period.
- Fetal monitoring should be continual. Fetal heart tones should normally be between 120 and 160 beats per minute at about 10 to 12 weeks' gestation. The obstetrics team, if available, should perform fetal monitoring so that the trauma team is free to resuscitate the mother.
- If fetal distress is evident, prepare for a stat cesarean section.
- If the pregnant mother is moribund and there is a possibility that the fetus may be viable, consider preparation for a stat cesarean section, possibly to be done in the Emergency Department. This may also be considered if the mother is very recently (minutes) postmortem. DePace and colleagues,[11] in their literature review, have found over 150 cases of fetal survival following postmortem cesarean section.
- In the event of fetal death, appropriate support personnel should be available to the mother, the family, and significant others to support them through the grieving process.

REFERENCES

1. Jackson F: Accidental injury, the problems and the initiatives. In Buschbaum HJ, editor: *Trauma in pregnancy*, Philadelphia, 1979, Saunders.
2. Baker D: Trauma in the pregnant patient, *Surg Clin North Am* 62:275-289, 1982.
3. American College of Surgeons Committee on Trauma: *Advanced trauma life support instructor manual*, Chicago, 1984, American College of Surgeons.
4. Esposito TJ: Trauma during pregnancy, *Emer Med Clin North Am* 12:167-197, 1994.
5. Lavery JP, Staten-McCormick M: Management of moderate to severe trauma in pregnancy, *Obstet Gynec Clin North Am* 22:69-90, 1995.
6. Buschbaum HJ, editor: *Trauma in pregnancy*, Philadelphia, 1979, Saunders.
7. Santos O: The obstetrical patient for non-obstetrical surgery, *Curr Rev Nurse Anesthetists* 9:66-71, 1984.
8. Barrett S: Trauma during pregnancy, *Prog Crit Care Med* 1:248-272, 1984.
9. Olson WR, Hildreta DH: Abdominal paracentesis and peritoneal lavage in blunt abdominal trauma, *J Trauma* 11:824, 1971.
10. Rothenberger D, and others: Blunt trauma: a review of 103 cases, *J Trauma* 18:173-177, 1978.

11. Moylan J: Trauma and pregnancy. In Gleicher M, editor: *Principles of medical therapy in pregnancy,* New York, 1985, Plenum Press.
12. DePace NL, Betsch JS, Kotler MN: Postmortem cesarean section with recovery of offspring, *JAMA* 248:971-973, 1982.

SUGGESTED READINGS

Auerbach PS: Trauma in the pregnant patient. In Meislin H, editor: *Priorities in multiple trauma,* Germantown, Md, 1980, Aspen Systems.

Deitch E, Rightmire D, Clothier J: Management of burns in the pregnant woman, *Surg Gynecol Obstet* 161:1-4, 1985.

Higgins S, Garite T: Late abruptio placentae in trauma patients: implications for monitoring, *Obstet Gynecol* 63 (suppl):105-109, 1984.

Pearse C, Magrina J, Finley B: Use of MAST suit in obstetrics and gynecology, *Obstet Gynecol Surg* 37:416-422, 1984.

Smith LG: Assessment and initial management of the pregnant trauma patient, *J Trauma Nurs* 1:8-20, 1994.

CHAPTER 25

Trauma in the Elderly

Catherine Mitchell McGrath

As a result of increasingly better living conditions, lifestyles, and medical advances in the last 200 years, there is a dramatic increase in the number of citizens over the age of 60 in our country and in most of the industrial nations of the world. In 1991 the elderly population accounted for 12.7% of the population; in 2050, the elderly are projected to constitute 23%.[1] Thus with increasing health, mobility, and activity in a person's later years, we are seeing an increasing number of elderly trauma patients. The approach that we take to elderly patients, with consideration of the normal physiologic changes that occur with aging, varies from the approach to the younger adult. Although the principles of trauma resuscitation remain the same, it is essential that we understand the normal changes of aging, anticipate different reactions to stress of injury and therapy, obtain detailed histories to get a complete picture of what may be a very complicated set of circumstances, and alter our approach given the clinical and historical information that we have collected.

Although they suffer fewer injuries, the mortality rate from trauma is highest in the over-60 age group. Society has not kept up with the activities of senior citizens, and we continue to create living and traveling conditions that do not protect the safety of the elderly. Traffic signs and road construction, particularly in cities, have caused so much congestion that they challenge even the quick reactions of the young. All these obstacles can create hazards for an elderly person who is trying to maintain independence with declining acuity of sensory capabilities.

Poor vision, hearing, dizziness and syncope, and slowing of reflexes, as well as the physical limitations from musculoskeletal changes, make the elderly person prone to injury. Thus the normal changes of aging may not only color our examination, they may also contribute as a cause of injury.

NORMAL PHYSIOLOGIC CHANGES WITH ADVANCING AGE

The rate at which a person ages depends on many things. Family background, life history, medical history, medication and drug and alcohol use, nutrition, and social well-being all contribute to the onset and degree of physiologic changes of aging. The overall health of the geriatric patient is determined by preexisting illness and the extent of physiologic degeneration. The ability to withstand the stress of critical illness is related to the normal biologic degenerative process, which decreases the organs' functional reserve.

Defining "aged" is really impossible, since some 70 year olds may be physiologically younger than a 55 year old, depending on the above-mentioned factors. The physiologic changes that we should anticipate as a normal part of aging include the following:

Cardiovascular changes

- Vasculature becomes less elastic and sympathetic response is slowed.
- Decrease in cardiac contractility causes a normally lower stroke volume and cardiac output.
- Likelihood of atherosclerosis increases and can significantly impair the elderly trauma patient's response to shock.
- Compensatory mechanisms tend to be less effective.

Respiratory changes

- Decrease in lung field size and compliance (may alter the ability to provide adequate ventilation).
- Blood flow to the lung is decreased.
- Muscles used for respiration become weaker.
- Kyphosis, thorax shortening, and increased chest wall stiffness increase respiratory effort.
- Vital capacity is diminished and gas exchange impaired.
- Decreased gag and cough reflexes increase risk of aspiration and pneumonia.

Renal changes

- Decrease in kidney mass.
- Decrease in the number of functioning glomerular and renal tubules.
- Decreased ability of the kidney to dilute and concentrate urine.
- Decreased ability of the kidney to excrete acid or alkaline urine or drugs.
- Inability of the kidneys to retain water in the presence of hypovolemia.
- Excretion of ADH (antidiuretic hormone) and diminished activation of the renin-angiotensin system. The elderly patient who develops acute renal failure as a complication of prolonged hypoperfusion from shock has a poorer outcome than a person of lesser years.

Liver changes

• Decreased total liver blood flow may contribute to adverse drug reactions, especially with polypharmacy.
• Liver dysfunction may adversely affect metabolism of medications or increase drugs' toxic effects.
• Compromised liver function may increase risk of coagulopathy, because several factors important in blood clotting are produced in the liver.

Gastrointestinal system changes

• Diminished ability to swallow, impaired esophageal motility, and delayed stomach emptying of liquids may predispose the elderly to aspiration.

Immune system changes

• Decreased antibody production in response to antigens.
• Decreased inflammatory response.
• Increased multisystem failure and sepsis from infectious complications.

Musculoskeletal changes

• Osteoporotic changes
• Joint stiffness secondary to arthritic and other inflammatory conditions; this can significantly affect the flexibility of the patient and may be a contributor to the cause of the injury and create a situation in which routine splinting and securing techniques may not be acceptable.
• Bone density and mass are lost at a rate of 3% to 9% per decade.
• Joints and ligaments become less elastic.
• Minimal to moderate trauma can result in fractures and dislocations.
• Cervical degenerative changes begin at age 40; chronic changes may make x-rays more difficult to interpret for signs of trauma.

Special concern for the cervical spine must be exercised with positioning for transporting and airway protection. If the patient must be turned to accommodate vomiting or if endotracheal intubation is attempted, maintaining the anatomic position that is normal for that patient is very important. Proper padding of the bony prominences is essential to prevent skin breakdown. Often these patients will not notice the pressure because of decrease in pain perception, and the responsibility falls on the trauma team to anticipate such complications and avoid them.

Neurologic and cognitive changes

It is important to remember when interviewing the elderly patient that intelligence does not change with aging; however, the speed of processing thoughts slows with age. Do not confuse slow answers with incorrect information. The patient may think that he or she is not as smart as he or she once was because of this change; patience and clear communication are very important (Fig. 25-1). Although memory may be less acute, unless there is or-

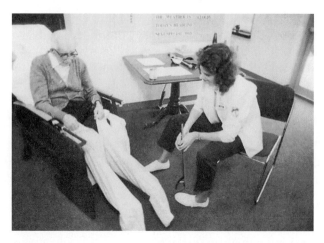

Fig. 25-1 Rehabilitation of the elderly trauma victim is often lengthy and requires patience on the part of the patient and the therapist.

ganic neurologic disease, the patient should be interviewed first before the family member is interviewed, whenever possible.

- Decreased cerebral blood flow
- Decrease in volume of brain tissue and increase in amount of intracranial dead space (allowing increased hemorrhage before symptoms become evident)
- Shortened attention span
- Poor short-term memory
- Decrease in psychomotor processing speed
- Alteration in special senses; the special senses (vision, hearing, strength of voice, touch, taste, smell) undergo alterations that cause slowing or dimming of those senses
- Decreased visual acuity (look for glasses)
- Decreased hearing (ask about hearing aids; stand in front of patient so that he or she will be able to hear you well and also be able to lip-read)
- Decreased touch/sensation; the patient may have a higher tolerance for pain that may mask minor injuries; the elderly tend to suffer more burns because of this change, because they often cannot feel the burning sensation until injury is significant
- Changes in vocal strength; patient may appear "dim," or not responsive
- Decreased sense of smell; patient may not recognize dangerous situations, such as carbon monoxide or smoke in the air, gas leaks, toxic fumes, and other toxic materials

Social changes

When the elderly population moves out of the workplace and into retirement, a perception of decreased "worth" is frequently associated with that

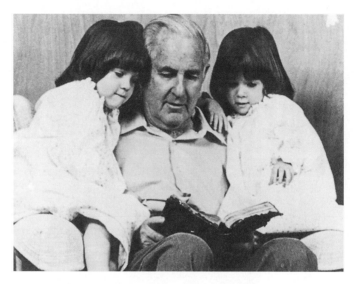

Fig. 25-2 Consideration of the grandparents' role in the family assists the caregiver in encouraging the patient's recovery.

move. As spouses, companions, and friends become infirm and die or are not available for companionship and support, a feeling of dependency, loss of control of life choices, and loneliness cause real problems for the elderly. Loss of mobility or fear of additional injury may result in admission to an elder care facility. The families of older patients are affected by injury. Many become primary caregivers for those incapacitated by their injuries or become over protective of those living independently (Figs. 25-2 and 25-3).

In some situations, elder abuse may be a factor. This possibility should be considered when evaluating the history, mechanism of injury, and pattern of injuries.

SPECIAL CONCERNS IN RESUSCITATION OF THE ELDERLY TRAUMA PATIENT

In addition to the specific conditions just discussed, there are some general things to remember about resuscitation of the aging person. The wide variety of prior functional levels that exists with each individual person may color the assessment findings, and considering these differences is important in doing a complete evaluation of the patient's status. Generally speaking, experts believe that aggressive early resuscitation is indicated and results in better long-term outcomes.

Fluid resuscitation in the elderly presents a particularly difficult problem, since we know from experience that they do not tolerate hypovolemia well,

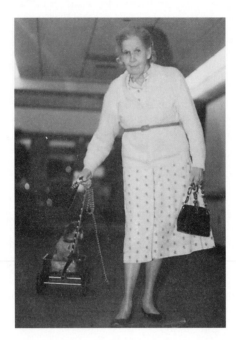

Fig. 25-3   Return to social activity and contribution is the ultimate goal of elderly trauma victim resuscitation.

they do not compensate for fluid loss well, and they are also unable to tolerate fluid overload well. It is important to monitor the response to blood loss and recognize that the older patient will not compensate on his or her own, thus decreasing the amount of time in which the trauma team must intervene with fluid support to prevent or treat shock. In addition to monitoring vital signs and urinary output, invasive monitoring may be used more aggressively in the elderly patient to maintain close scrutiny of the patient's response to fluid resuscitation. A traumatically injured patient who is resuscitated from shock but develops pulmonary edema and cardiac problems from fluid overload is a difficult one to manage. Emphasis must be put on *careful* monitoring of the patient's fluid status by the trauma team throughout the resuscitation.

Obtaining adequate information from witnesses at the scene and from ambulance personnel is essential in evaluating the patient's response to injury and to the prehospital treatment that has been administered before coming to the hospital. Good documentation by the ambulance personnel, as well as careful record keeping from the time that the patient enters the Emergency Department, will answer the basic question that the trauma team should be asking: Is the patient getting worse or is the patient getting better?

ASSESSMENT

Cardiovascular
- Blood pressure may not be an accurate indicator; prior dysfunction, medication or compensation may alter what we generally consider "normal" response to shock.
- Close monitoring is needed to identify trends and responses in cardiac response to resuscitation.
- Although arrhythmias may be more common in the elderly, clinical personnel must first rule out hypoxemia and cardiac injury as the cause and not assume that they were preexisting conditions.
- Consider dual diagnosis if the patient demonstrates signs of cardiac dysfunction:
  Did myocardial infarction occur and cause the accident?
  Did low-flow state induce myocardial infarction?
- Complete cardiac work-up with serial electrocardiograms and enzyme evaluation is recommended.

Pulmonary
- Arterial blood gases normally show a moderate decrease in O_2 tension; otherwise the parameters are the same as for younger patients; serial monitoring to identify trends is important.
- Decrease in chest expansion ability, vital capacity, and ability to cough can be anticipated as normal and should not be mistaken for chronic obstructive pulmonary disease.

Neurologic
- Changes in vision, hearing, and touch may alter assessment findings.
- Sensory overload, short-term memory loss, or senile dementia may alter evaluation of cognitive function.
- Careful assessment should be made to determine the presence of intracranial bleeding; the elderly are more prone to bleeding (the young tend to develop cerebral edema with the same type of injury).

Renal
- Inappropriately high urine output with hypovolemia caused by inadequate compensation may be present.
- Decreased renal blood flow causes decreased glomerular filtration rate and impaired water reabsorption.
- Urinary catheter is essential as an assessment tool, but in the elderly it carries a higher risk of infection; asepsis must be strict.

THERAPEUTIC INTERVENTIONS

Airway
- Cervical spine protection may be difficult because of osteoporosis, particularly during endotracheal intubation; avoid hyperextension of the neck.

- Tissues of the airway are fragile and prone to injury with intubation.
- The oral cavity should be inspected to ascertain the presence and location of artificial teeth.
- Asepsis is important to minimize the risk of pneumonia.

Breathing

- Mechanical ventilation should be started early to support ventilation.

Circulation

- Prolonged hypovolemia is worse than fluid overload. Central venous pressure monitoring and conventional noninvasive monitoring for shock are very important. Withholding fluids for fear of causing overload is a very dangerous risk.

POLYPHARMACY

Multiple medications have created a mounting problem in the elderly, as they attempt to address changes in function with medicines. Often the patient will "doctor shop" and may be taking a number of unsupervised medications, both prescription and over the counter. It is very important to get a good medication history, especially for the current 24 hours, to be able to reliably administer necessary medications for resuscitation and to be able to anticipate interactions among medications. Getting this information may be difficult on the occasion of a traumatic injury, but previous hospital records should be sought in addition to family information and documentation by ambulance personnel if the patient is unable to provide it. Consultation with a pharmacist during the resuscitation may be necessary to sort out the interactions of many drugs, and it is a good idea to make provisions for the availability of a pharmacist to the trauma team.

GENERAL NURSING CONSIDERATIONS

As with all trauma patients, provision of comfort during resuscitation takes a low priority when lifesaving procedures are necessary, but remember that the elderly patient may have skeletal changes that make positioning on backboards, stretchers, and radiology tables particularly painful. Because of normal losses of subcutaneous fat, bony prominences should be padded, if possible, particularly when the patient is going to remain in one position for an extended time. Speaking to the patient regularly will not only help your ongoing assessment of their neurologic status and level of consciousness, but will also give the patient the opportunity to express concerns, identify painful areas, and ask questions. Be sure to observe the patient's responses during conversation to recognize confusion or possible misinterpretation of information. Also, talk to the patient and explain procedures before they are performed.

Because of possible injury or normal changes to the thermoregulation system and because of peripheral vascular changes, the elderly patient may become chilled sooner than would a younger adult. Dehydration and poor nutrition and inactivity may exacerbate this problem. Mildly hypothermic geriatric patients are confused and less communicative than usual. They may display a flat affect, appear senile, and exhibit poor judgment and coordination. (See also the heat loss reducing techniques described in Chapter 27 of this manual.) Providing warm blankets when care allows will not only prevent heat loss, but will also make the patient feel more secure and well cared for.

Emergency and trauma nurses should be involved in injury prevention efforts aimed at the elderly population. One-to-one teaching and group educational programs can assist in preventing falls and motor vehicular injuries.

REFERENCE

1. US Bureau of the Census: *Current Population Reports, Special Studies, Sixty-five plus in America,* Washington, DC, 1992, US Government Printing Office.

SUGGESTED READINGS

Birchenall JM, Streight ME: *Care of the older adult,* ed 3, Philadelphia, 1993, JB Lippincott.

Burke M: Motor vehicle injury prevention for older adults, *Nurse Pract* 19(2):26-28, 1994.

Davis AE: Hip fractures in the elderly: surveillance methods and injury control, *J Trauma Nurs* 2(1):15-21, 1995.

Dubin S: Geriatric assessment, *Am J Nurs* 96(5):Nurse Pract Extra Ed: 49-50, 1996.

Knies RC: Assessment in geriatric trauma: what you need to know, *Int J Trauma Nurs* 2:85-91, 1996.

Rauen CA: Too old to live, too young to die: multiple organ dysfunction syndrome in the elderly, *Crit Care Nurs Clin North Am* 6(3):535-542, 1994.

Santora TA, Schinco MA, Trooskin SZ: Management of trauma in the elderly patient, *Surg Clin North Am* 74(1):163-186, 1994.

Stamatos CA: Geriatric trauma patients: initial assessment and management of shock, *J Trauma Nurs* 1(2):45-54, 1994.

CHAPTER 26

Interpersonal Violence

Deborah A. D'Avolio

Domestic violence has serious implications for the healthcare professional. Emergency providers are in an ideal position to offer both physical and psychologic interventions while they are caring for victims of violence. A popular misconception is that patients do not want to tell healthcare providers about the violence in their lives. Clinicians with experience in this area have found that patients are relieved to have the opportunity to talk about the trauma they are experiencing.

The statistics on the prevalence of abuse and trauma are staggering. Given these figures, it is very likely someone whom the medical professional treats is at risk or has already been a victim of abuse. Injuries are one of the leading causes of death for women in the United States. Many injuries to women result from violent acts, including homicide, physical and sexual assault, and suicide. Physical assaults by someone known to the victim are the leading cause of injury to women. An estimated 1.8 million women are assaulted each year by the men with whom they share a household or consider their partners, and as many as 30% of women receive treatment for their injuries in emergency departments. Domestic violence affects many more women than men.[1]

Identifying domestic violence has been an area that healthcare providers have at times avoided for several reasons: lack of time, lack of comfort with the topic, lack of training, and fear of offending the patient.[2] Other research has shown that response of healthcare providers caring for victims of violence has been at best nontherapeutic and in many cases nonexistent.[3] Domestic violence has been underappreciated by society, is frequently unrecognized by providers, and has been given a low priority.[3] Accredited Emergency Departments are required by the Joint Commission on Accreditation of Healthcare Organizations to have policies, procedures, and education for the staff on the care of victims of domestic violence.[4] Clinical personnel should become familiar with their healthcare institutions' systems to provide the necessary support and intervention for victims of violence.

Domestic violence has been defined in many ways; there are many legal definitions. Most of the victims are women; therefore, in this chapter, the patient will be referred to as a woman. But personnel must realize that domestic violence can also happen to men. Battering can occur in all combinations of relationships. Women of all cultures, educational levels, races, incomes, and ages are battered by husbands, boyfriends, lovers, and partners. Women who leave a violent relationship are also at risk of battering. Leaving the violent partner can sometimes escalate the violence.

Domestic violence includes partner abuse, teen dating violence, spouse abuse, child abuse, family violence, and elder abuse. Violence in adolescent dating relationships is often unrecognized because of lack of awareness. Domestic violence is a pattern of behaviors that includes physical, psychologic, and sexual assaults. Behaviors, including withholding of economic resources, can intimidate and coerce the victim. Some examples are physical assault, the threat of harm, isolation from family and friends, controlling behaviors, degrading behaviors, name calling, and sexual assault. At times, the abuser may threaten to abuse the victim's children or commit abusive acts against the children as a form of power and control over the victim. Intimidation and attacks against pets or property are forms of control that inflict fear on the victim. In some states, the threat of harm and acts of intimidation are considered domestic violence. Each state has different definitions and legal remedies. Several states have mandated reporting laws, requiring healthcare providers to report to authorities when they care for patients who are victims of domestic violence. Healthcare providers must be familiar with the laws of the state in which they practice.

ASSESSMENT, IDENTIFICATION, AND INTERVENTION

Victims of violence may present to any clinical setting, including emergency departments, trauma centers, HMOs, clinics, and private medical offices, and they may present in various ways. All patients at each visit to a healthcare setting should be assessed for interpersonal violence by asking a few key questions, such as: (1) Does anyone try to control you? (2) Does anyone make you feel afraid? (3) Has anyone threatened you? If clinical personnel wait for a "classic presentation," many opportunities will be lost to provide support and intervention that can be life-changing and at times life-saving.

Almost any type of injury or trauma can be a result of domestic violence. The injuries can range from simple soft-tissue contusions to gunshot wounds. Recent research has shown that often chronic presentations without evidence of pathology—headaches, abdominal pain, pelvic pain, and back pain—can be attributed to interpersonal violence. Vague, nonspecific complaints can be manifestations of battering.

Special populations

Pregnant women can be at increased risk for domestic violence. Pregnancy is often a positive time in a woman's life. A controlling, manipulative abuser can feel threatened with this positive focus, and the abuse may increase. Studies point to violence as the cause of miscarriages and multiple abortions. Abused women are twice as likely to delay prenatal care until the third trimester of pregnancy.[5] All pregnant patients should be screened for violence at every prenatal visit.

With our aging society, domestic maltreatment of the elderly is now recognized as a significant problem. In the 1981, U.S. Select Committee on Aging 500,000 to 1.5 million cases of elder abuse were suggested to occur annually in the United States. Healthcare providers in all settings are in an ideal position to detect abuse and neglect of the elderly. There are six types of elder abuse: physical abuse, physical neglect, psychologic abuse, psychologic neglect, material abuse, and violation of personal rights or exploitation. It is necessary for healthcare providers to know about the adult protective service systems and the reporting laws in their state. Laws vary from state to state, and healthcare providers must know necessary information related to the reporting law: the patient's age, which events are reportable, the required timeliness of filing a report, the necessary forms, when an investigation should begin, and the penalty for failure to report. Reports may be written or verbal.

The disabled are another population that is at risk for maltreatment. Usually the disabled patient depends on another adult, and the victim and the perpetrator generally live together. Again, clinical personnel must know about the reporting law in the state in which they practice.

Child abuse and neglect is a complex problem that can be defined as harm to a child by a caregiver that results in injury or harm. Healthcare providers are legally responsible for reporting their suspicions of abuse to the authorities. Child abuse and neglect create long-standing emotional and physical costs.

The four types of child abuse are physical, emotional, sexual, and neglect.

ASKING QUESTIONS

Clinical personnel should include questions about abuse in routine triage and exams. Assessment for interpersonal violence has to be conducted in privacy. A few minutes alone with the patient is part of normal practice in the healthcare setting. Family members or significant others can remain in the waiting area during the initial patient evaluation. An environment of safety has to be created to help the patient talk freely. All patients should be interviewed in a quiet, private area where their confidentiality can be ensured. The question of abuse should be included in routine screenings (past medical history, medications, allergies).

An essential part of a triage assessment is a violence assessment, in which these questions are asked:

- Is someone you know hurting you?
- Are you afraid of the person you have a relationship with?
- Some of the women for whom I care have injuries similar to yours, and they have been hurt by someone they care about. Did someone hurt you?

Clinical personnel should conclude with a supportive statement and let the patient know that there are people and places that can help. The patient should be reassured that she is not alone and that there are many people in the same situation. The patient does not deserve to be hurt, and resources are available to battered women and their children.

Disclosure can at times put the patient at increased risk, and she may decline intervention or services. If there is disclosure and the patient declines intervention, clinical personnel can use this visit as an opportunity to inform the patient of the resources in the healthcare setting and in the community. A therapeutic relationship of trust can be established. Women have returned to the healthcare setting uninjured to access the services that were offered. It is important to let the patient know that confidentiality will be maintained within the limits of state law. If there is mandated reporting in the state, the implications should be discussed with the patient. The patient should be informed that the healthcare provider is a mandated reporter and that services will be provided to keep both her and the children safe.

Physical examination and documentation

A thorough physical examination must be conducted. The injuries must be evaluated and described. A body map is helpful to describe and document the injuries. A careful evaluation and description of the injuries should include the type, number, size, and location. Assessment for other injuries, such as sexual assault, is also essential. The sexual assault procedures of the healthcare facility should then be followed. In cases in which domestic violence is suspected and the patient does not disclose, clinical personnel should document whether the pattern of injury is consistent with the history that the patient provides. Also personnel should include that they offered services and/or resources and that the patient declined.

Safety and lethality assessment

It is essential to ensure safety of the patient and the staff at all times. If the person who is battered is at risk of further injury in the healthcare setting, notify hospital security of the potential risk.

Assess the patient's needs:

- Does she want clinical personnel to notify the police?
- Is she safe to return home?
- Does she want to go to a shelter?

All victims of violence should be assessed for risk of homicide or serious injury. There are several risk factors for serious injury. Questions to consider are:

- Have threats been made to kill the victim, the children, or other family members?
- Does the abuser have a history of drug and or alcohol abuse?
- Has the abuser been arrested before?
- Is the abuser stalking the victim?
- Has the abuser been involved in violent relationships in the past?
- Does the abuser own a gun or a knife? (The possession of a gun or a knife is a serious risk.)
- Is the victim afraid that she will be killed?

Clinical personnel should tell the patient that they are very concerned about her safety and that she is at risk. Many times, discussing this abuse with someone will help the patient realize the seriousness of her situation. If the lethality assessment is high, it is critical that the patient be provided with referrals to local emergency shelters, police, and legal advocacy.

Clinical personnel should assess for suicide and homicide. A battered woman should be asked if she is thinking of harming herself. It should be a direct question. If there is risk, the patient should be provided a safe environment and an emergency psychiatric evaluation. Homicidal ideation will also warrant an emergent psychiatric evaluation. If the patient has a plan, the practitioner may have a legal duty to breach confidence and warn a third party.

SAFETY PLANNING

Many patients will decide to return to their homes. Clinical personnel should review with patients some of the basic elements of safety planning:

- The patient should review and list several safe places that she can go if she decides to leave home.
- The patient should have important phone numbers available and know how to access emergency help, such as 911.
- The patient should talk to a trusted person about the violence and ask that person to call the police if any suspicious events or sounds should take place in or around the home.
- The patient should leave extra car keys, clothes, money, and copies of important documents with a trusted person.
- The patient should review escape routes with a support person.
- The patient should review safe places to go and persons to call with older children in the family.
- The patient should discuss safety measures, such as changing phone numbers and locks on the windows and doors.
- The patient should review safety procedures when going to and from work.

RESOURCES AND REFERRAL

Appropriate referrals and resources—counseling, internal and external agencies, and a list of therapists who have experience with victims of violence—must be available to share with patients. Many communities have services for victims of domestic violence. Battered women's service groups provide counseling and advocacy for victims of domestic violence. The battered women's support network will review with her more in-depth safety options if she returns to the abuser, or if she decides to leave. Battered women advocacy programs provide a wide variety of services. Many states have agencies that provide resources to victims of abuse, including elder, disabled, and child abuse. Most police departments have officers who are specially trained to respond to victims of violence. When providing this information, medical providers should tell women that the services are confidential and usually free. If there is a charge, it is nominal.

LEGAL INTERVENTION

Civil protection orders are available to battered women in every state. The civil order can be used to provide legal protection for battered women and their children. The restraining orders prohibit the abuser from further acts of violence. Clinical personnel should be aware of the state's laws and understand what is available.

Violence against specific age groups or special populations is addressed in each of the states' laws. Elder abuse, child abuse, and disabled abuse usually require mandated reporting by healthcare personnel. Again, clinical personnel should check state laws.

Personnel should document the treatment, referrals, and safety planning provided while caring for patients. If the patient declines services, this statement must be included in documentation. It is the patient's choice; only he or she can decide when the time is right to leave the relationship.

SUMMARY

The healthcare provider's main role is to support the patient and provide a linkage with special services. The patient is not responsible for the abuse. Clinical personnel should provide resource and referral information. Complex issues and challenges arise when providing care for persons who experience interpersonal violence. Collaboration with the advocacy community will help the healthcare provider become more knowledgeable. An advocacy model that links the healthcare system with domestic violence advocates provides an integrated community response. Many states have a domestic violence coalition or resource center that can provide information, training, support, and connections to other violence resources.

The emergency healthcare provider may be the first person to encounter a victim of violence and must be prepared to offer support and intervention.

The healthcare provider's actions have tremendous impact in profound ways that he or she may never fully know. Domestic violence can often be a hidden trauma; effective intervention can be life-changing and life-saving.

REFERENCES

1. Centers for Disease Control and Prevention, Office of Women's Health, Women's Health Page: *Violence and injury* (on line), available through www.cdc.gov/od/owh/whvio.htm, 1997.
2. Sugg NK, Inui T: Primary care physicians' response to domestic violence: opening Pandora's box, *J Am Med Assoc* 267(23), 3157-3160, 1992.
3. Campbell J, and others: Battered women's experiences in the emergency department, *J Emerg Nurs* 20:280-288, August 1994.
4. Joint Commission on Accreditation of Healthcare Organizations: *Accreditation manual for hospitals, Volume 1: Standards,* Oakbrook Terrace, Il, 1992, JCAHO.
5. McFarlane J, Parker B, Soeken K, Bullock L: Assessing for abuse during pregnancy: severity and frequency of injuries and associated entry into prenatal care, *J Am Med Assoc* 267:3176-3178, 1992.

SUGGESTED READINGS

Campbell J, Humphreys J, editors: *Nursing care of survivors of family violence,* ed 2, St Louis, 1993, Mosby.
Ernst AA, Nick TG, Weiss ST, and others: Domestic violence in an inner-city ED, *Ann Emerg Med* 30(2), 190-197, 1997.
Lynch SH: Elder abuse: what to look for, how to intervene, *Am J Nurs* 97(1), 27-32, 1997.
Lumley VA, Miltenberger RG: Sexual abuse prevention for persons with mental retardation, *Am J Ment Retard* 101(5), 459-472, 1997.
Warshaw C, Ganley AL: *Improving the health care response to domestic violence: a resource manual for health care providers,* San Francisco, 1995, Family Violence Prevention Fund.

PART V

Clinical Skills and Procedures

CHAPTER 27

Skills for Trauma Management

Greg Schneider

DIGITAL (TACTILE) INTUBATION

Digital or tactile intubation is an alternative method of endotracheal intubation that may be used when the vocal cords are visibly obstructed by blood or emesis, when the head and neck must be maintained in alignment, when traditional laryngoscopic intubation has been unsuccessful, or when the patient is entrapped and direct access and/or visualization is not possible.

Equipment

Appropriate size endotracheal tube
Appropriate size malleable stylette
Gloves
Suction
Bag valve resuscitator and mask

Preparation for procedure

- Someone should be ventilating the patient using an oropharyngeal or nasal tube airway and a bag-valve-mask device.
- Prepare the endotracheal tube by inserting the stylette and forming it in the shape of an open-ended J at the distal end of the tube.
- Face or straddle the patient.

Procedure

1. While facing or straddling the patient, insert the index and middle fingers of a gloved, nondominant hand alongside of the patient's tongue, moving the tongue out of the way as the fingers are advanced to the anterior pharyngeal region.
2. Advance the fingers until the epiglottis or opening of the trachea can be palpated.
3. Grasp the endotracheal tube in the dominant hand and insert it into the patient's mouth.

4. Advance the tube to the posterior pharyngeal area until the tip of the tube can be felt by the fingers of the nondominant hand.
5. Slip the tube into the trachea.
6. Remove the stylette, attach a bag valve resuscitation, and ventilate the patient while observing for chest rise and listening for breath sounds bilaterally.
7. Secure endotracheal tube in place and assure appropriate insertion depth.

INTUBATION USING LIGHTED STYLETTE

Lighted stylettes provide another means of assisting with endotracheal intubation. The technique is a nonvisual insertion that uses transillumination of the trachea to guide placement of the endotracheal tube. This technique may be used as an aid to a digital intubation. The tip of the stylette contains a bright fiber-optic light. A lighted stylette may be useful in patients in whom direct visualization is difficult or access is limited, who have cervical spine injury, or who have severe facial trauma accompanied by ongoing blood loss that obliterates the field.

Equipment

Appropriate size endotracheal tube
Lighted stylette
Gloves
Suction
Bag valve resuscitator and mask

Procedure

1. The lighted stylette is inserted into the endotracheal tube and lined up with the corresponding numerical markings of the endotracheal tube.
2. The stylette has a marking at its distal end indicating a point where the stylette is bent into a 90-degree ($\pm$20 degrees) angle.
3. The ETT and stylette are advanced through the oropharynx and into the trachea. Observe for transillumination of the lighted stylette through the tissue of the anterior neck as the tube is advanced. If the light beam is bright, clear, and easily seen, the ETT is likely advancing into the trachea. A dim and poorly seen light indicates likely insertion into the esophagus.
4. Confirm endotracheal tube placement with lung auscultation; and observe for chest expansion, misting of the tube, end tidal CO_2 detection, no air over the epigastrum and chest x-ray. The lighted stylette may provide an additional means of confirming endotracheal tube placement in a patient already intubated by other means. The light allows clinical personnel to see the direction of the endotracheal tube.
5. The lighted stylette will begin flashing (after 30 seconds) when the recommended insertion time has been exceeded.
6. Secure the endotracheal tube in place and assure appropriate insertion depth.

NEEDLE CRICOTHYROTOMY

Needle cricothyrotomy should be considered in patients who have a complete upper airway obstruction and in whom conventional means of airway management have been unsuccessful. The technique involves inserting an over-the-needle catheter into the trachea and ventilating the patient until a more adequate airway is obtained.

A needle cricothyrotomy provides ventilation for 30 to 40 minutes, at most, and should only be considered a temporary measure until a more adequate airway is obtained.

A needle cricothyrotomy is an advanced airway skill reserved for emergent airway management when other methods of airway management have failed. It is most frequently used for children less than 12 years old because of the low tidal volumes generated by the catheter and jet insufflation technique.

Indications

Complete upper airway obstruction because of
- Pharyngeal and epiglotic edema or obstruction
- Facial trauma and/or neck trauma with airway compromise
- Inability to remove foreign body with abdominal thrusts or forceps
- Inability to obtain and maintain adequate airway with conventional means
- Inability to ventilate with bag-valve mask

Contraindications

- Any airway impairment that can be corrected by more conventional techniques such as use of oropharyngeal or nasopharyngeal airway; endotracheal intubation; or bag-valve mask ventilation.

Equipment

12 or 14 gauge, 8.5 cm over-the-needle catheter
5 to 10 ml syringe
3.0 mm pediatric endotracheal tube adapter
Oxygen tubing
Betadine swab
Y connector
Tape
Bag-valve-mask resuscitation
Suction with appropriate catheter(s)

Procedure

1. Position patient supine.
2. Palpate cricothyroid membrane (located on the anterior neck between inferior margin of the thyroid cartilage and superior margin of the cricoid cartilage (Fig. 27-1).
3. Prep the area with Betadine.

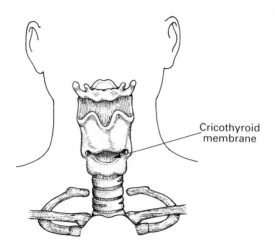

Fig. 27-1   Cricothyroid membrane.

4. Open sterile packages on sterile field.
5. Put on sterile gloves.
6. Assemble the 10-, 12-, or 14-gauge catheter with a 5- or 10-ml syringe.
7. Identify the cricothyroid membrane (as in step 2) and stabilize the thyroid cartilage with nondominant hand.
8. Puncture the skin in the midline directly over the cricothyroid membrane.
9. Direct the needle at a 45-degree angle caudally.
10. Carefully insert the needle through the lower half of the membrane, aspirating the syringe as hand advances (air return into the syringe signifies entry into the lumen of the trachea).
11. Withdraw the stylette while gently advancing the catheter downward.

NOTE: Do not force catheter, or puncture of the posterior wall of the trachea may occur.

---

12. Attach catheter hub to a 3.0-mm pediatric endotracheal tube adapter.
13. Connect Y connector to 3.0-mm pediatric endotracheal tube adapter.
14. Administer oxygen at 15 liters per minute (50 psi).
15. Tape catheter in place.
16. Use a 1:4 technique for jet insufflation; hold finger over open end of Y connector for 1 second, then leave connector open for 4 seconds for exhalation of air; repeat sequence until a more definitive airway can be established.
17. Observe lung inflations; auscultate for adequate ventilation (other lung injuries may become apparent at this time).

SURGICAL CRICOTHYROTOMY

Surgical cricothyrotomy should be considered in patients older than 12 years of age when a complete upper airway obstruction is present and conventional means of airway management have been unsuccessful. Surgical cricothyrotomy provides effective airway control and allows for oxygenation and ventilation of the patient. A surgical cricothyrotomy is an advanced airway skill reserved for emergent airway management when other methods of airway management have failed. This technique is more complicated than a needle cricothyrotomy and should be performed by a clinician specifically trained to establish a surgical cricothyrotomy.

Indications

Complete upper airway obstruction with the following complications:
Inability to effectively visualize anatomic structures because of facial trauma, pharyngeal or epiglottic edema or obstruction, or other structural anomaly.
Inability to remove a foreign body with abdominal thrusts or forceps.
Inability to obtain and maintain an adequate airway by conventional means.
Inability to ventilate with bag-valve mask.

Contraindications

Any airway impairment that can be corrected by more conventional means such as suctioning, nasopharyngeal or oropharyngeal airways, endotracheal intubation, or bag-valve-mask ventilation.

Equipment

Appropriate size endotracheal tube such as tracheostomy tube, cuffed endotracheal tube, or commercially available surgical airway kit (Mini Trach II)
10-cc syringe
Hemostats
Retracting device such as trach hook, small rake retractors, or tracheal spreaders
#10 and #11 scalpel blade and handle
Betadine
Suction with appropriate catheters
Trach tape or adhesive tape
Bag-valve resuscitator
Sterile 4 × 4 sponges

Procedure

1. Position patient supine with neck in a neutral position.
2. Palpate the cricothyroid membrane (located on the anterior neck between the inferior margin of the thyroid cartilage and the superior margin of the cricoid cartilage.
3. Prep the area with Betadine.
4. Open sterile packages onto a sterile field.

5. Put on sterile gloves.
6. If the patient is conscious, consider a local anesthetic.
7. Identify the cricothyroid membrane and stabilize the thyroid cartilage.
8. Make a vertical or horizontal incision through the skin over the cricothyroid membrane and sharply dissect through the cricothyroid membrane.
9. Insert the scalpel handle or available retracting device into the incision and rotate at least 90 degrees to open the airway.
10. Insert the appropriate sized, cuffed tube into the cricothyroid membrane incision and direct it caudally into the trachea.
11. Inflate the cuff and begin ventilating the patient.
12. Confirm placement by lung auscultation, and observe for chest expansion, misting in the tube, end tidal CO_2 detection, no gurgling over epigastrium and chest x-ray.
13. Secure the tube in place.

SPINAL IMMOBILIZATION

Cervical and complete spinal immobilization must be considered simultaneously with airway management as one of the first priorities of care in the management of the injured patient. The responsibility of "doing no harm" cannot be overemphasized. Extreme caution and a high index of suspicion are recommended when handling trauma patients before cervical spine injury has been ruled out.

Equipment

Semirigid cervical collar (preferably with window in anterior portion, which allows for evaluation of trachea and carotid pulse) or other commercially available cervical immobilization device
Long spine board with straps
Blankets, towels for padding
2- or 3-inch adhesive tape
   Equipment used to immobilize the neck may be as varied as the situation in which the items are being used. If equipment is being applied in the hospital or in the field by prehospital rescue personnel, many commercial devices are available. However, if cervical spine immobilization is indicated in the absence of this equipment, common available materials are adequate for achieving the necessary stabilization. The best cervical spine stabilizers are a pair of trained hands; the presence of trained personnel may not be practical for the duration of care, or personnel may not be available in adequate numbers.

Procedure

1. Stabilize the patient's head; tell the patient not to move the neck or turn the head.
2. Assess airway; ensure patency by using jaw thrust or chin lift; do not hyperextend neck. If endotracheal intubation is necessary, maintain manual in-line stabilization during endotracheal tube placement.

3. Evaluate cervical spine by observation: palpate each spinous process. Note deformity, crepitus, pain, and instability (talk to the patient; also remember to inform the patient of each step of the procedure to enlist his or her co-operation and to alleviate anxiety and movement).
4. Gently apply in-line manual stabilization by placing one hand on either side of the head and stabilizing head and neck in a neutral vertical position. (Once manual, it must be maintained until complete immobilization of the neck and spine has been achieved, spine injury has been ruled out by radiographs.)
5. Direct other members of the team in body positioning, spine board placement, and patient movement. The patient is logrolled with strict inline manual stabilization onto the spine board. The person maintaining in-line stabilization is the team leader and directs all movement of the patient.

NOTE: Do not attempt to logroll without assistance.

---

6. Secure the patient to the board by:
   • Fastening chest, hip, and leg straps across the patient, snugly attached to handles or cutouts in board. (Remember to undress patient completely, if possible, or at least empty pockets and remove any sharp or bulky items that may cause soft-tissue pressure areas: pad bony prominences liberally.)
   • Securing straps diagonally from pelvis to chest
   • Padding behind the head and neck to support cervical spine (always maintaining the neutral, vertical position of the manual stabilization)
   • Securing the patient's head to the spine board using 2- or 3-inch tape applied above the eyebrows and across the chin; this tape must be secured snugly to both sides of the spine board.
   • Caution must be exercised to prevent any of the securing devices from interfering with respirations or emesis.
7. When satisfied with absolute immobility of patient's cervical spine, release manual stabilization.
8. Be prepared to logroll the patient using the backboard if vomiting occurs; have suction at hand.
9. Be sensitive to the frightening nature of this procedure; maintain a dialogue with the patient to explain each new move and to evaluate changes in neurovascular status and cognizant function.

Criteria for evaluating cervical spine

Cervical collar should remain in place if:
   • Patient complains of pain, weakness, or parasthesias suggestive of acute cervical injury
   • Patient complains of neck pain, tenderness, spasm, or limited range of motion

- Patient is unreliable because of altered mental status from injury, alcohol, or other drugs
- Impaired communication because of language barrier, aphasia, developmental delay, or dementia
- Patient has preexisting cervical injury
- Patient has distracting pain from other injuries or long-bone fractures
- Patient's neurologic exam reveals deficit
- Patient is in shock following blunt trauma

If the above criteria are not present, the clinician may elect to remove the collar and completely examine the patient's neck. The clinician may clear the cervical spine by examination if no signs or symptoms of injury exist.

In the presence of any of the above criteria along with or without physical findings, the patient should have radiographic evaluation. A complete radiographic evaluation includes a lateral, an AP, and an odontoid view of the cervical spine. Despite normal radiographic evaluation, the cervical collar should remain in place with comatose or chemically relaxed patients.

NEEDLE THORACENTESIS AND FLUTTER VALVE

Needle thoracentesis is a procedure for the treatment of a patient whose condition is deteriorating rapidly because of life-threatening tension pneumothorax. It should be used when chest tube insertion is not an immediate option because of limited time or lack of available skill or equipment. The procedure involves relieving the trapped air in the pleural space and allowing for decompression of positive pressure within the pleural space. This may be accomplished with an over-the-needle catheter, allowing the air to escape passively via the catheter or a simple one-way valve (flutter valve) attached to the catheter.

Indication

- Tension pneumothorax

Equipment

Prep solution (Betadine)
14-gauge over-the-needle catheter of adequate length to reach pleural space
3-inch collapsible tubing for flutter valve (Penrose drain or Heimlich valve)
Suture ties or small rubber band

Procedure

1. Evaluate the patient's respiratory status and skin color: look at chest excursion, auscultate for absence of breath sounds on affected side, observe for tracheal deviation away from affected side, look for distended neck veins to determine the presence of tension pneumothorax.
2. Administer oxygen per bag-valve mask or nonrebreather mask.
3. If the patient is intubated, confirm correct tube placement and insertion depth before needle decompression.

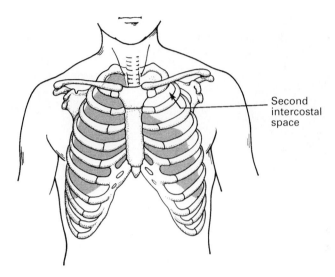

Fig. 27-2   Needle thoracentesis.

4. Prep insertion area (second intercostal space, midclavicular line) with antiseptic solution.
5. If time allows, inject local anesthetic into the insertion site.
6. Insert the needle into the second intercostal space, riding just over the top of the third rib to avoid the intercostal neurovasculature that lies on the inferior borders of the ribs (Fig. 27-2).
7. Puncture the parietal pleura (a hissing sound should confirm proper venting if using a needle and flutter valve).
8. Leave the catheter in place. If using a flutter valve, no dressing is necessary. (Intubated patients receiving positive pressure ventilation do not necessarily require a flutter valve.)
9. Leave the catheter in place until a chest tube is inserted.
10. Obtain a chest radiograph (preferably an upright view) to confirm relief of the tension pneumothorax.

CHEST TUBE PLACEMENT AND CHEST DRAINAGE

Chest tubes are placed so that air and blood can be removed from the intrathoracic cavity. The procedure involves placing a chest tube through the appropriate intercostal space so that air can be removed and the pneumothorax or tension pneumothorax can be relieved or so that blood and fluid can be drained by gravity drainage or with the assistance of suction.

The accumulation of blood and air in the pleural cavity along with the loss of negative pressure causes the lung to collapse. Once a chest tube is inserted through an intercostal space into the pleural cavity, air, blood and/or fluid is drained by gravity or suction into a drainage collection device, and negative pressure is restored.

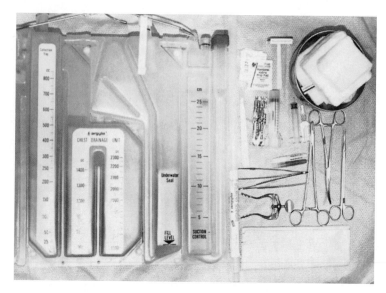

Fig. 27-3 Equipment for chest tube thoracostomy and drainage collection.

Indications

- Hemothorax
- Pneumothorax
- Tension pneumothorax
- Empyema
- Open pneumothorax

Equipment (Fig. 27-3)

Closed chest drainage system with autotransfusion capabilities
Betadine
Prep sponges
Two large, curved Kelly clamps
Syringes, 6 ml and 10 ml
18- and 25-gauge needles
Scalpel and blade
Lidocaine 1%
Suture to secure chest tube
Suction
Sterile water
Suture for wound approximation
Chest tube (usually 32, 36, or large enough to collect large quantities of blood)
Sterile gloves
Occlusive dressing material
Sterile drape

Needle holder
Benzoin
Wide adhesive tape

Preparation for procedure

1. Prepare the patient by explaining the procedure.
2. Evaluate the patient's respiratory status. Observe for respiratory rate, respiratory effort, skin color, tracheal deviation, distended neck veins, chest expansion, and auscultate breath sounds.
3. Monitor the patient's vital signs throughout the procedure.
4. Administer oxygen via the appropriate route.
5. Administer analgesia, as prescribed.
6. Chest drainage systems vary among manufacturers.

In general, the water seal and suction control chambers require sterile water. Low suction should be applied. The tubing connection to the patient should be clamped before insertion to prevent unnecessary exposure or loss of blood from the pleural space. Once connected to the closed chest drainage system, the tubing should not be "milked" or "stripped."

Procedure

1. The most advantagous and more cosmetically appealing site for chest tube insertion is the midaxillary, fifth intercostal; this position allows for adequate removal of air and/or blood.
2. Assist the physician as necessary with the procedure:
   • The site is prepped with Betadine and draped with sterile towels.
   • The skin and periosteum are infiltrated with lidocaine.
   • Using a scalpel, a 2- to 3-cm transverse incision is made through the skin.
   • Using a scalpel, sharply dissect through the subcutaneous tissue over the superior edge of the fifth rib.
   • Carefully puncture the tip of the Kelly clamp, and dissect through the pleura. If there is a pneumothorax, air will rush out through the punctured pleura.
   • Explore the intrathoracic area with a sterile, gloved index finger of the dominant hand to free adhesions, clots, or lung tissue.
   • Place the Kelly clamp over the perforation on the distal end of the chest tube so that the tip is firm. This aids in the insertion of the chest tube through puncture placed in the pleura.
   • Progress the distal tip of the tube into the thoracic cavity, ensuring that the tube is advanced past the most proximal fenestration.
3. After the tube is determined to be in the proper place, secure it, using suture attached to skin.
4. Close the skin edges with nonabsorbable suture.
5. Apply an occlusive dressing around the tube.
6. Cover the dressing with wide adhesive tape.

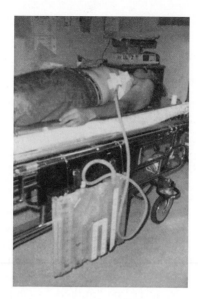

Fig. 27-4 Chest tube in place, attached to Pleur-Evac unit.

7. Attach the tube to a closed chest drainage system. The chest drainage system should be adaptable for autotransfusion (Fig. 27-4).
8. Maintain the chest drainage system below the level of the chest to facilitate the flow of drainage and prevent reflux back into the chest.
9. Record the amount of blood that returns initially and any subsequent drainage on both the collection chamber and the trauma flow sheet.
10. Obtain a chest x-ray to ensure proper positioning of the chest tube.

Troubleshooting

The assessment of air leaks allows the clinician to monitor lung expansion, tube placement, the integrity of the closed chest drainage system, and potential injury of the trachea or esophagus. The water-seal chamber directly reflects the change of pressure within the pleural space. Fluid in the water-seal chamber will normally fluctuate with inspiration and exhalation.

Initially, fluctuation of fluid in the water-seal chamber reflects the removal of air from the pleural space. Any ongoing fluctuations or vigorous bubbling suggests potential tracheal or bronchial injury, leak in the chest drainage system itself, or improper tube placement.

To help determine the location of a leak, first occlude the chest drainage tubing proximally to the patient. Immediate cessation of bubbling in the water-seal chamber indicates a problem with tube placement, the dressing site, or ongoing leak from the pleural space. Working distally from the chest tube toward the chest drainage device, intermittent occluding of the system will isolate the problem between the area occluded and the drainage system.

Any continued bubbling at the end of the tubing indicates a leak within the closed chest drainage system.

Loss of chest tube patency indicates a mechanical or blood clot occlusion. Examine the tubing to determine any kinks in the line. Suspected clots may be dislodged by gently squeezing the drainage tubing in a proximal to distal direction from the patient. The only indication for squeezing the drainage tubing is to dislodge a suspected clot.

AUTOTRANSFUSION

Autotransfusion is the collection and reinfusion of a patient's shed blood from his or her pleural cavity. The blood is collected in an autotransfusion collection device, then reinfused into the patient. In the absence of type-specific or crossmatched blood, autotransfusion is readily available, warm, and perfectly crossmatched.

There are several types of autotransfusion setups. The clinician should be familiar with the type of equipment used at his or her own facility.

Generally speaking, only blood collected from the thoracic cavity is used for autotransfusion. Patients with injuries that include thoracoabdominal communication, such as with a diaphragmatic tear, are candidates for autotransfusion in the emergent setting. Any collected blood with obvious fecal material, clots, or coagulopathies should not be reinfused. The reinfusion of contaminated blood may result in an adverse effect, such as sepsis or worsening of a coagulopathic state.

Indications

• Massive hemothorax
• Myocardial rupture
• Great vessel rupture
• Other chest trauma where there is
    Nonavailability of banked blood
    History of transfusion reactions
    Refusal of blood for religious reasons

Contraindications

• Wounds over 4 hours old
• Contamination of blood by outside sources, gastrointestinal tract contents, or cancer cells
• Mediastinal, pericardial, pulmonary, or systemic infection
• Coagulopathies

Procedure

The autotransfusion procedure will vary, depending on the type and brand of equipment used (Fig. 27-5). However, some basic principles apply, regardless of which type of equipment is used:

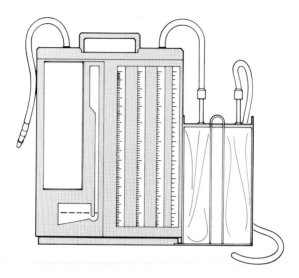

Fig. 27-5 Autotransfusion equipment.

- Set up as if doing regular chest drainage.
- Blood that is collected in the autotransfusion unit must be reinfused within 4 hours from the start of the collection.
- When the collected blood is being transfused, be sure to switch the patient's chest tube to another autotransfusion unit or to a regular blood chest drainage unit.
- Attach a blood filter to bag of collected blood before reinfusion.

EMERGENCY THORACOTOMY

Emergency thoracotomy is a much-debated topic. Indications for emergency thoracotomy exist based upon patient benefit and long-term outcome. The most appropriate candidates with the best outcomes are patients with cardiac-specific, penetrating trauma.

Emergency thoracotomy may be beneficial in cases of penetrating wounds to the heart, repeat pericardial tamponade not relieved by pericardiocentesis, crush injuries to the chest, or any other incident for which ready access to the intrathoracic cavity is needed. Note that this procedure should be performed only by a skilled physician.

Equipment (Fig. 27-6)

Surgical prep solution
Scalpel and blades
Large, heavy scissors
2 large Kelly clamps

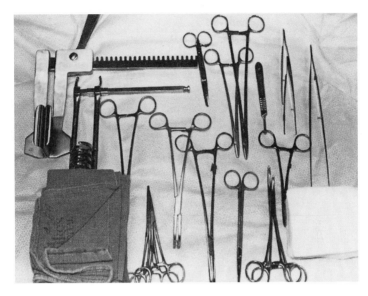

Fig. 27-6   Minimal equipment for emergency thoracotomy.

Suture material
Rib spreaders
Two aortic clamps
Two needle holders
Four mosquito clips
Sterile gloves
Prep solution
Large-bore suction needles

Criteria

Loss of vital signs (respiratory effort, auscultated heartbeat, motor function, or pupillary activity) en route to the hospital, in the Emergency Department, and/or less than 5 minutes of CPR that is unresponsive to volume resuscitation, airway management, or chest decompression.
Cardiac-specific, penetrating injury.
Persistent pericardial tamponade unrelieved with pericardiocentesis.
Adequate support services to manage the patient once resuscitated, (i.e., appropriately trained surgical staff, operating room, ongoing critical care capabilities).

PERICARDIOCENTESIS/PERICARDIAL WINDOW

Pericardiocentesis is performed to relieve a pericardial tamponade.

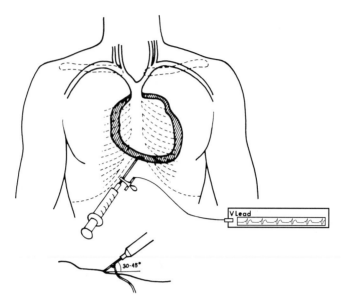

Fig. 27-7 Pericardiocentesis. (From Budassi SA, Barber J: *Mosby's manual of emergency care,* ed 3, St Louis, 1990, Mosby.)

Equipment

16-gauge spinal or cardiac needle
50-ml syringe
Alligator clips
Kelly clamp
ECG machine
3-way stopcock
Local anesthetic
Antiseptic solution
Sterile gloves
Small basin

Procedure

1. Prepare the patient's chest at the left inferior costal margin and the xyphoid.
2. Administer local anesthetic to the area.
3. Attach one end of the alligator clip to the hub of the needle and the other end of the alligator clip to the V lead of the ECG machine.
4. Attach the needle to the syringe via the three-way stopcock.
5. Run the ECG machine off the V-lead setting.
6. Advance the needle in subxyphoid approach between the left inferior costal margin and the xyphoid at 30- to 45-degree angle to the body, advancing toward the tip of the left scapula.

7. Gently aspirate the syringe as the needle is advanced.

   If blood returns and there is no ST segment elevation on the ECG, the needle probably entered the pericardial sac. If an ST-segment elevation appears on the ECG, the needle has pierced the epicardium. In this case, withdraw the needle slowly until the ST segment returns to normal.

   If the needle has gone all the way through to the myocardium, a pulsation may be felt up through the needle into the syringe.

8. When blood is being withdrawn from the pericardial sac, attach a Kelly clamp to the needle at the level of the skin to avoid accidental advancement of the needle (Fig. 27-7).

NOTE: Blood that is withdrawn from the pericardial sac may not clot because it has been defibrinated in the sac.

Complications

- Laceration of a coronary artery
- Laceration of a lung
- Laceration of a ventricle
- Cardiac dysrhythmias
- Increased tamponade

Pericardial window

A *pericardial window* is a small incision made just under the xyphoid. The tissue is dissected until the apex of the heart can be directly visualized. A segment of pericardium is lifted with forceps; and a small, square incision is made, creating a window from which pericardial fluid can drain. A pericardial window is generally performed in an operating room.

INTRAOSSEOUS INFUSION

An *intraosseous infusion* is the administration of IV fluids and drugs directly into the bone marrow.

Intraosseous cannulation

The intraosseous administration of fluids and medications is a safe and effective procedure in children under 6 years of age. It may be used when the child is in hypovolemic shock, cardiopulmonary arrest, or status epilepticus. Intraosseous infusion can also be used when administration of fluids or drugs is critical to the survival of a child and the establishment of an IV cannot be accomplished. Catecholamines, colloids, crystalloids, blood products, antibiotics, calcium, heparin, lidocaine, atropine, sodium bicarbonate, and digitalis have been successfully infused by the intraosseous route.

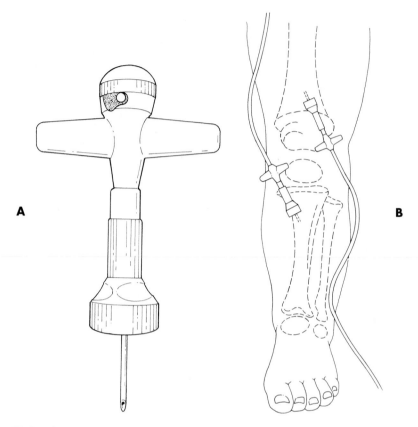

Fig. 27-8 **A,** 1-gauge disposable Illinois Sternal bone marrow aspiration needle. **B,** Recommended sites for intraosseous infusion. (**A,** From Sheehy SB: *Mosby's manual of emergency care,* ed 3, St Louis, 1990, Mosby.)

Contraindications

The following sites for interosseous perfusion are to be avoided:
- Burn site
- Fractured extremity

Equipment

Betadine swabs
Intraosseous needle (or bone marrow biopsy needle, Fig. 27-8, *A*)
Sterile gloves

Procedure

1. Locate the anterior medial surface of the tibia, 1 to 3 cm below the tibial tuberosity (Fig. 27-8, *B*).
   Other (optional) sites are the distal anterior femur, the medial malleolus, and the iliac crest.

2. Prepare the area with Betadine.
3. Using an osseous needle, advance intraosseus needle through the skin, fascia, and bony cortex with a rotating, boring motion.
    It will become apparent that the needle is in the bone marrow when a popping sensation occurs, followed by a sudden absence of resistance, when the needle can stand upright without manual support, and when fluid flows freely through the needle.
4. Aspirate, using a syringe.
    If bone marrow is returned, the needle has been placed correctly. If bone marrow is not returned, try running fluid into the needle.
5. After needle is in place, tape it and infuse solutions or medications.
6. Observe for infiltration on local irritation.

DIAGNOSTIC PERITONEAL LAVAGE

Diagnostic peritoneal lavage (DPL) is a rapid diagnostic procedure that may be used to determine intraperitoneal hemorrhage when results of a physical examination are equivocal, the patient is unstable with unidentified blood loss, is unable to participate in abdominal evaluation, or requires emergency surgery with general anesthesia for other injuries. Diagnostic peritoneal lavage is sensitive and relatively accurate for the presence of abdominal injury but not specific with regard to the type or extent of organ injury.

Diagnostic peritoneal lavage involves the placement of a catheter through the abdomen, into the peritoneum, and evaluating the gross aspirate. Crystalloid fluid may be infused and then retrieved for evaluation of blood, RBCs, WBCs, amylase, bacteria, and fecal matter.

Indications

Peritoneal lavage is indicated for confirmed or suspected blunt (nonpenetrating) abdominal trauma, especially for those patients who have
  • Unstable vital signs with unidentified blood loss
  • Head injury requiring emergency operative management
  • Equivocal physical exam
  • Inability to participate in abdominal evaluation because of spinal cord injury, mental status changes, or drug intoxication
  • Physical signs of abdominal trauma (steering wheel bruises, abrasions, fractured lower ribs, or fractured pelvis)

Contraindications

Peritoneal lavage is *not* indicated for the following conditions (exceptions are based on physician judgment):
  • Penetrating abdominal trauma
  • Several abdominal scars that may suggest the possibility of intraabdominal adhesions from previous surgical procedures
  • Abdominal wall hematoma that may result in false-positive reading

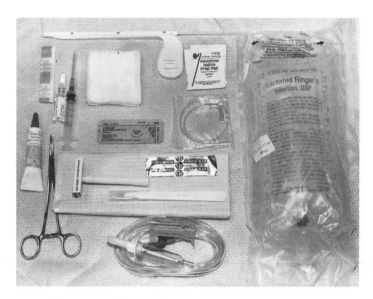

Fig. 27-9 Basic equipment for peritoneal lavage.

- Evisceration
- Morbid obesity

Equipment (Fig. 27-9)

Foley catheter to straight drain	Betadine prep swabs
Razor	Sterile fenestrated drape
Sterile gloves	1% lidocaine *with* epinephrine
6- and 20-ml syringes	11 scalpel
Peritoneal dialysis catheter	Curved Kelly clamp
Large-bore IV or irrigation tubing	1000 ml warmed Ringer's lactate or
Antibiotic ointment	saline IV solution in plastic bag
Three red top laboratory tubes	4-0 nylon suture with needle
Sterile 4 × 4 sponges	Two capillary tubes

Procedure

Three methods of peritoneal lavage may be selected: closed (percutaneous), semiopen, and open. Advantages and disadvantages of each method exist. An open procedure is performed as follows:

1. Place Foley catheter and drain urinary bladder.
2. Place nasogastric tube.
3. Observe for gravid uterus; obtain good history (physician may elect not to proceed if pregnant).
4. Prep anterior abdominal wall (shave, cleanse with Betadine, and drape with sterile towel); maintain sterile field throughout.
5. Maintain absolute hemostatis throughout.

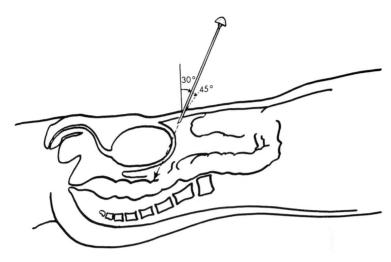

Fig. 27-10 Distended bladder may be perforated by trochar for peritoneal lavage.

6. Assist the physician as necessary with procedure:*
    - Inject 1% lidocaine with epinephrine in a subcutaneous wheal (2 to 3 cm below umbilicus).
    - Make a "nick" incision through the skin and subcutaneous adipose tissue.
    - Continue dissecting down to linea alba, using curved Kelly clamp.
    - Once the peritoneum is visualized, it is elevated, and a small incision is made through the peritoneum with a scalpel (Fig. 27-10).
    - Slide the catheter off the trocar and into the peritoneal cavity.
    - Connect the 90-degree angle plastic tubing (found in kit).
    - Connect free end to 20-ml syringe and aspirate for presence of blood, bile, feces, fiber, or urine.
        If aspirate contains more than 10 ml of bright red blood, the procedure is considered positive and should be immediately discontinued.
        If aspiration is negative, infuse 1000 ml of *warmed* Ringer's lactate or normal saline solution (10 to 20 ml/kg in a child) over 10 to 15 minutes.
    - Once the fluid is in the peritoneum, manipulate patient's abdomen from side to side or roll patient from side to side if condition permits, to mix solution with any free material in the cavity.
7. When it is time to drain the fluid, lower the bag (be careful not to put any tension on the tubing into the abdomen).

---

*This technique is known as the *nick technique.* The physician may elect to perform a *minilap technique,* in which a small surgical incision is made and the anterior peritoneum visualized, elevated, and nicked with a scalpel before catheter insertion.

8. Place bag below the level of the patient.
9. Allow fluid to drain from the patient's peritoneal cavity by gravity back into the bag.

Positive findings

- Aspiration of greater than or equal to 10 cc gross blood
- Aspiration of feces, bile, intestine, or bacteria
- Lavage fluid is grossly bloody
- RBC greater than 100,000 cells/mm
- WBC greater than 500 cells/mm
- Amylase greater than 175 U/100ml
- Lavage fluid return through Foley catheter, gastric tube, or chest tube

Controversies

Several methods exist for evaluation of the abdomen for injury and determining the need for laporotomy. Physical examination remains the mainstay, but in patients with mental staus changes and unconsciousness, physical examination is limited. Abdominal CT scan, diagnostic peritoneal lavage, and abdominal ultrasound are additional tools to evaluate the patient for intraabdominal and retroperitoneal injuries. Abdominal CT provides excellent examination for hemorrhage in the intraabdominal and retroperitoneum and for hollow viscous and diaphragmatic injuries. Diagnostic peritoneal lavage is a more rapid procedure that is best suited for early evaluation of intraabdominal hemorrhage. It has limitations in the early detection of hollow viscous injuries, diaphragmatic injuries, and retroperitoneal injuries. Abdominal ultrasound is more specific than DPL and may be done rapidly at the bedside, but it can be operator dependent.

EXTREMITY SPLINTING

An injured limb is splinted to prevent further injury to the possibly fractured bones, damaged soft tissue, and neurovascular structures involved and also to reduce pain. Some simple principles can greatly reduce the discomfort and risk of complication from the injury. These principles should be considered when treating extremity trauma:

- Immobilize (splint) joint above and below injury
- Elevate injured part above level of heart
- Apply ice for first 48 hours; then apply heat
- Continuously reevaluate neurovascular status distal to injury
- Splint extremity in position of function, if possible.

Indications

- Known or suspected extremity trauma that causes the patient pain or dysfunction or demonstrates swelling, ecchymosis, neurovascular compromise, or deformity

- Trauma that causes bleeding or effusion of fluid into a joint, rendering it symptomatic, as above

Contraindications

When the patient is comfortable in the position in which he or she is found and is without neurovascular compromise, or if manipulation of the limb may cause further damage, supportive padding around the injured limb is adequate until surgical correction is available.

Equipment (options)

Soft splints (pillows, rolled towels, blankets)
Hard splints (padded boards, metal splints)
Air splints (inflatable plastic bladders or negative-pressure bead splints)
Traction splints (provide traction as well as immobilization)
2-inch adhesive tape

Kerlix or roller gauze
Generous amounts of padding (ABDs, towels, soft foam rubber)
Cravats or triangular bandage
Straps
Large safety pins
Spine board

Procedure

1. Evaluate the neurovascular status of the extremity.
2. Keep the patient informed throughout the procedure.
3. Choose the type of splint appropriate for injury (it must be large enough to splint the joint above and the joint below the injury).
4. Secure the splint on the extremity in a position of function or least manipulation, padding bony prominences well.
5. When lifting an injured limb onto a splint, be certain to adequately support both ends of the injured limb (distal and proximal) to reduce mobility (this takes two hands).
6. Leave part of the extremity distal to the injury (e.g., fingers on a forearm injury) exposed to allow for reassessment of the neurovascular status.
7. Elevate injured part, preferably above the level of the heart, to reduce edema.
8. Apply well-insulated ice pack to the injury.
9. Repeat neurovascular evaluations for color, pain, temperature, swelling, capillary refill, sensation, and function frequently.

TRACTION SPLINTING DEVICES

There are several devices for splinting injured femurs that not only offer immobilization but also a means of applying traction to the distal part of the leg, reducing muscle spasm, pain, and deformity.

Indications

- Midshaft femur fracture
- Proximal tibia fracture

Contraindications

- Hip fractures
- Pelvic injuries
- Middle or lower tibial fractures
- Ankle or foot injuries
- Most knee injuries

Procedure

The procedure outlined here is for the HARE traction splint. Other similar devices are available. Clinical personnel should refer to product literature for specific directions for use.

1. Remove traction splint from case, and loosen collet sleeves to release for lengthening.
2. Position traction splint parallel to injured leg; adjust length to allow 8 to 10 inches past the foot, measuring from position of ischial tuberosity.
3. Tighten collet sleeves to lock.
4. Fold down heel stand until it locks at 90-degree angle; position about 5 inches from end of splint (flexion of the fracture and pain result from not using this stand to provide elevation of the foot).
5. Position Velcro support straps according to patient's size, with 2 above the knee and 2 below; to keep the Velcro out of the way until needed, wrap it under the splint and hook it on itself (Velcro tends to stick to blankets, carpet, and the like).
6. Place the ankle straps under the patient's ankle, padding heel and ankle as necessary to assure fit.
7. Place one hand under the ankle and one hand under the knee, and apply gentle, manual traction (when manual traction is on, it must *not* be released until the entire traction splint has been applied and secured) such as the traction splint (Fig. 27-11).
8. Have an assistant place the splint under the injured leg with the half-ring positioned just below the buttock, against the ischial tuberosity; continue to maintain manual traction.
9. When the leg is lowered onto the splint, attach the ankle hitch into the S hook; twist knurled knob on splint to apply traction, and tighten until the strap is snug. Ask the patient for feedback regarding pain relief and comfort.
10. Fasten the Velcro straps around the leg. If the patient has an open wound, dress it with a sterile dressing first; Velcro straps can hold the dressing in place and may be tightened if direct pressure is needed (Fig. 27-12).
11. Support the leg in the area beneath the splint to ensure stable positioning.
12. Reassess neurovascular status in the limb; make strap and stabilization adjustments, as necessary.
13. Inform and comfort to the patient.

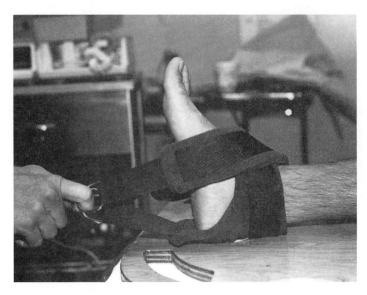

Fig. 27-11   Traction harness for traction splinting devices must be evaluated for fit, function, and provision of adequate blood flow to foot.

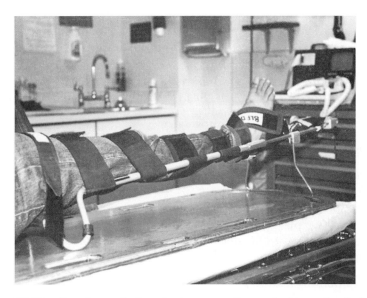

Fig. 27-12   Traction splinting device correctly applied to patient's leg.

When properly applied, the traction device will alleviate a great deal of muscle spasm and pain. Patient comfort (or discomfort) is an important indicator of accurate placement and effectiveness of the splint. Clinical personnel should never release the traction on the splint without first providing manual traction to maintain tension on the muscles.

HELMET REMOVAL

Various helmets are available for those sports in which head protection is recommended. Motorcycling, bicycling, kayaking, ice hockey, football, and auto racing are just a few. The careful removal of this gear is imperative for protection of the cervical spine.

Procedure

A quick examination of the helmet to determine its construction before attempting removal may save time, effort, and risk to the patient. Some sport helmets have air bladders that can be deflated to make space in the helmet, some have removable parts, and some are made of molded plastic that can be safely cut with a cast saw. Creating enough space to allow hands for cervical spine immobilization is the objective in altering the helmet, and all procedures should be explained to the patient as removal progresses.

1. Never attempt to remove a helmet alone; airway protection can be achieved with most helmets in place, and the potential for complicating an injury with a difficult removal is great.
2. One person should apply in-line stabilization by placing one hand behind the head, resting on the occiput, and the front hand on the angles of the mandible, thumb on one side, fingers on the other (this person is in control of the head and neck).
3. The second person should then remove the helmet by pulling laterally on the sides and sliding it off in caudad maneuver. If the helmet has full face protection, special consideration must be given to the eye and mouth covering, which must be removed first. If it cannot be removed, tilt the helmet (not the head) back to pass the face protector over the patient's nose.

EYE IRRIGATION USING MORGAN THERAPEUTIC LENS

The Morgan therapeutic lens (MorTan) is a specially designed lens that is placed on the eye and used to provide continuous ocular lavage or medication (Fig. 27-13). It is a scleral lens that is made of polymethyl methacrylate plastic. The tubing is made of soft silicone plastic and has a female adapter at the distal end that can be connected to standard IV tubing.

Equipment

Morgan therapeutic lens
Ocular anesthetic drops
4 × 4 gauze sponges
Warmed saline solution in IV bag
Standard IV tubing
Towels, absorbent pads, or drainage basin

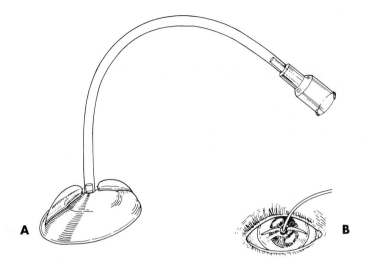

Fig. 27-13   **A,** Morgan therapeutic lens. **B,** Lens in place for continuous irrigation.

Procedure

1. Explain what you are about to do to the patient.
2. Instill anesthetic ocular medication.
3. Ask the patient to look down.
4. Retract the upper eyelid.
5. Grasp the lens by the tubing and the small, finlike projections.
6. Slip the superior border of the lens up under the eyelid.
7. Have the patient look up.
8. Retract the lower eyelid, and place lower border of the lens beneath it (Fig. 27-13, *B*).
9. Have the patient turn his or her head toward the affected side.
10. Place a folded towel or absorbable pad under the patient's head to collect irrigation solution.
11. Attach the female adapter at the end of the lens tubing to a syringe filled with the solution of choice, and instill the solution at the desired rate to IV tubing that is connected to the solution of choice in an IV bag instilled at a selected drip rate.
12. To remove the lens, follow steps 3 through 8 in reverse order.
13. Dry the patient's face and eye area with a dry towel.
14. Dispose of the lens.
15. Follow additional orders for ophthalmic medications and eye dressings.
16. Patients should be carefully maintained for further eye irritation during irrigation.

NOTE: Use caution to avoid corneal abrasion during insertion of the lens.

PREVENTING HEAT LOSS IN TRAUMA PATIENT

Hypothermia occurs to some degree in nearly every victim of major trauma. When clinical personnel approach the trauma patient with many hands and deliver many volumes of cold oxygen, cold fluid replacement, cold irrigations, and a cold environment, they add to the patient's already hypothermic condition. Rewarming a patient who has become cold from blood loss, exposure, dehydration, and organ failure is a difficult and sometimes unsuccessful effort. *Preventing* heat loss is much more efficient than attempting to rewarm. Practicing a few techniques can avert a complicated situation. Anticipation of heat loss in *all* trauma patients prepares caregivers for preventing loss of precious body heat. The environments where we resuscitate and manage injured patients directly affect the degree of heat loss. Often, exposure during transport and in radiologic suites may enhance heat loss unless adequate measures are taken to prevent the loss.

The following is a list of methods of preventing heat loss:
- Removal of wet clothing
- Placement of a wool blanket under the patient (this is most easily accomplished when the patient is placed on the backboard)
- Use of head coverings (caps made of Mylar or stockinette work well)
- Administration of warm O_2
- Warm fluid replacement
- Use of warm irrigating solutions for wound cleansing, nasogastric lavage, bladder irrigation, diagnostic peritoneal lavage
- Covering the patient with warmed blankets and commercially available devices between exams and procedures (Mylar chest aprons and leggings are also available)
- Administration of fluid and blood through an infuser/warmer

Continuous temperature monitoring with a deep rectal probe, esophageal probe, or bladder catheter-tip monitor is an important element in monitoring vital signs.

MAST (Medical Anti-Shock Trousers)

The pneumatic antishock garment (PASG) is a useful tool for stabilizing pelvic fractures, tamponading exsanguinating hemorrhage, and stabilizing lower extremity fractures. The PASG was once believed to autotransfuse a patient. Data collection and outcome-based research have shown this not to be true. The PASG does not improve a patient's mortality or morbidity when used for management of hypovolemia. When applied, the PASG may transiently change a patient's blood pressure. The indications for use and application may vary among clinical practice areas.

Indications

- Stabilization of pelvic fractures
- Tamponade for exsanguinating hemorrhage
- Stabilization of lower extremity fractures

Contraindications
Absolute contraindications

- Presence of existing pulmonary edema
- Circulatory instability secondary to myocardial insufficiency
- Possible ruptured diaphragm
- Tension pneumothorax

Relative contraindications

These conditions warrant careful consideration and projection of the patient's ultimate outcome if the hypovolemic shock is not corrected:
- Pregnancy (may apply and inflate just leg panels)
- Intrathoracic hemorrhage
- Impaled object
- Intracranial injury

Application and inflation procedure

1. Continuously monitor patient's vital signs. Specifically note vital signs following the inflation or deflation of any section of the PASG.
2. Unfold and lay out the PASG flat alongside the patient.
3. Ideally the PASG should be positioned on a long spine board and the patient subsequently logrolled onto the spine board. When a long spine board is already in place, the patient should be logrolled and the PASG positioned underneath the patient.
4. Apply and secure the leg panels followed by the abdominal panel, noting the color-coded Velcro straps. Avoid wrinkles in the suit.
5. Attach inflation hoses from the pump to the corresponding connections on the PASG. Keep all stopcocks open at this time.
6. Inflate the leg sections first. Close the stopcock for the abdominal section, and close leg panel stopcocks once the desired inflation has been achieved.
7. The leg panels should be inflated based on patient comfort, desired immobilization, and/or tamponade of external hemorrhage.
8. Open the abdominal panel stopcock and inflate. Close the abdominal panel stopcock once the desired inflation has been achieved.
9. The abdominal panel should be inflated based upon patient comfort, desired immobilization, and/or tamponade of external hemorrhage.
10. Do not overinflate any compartment. The compartments should not be taut, bulging, or stretching the Velcro closures.
11. Always monitor vital signs along with the circulation, sensation, and mobility of the lower extremities.

Deflation and removal of PASG

Deflation and removal of the PASG should only be carried out when an adequate IV access has been established. The patient may be x-rayed through the PASG; therefore it should never be taken off for that reason. The patient can easily be transported in the PASG. If the patient is en route to surgery, it is recommended that the PASG remain in place.

1. Deflate the abdominal panel slowly, monitoring the patient's blood pressure continuously
2. If a 5-mm blood pressure drop occurs, stop deflation and administer enough IV fluid to regain the dropped pressure, and reinflate the PASG
3. Slowly deflate the leg panels, one first and then other, using the same precaution as in step 2
4. If patient's blood pressure falls suddenly, reinflate the PASG. Begin the removal process again only after an adequate pressure has been reestablished and additional IV fluid has been administered or surgical intervention is under way

---

CAUTION: Sudden deflation of the PASG may result in profound shock. Exercise absolute caution and careful monitoring of the patient when the PASG is being removed.

Index

A

ABC's
  in abdominal trauma, 276
  in chest injury, 251-252
  in prehospital trauma resuscitation, 48
  in trauma initial assessment, 165-173
    airway in, 165-169
    breathing in, 169-170
    circulation in, 170-173
Abdomen
  in secondary survey, 179
  suture removal from, 80
Abdominal aorta trauma, 277
Abdominal trauma, 273-283
  anatomy in, 274
  blunt, 274-278
  genitals in, 280-282
  genitourinary system in, 278-280
  mechanism of injury in, 42
  nursing diagnoses for, 137
  pediatric, 353
  penetrating, 282-283
Abdominal wall bruise, 274, 275
Abducens nerve, 185
ABG; *see* Arterial blood gases
Abrasion, 81-82
Abruptio placentae, 357
Absorbable sutures, 80
Abuse, child, 354, 372
Acceleration forces
  in brain injury, 40
  in concussion, 204-205
Accessory muscles of respiration, 250
Accessory nerve, 186
Accessory vertebral process, 211
Accidental Death and Disability: The Neglected
  Disease of Modern Society, 3
Achilles' tendon rupture, 288-289
Acid-base balance
  arterial blood gas values in, 93-94
  chemistry profile in, 101-103

Acidosis
  arterial blood gases in, 94-95
  massive transfusion and, 73
  shock and, 61, 62
ACIP; *see* Immunization Practices Advisory
    Committee
Acoustic nerve, 186
Acromioclavicular dislocation, 314-315
ACS; *see* American College of Surgeons
Activated partial thromboplastin time, 100
ADH; *see* Antidiuretic hormone
Adhesive tape for wound closure, 80
Adjunct devices for fluid replacement, 70
Administrative components of trauma
    systems, 7-9
Adrenal glands in shock, 61
Adult respiratory distress syndrome, 337
Advanced Burn Life Support, 20
Advanced Cardiac Life Support, 19-20
Advanced Trauma Life Support Course, 15,
    19-20
Air bag, vehicle, 36
  in eye trauma, 234, 235
Air medical transport, 46
Air splint, 325
Airplane in patient transfer, 54
Airway
  in abdominal trauma, 276
  in burn injury, 336
  in chest injury, 251
  in geriatric trauma, 367-368
  in initial assessment, 165-169
  in pediatric trauma, 349-350
  in prehospital resuscitation, 48
  in stabilization for transfer, 55-56
Airway clearance, ineffective
  in chest trauma, 133-134
  in facial/EENT trauma, 132
Airway obstruction
  in burn injury, 334-335
  in mandible fracture, 231
Alanine aminotransferase, 106-107